T0325388

ANNALS *of* THE NEW YORK ACADEMY OF SCIENCES

EDITOR-IN-CHIEF
Douglas Braaten

ASSOCIATE EDITOR
Rebecca E. Cooney

PROJECT MANAGER
Steven E. Bohall

EDITORIAL ADMINISTRATOR
Daniel J. Becker

Artwork and design by Ash Ayman Shairzay

The New York Academy of Sciences
7 World Trade Center
250 Greenwich Street, 40th Floor
New York, NY 10007-2157

annals@nyas.org
www.nyas.org/annals

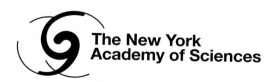

**The New York
Academy of Sciences**

Published by Blackwell Publishing
On behalf of the New York Academy of Sciences

Boston, Massachusetts
2011

ANNALS *of* THE NEW YORK ACADEMY OF SCIENCES

VOLUME
1246

ISSUE

The Year in Human and Medical Genetics

Inborn Errors of Immunity II

ISSUE EDITORS

Jean-Laurent Casanova,[a] Mary Ellen Conley[b] and Luigi Notarangelo[c]

[a]The Rockefeller University, [b]St. Jude Children's Research Hospital, and [c]Harvard University

TABLE OF CONTENTS

Ann. N.Y. Acad. Sci. ISSN 0077-8923

ANNALS OF THE NEW YORK ACADEMY OF SCIENCES
Issue: *The Year in Human and Medical Genetics: Inborn Errors of Immunity*

The establishment of early B cell tolerance in humans: lessons from primary immunodeficiency diseases

Eric Meffre

Department of Immunobiology, Yale University School of Medicine, New Haven, Connecticut

Address for correspondence: Eric Meffre, Yale University School of Medicine, 300 George Street, New Haven, CT 06511. Eric.meffre@yale.edu

Patients with primary immunodeficiency (PID) provide rare opportunities to study the impact of specific gene mutations on the regulation of human B cell tolerance. Alterations in B cell receptor and Toll-like receptor signaling pathways result in a defective central checkpoint and a failure to counterselect developing autoreactive B cells in the bone marrow. In contrast, CD40L- and MHC class II–deficient patients only displayed peripheral B cell tolerance defects, suggesting that decreased numbers of regulatory T cells and increased concentration of B cell activating factor (BAFF) may interfere with the peripheral removal of autoreactive B cells. The pathways regulating B cell tolerance identified in PID patients are likely to be affected in patients with rheumatoid arthritis, systemic lupus erythematosus, and type 1 diabetes who display defective central and peripheral B cell tolerance checkpoints. Indeed, risk alleles encoding variants altering BCR signaling, such as *PTPN22* alleles associated with the development of these diseases, interfere with the removal of developing autoreactive B cells. Hence, insights into B cell selection from PID patients are highly relevant to the understanding of the etiology of autoimmune conditions.

Keywords: B cell tolerance; B cell receptor; Toll-like receptors; receptor editing

Introduction

Autoimmune diseases affect about 5% of the population and are often characterized by the production of autoantibodies directed against self-antigens.[1] An important role for B cells in autoimmune diseases is demonstrated by the successful treatment of patients with rheumatoid arthritis (RA), type 1 diabetes (T1D), multiple sclerosis (MS), and other autoimmune syndromes with anti-CD20 monoclonal antibodies that eliminate B cells.[2–4] However, the underlying mechanisms that account for autoreactive B cells and autoantibody production in autoimmune diseases remain elusive. We developed a method that allows us to analyze the frequency of autoreactive clones in diverse B cell subpopulations by amplifying and cloning immunoglobulin heavy and light chain genes from single B cells. The reactivities of recombinant antibodies are then tested by two ELISA assays detecting polyreactivity and HEp-2 reactivity as well as in indirect immunofluorescence assays on slides coated with HEp-2 cells to detect antinuclear antibodies (ANAs).[5–7]

We review herein data demonstrating that central B cell tolerance is mostly controlled by intrinsic B cell factors regulating B cell receptor (BCR) and Toll-like receptor (TLR) signaling, whereas peripheral B cell tolerance seems to involve extrinsic B cell factors such as regulatory T (T_{reg}) cells and serum B cell activating factor (BAFF) concentrations.

Central B cell tolerance requires proper BCR signaling

Using a single cell PCR method, we found that random V(D)J joining in healthy donors generated a large number of autoreactive B cells that were removed at two discrete checkpoints.[5,8] First, a central checkpoint in the bone marrow between early immature and immature B cells removed most B cells expressing polyreactive and ANAs[5] (Fig. 1). Interestingly, we can assess the functionality of the central B cell tolerance checkpoint in a subject without a bone marrow sample simply by following the frequency of polyreactive and antinuclear clones in the new emigrant/transitional B cell compartment in

doi: 10.1111/j.1749-6632.2011.06347.x

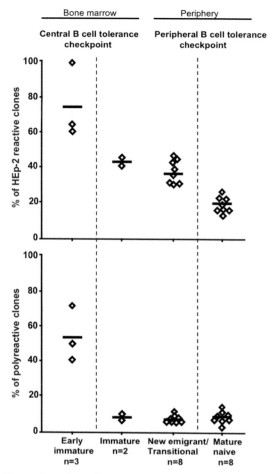

Figure 1. Early B cell tolerance checkpoints in healthy donors. Single CD34⁻CD19⁺CD10⁺IgM⁻ early immature B cells and CD34⁻CD19⁺CD10⁺IgM⁺ immature B cells from bone marrow and CD19⁺CD10⁺IgM⁺⁺CD27⁻ new emigrant/transitional and CD19⁺CD10⁻IgM⁺CD27⁻ mature naive B cells from peripheral blood of healthy controls were isolated by flow cytometry based on the indicated surface markers. IgH and IgL chain genes from single purified B cells were cloned, and the monoclonal antibodies were expressed *in vitro*.[7] The frequency of HEp-2 reactive antibodies (top panel) was determined by HEp-2 cell ELISA and indirect immunofluorescence on HEp-2 cells. The frequency of polyreactive antibodies (bottom panel) was determined by ELISA with ssDNA, dsDNA, insulin, and lipopolysaccharide as antigens. Polyreactive antibodies recognized at least two structurally diverse antigens and often all four. Each diamond represents an individual; the average is shown with a bar. The central and peripheral B cell tolerance checkpoints are indicated.

peripheral blood because bone marrow immature B cells and peripheral new emigrant/transitional B cells express similar antibody repertoire and reactivity uninfluenced by proliferation steps.[5,9] In ad-

dition, the frequencies of polyreactive and antinuclear clones are remarkably similar among the eight analyzed healthy donors who did not carry the *PTPN22* risk allele associated to the development of autoimmunity (Fig. 1).[10] Indeed, polyreactive clones ranged from 5.0% to 11.1% in new emigrant/transitional B cells from healthy donors, whereas the frequencies of antinuclear new emigrant B cells averaged 1.6% (0%–5.6%), reflecting the proper removal of polyreactive and antinuclear clones in the bone marrow (Figs. 1 and 2).[5,10] Hence, increased frequencies of polyreactive and/or antinuclear new emigrant/transitional B cells reflect an abnormal failure to remove autoreactive clones in the bone marrow, thereby revealing a defective central B cell tolerance checkpoint.[10] A second checkpoint at which additional autoreactive B cells were removed from the population was detected in the periphery of healthy donors at the transition between new emigrant and mature naive B cells (Fig. 1).[5,8] Indeed, anti-HEp-2 frequencies ranged from 30.0% to 46.2% in new emigrant/transitional B cells, which decreased to 16.7–26.3% in the mature naive B cell compartment, potentially reflecting counterselection of some autoreactive immature B cells that encounter peripheral autoantigens not expressed in the bone marrow environment (Fig. 1).[5,8]

We conclude that autoreactive B cells generated by random V(D)J recombination are eliminated at two distinct early B cell tolerance checkpoints in healthy donors, first in the bone marrow and then in the periphery.

Central B cell tolerance relies on proper BCR signaling

We analyzed the molecules and pathways that regulate the establishment of human B cell tolerance by studying PID patients. Many mouse models suggest that B cell tolerance is regulated by BCR signaling.[11] While it has been postulated that increased BCR signaling led to autoimmunity, new data in mice and humans suggest instead that decreased BCR signaling interfere with autoreactive B cell counterselection at immature B cell stages by failing to induce proper tolerance mechanisms.[10,12,13]

Indeed, we reported that patients with X-linked agammaglobulinemia (XLA)[12] who carry mutations in the *BTK* gene that encodes an essential BCR signaling component[14,15] display a high frequency of autoreactive new emigrant/transitional B

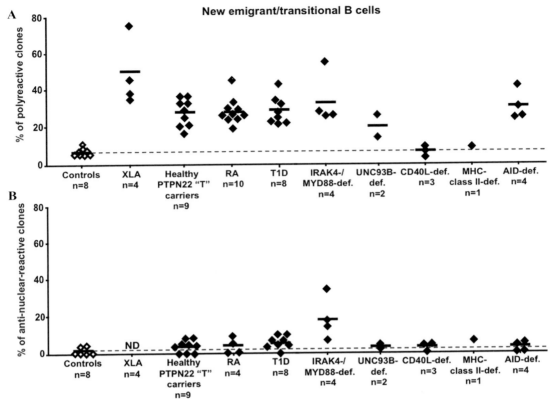

Figure 2. Central B cell tolerance requires proper BCR and TLR signaling. The frequencies of polyreactive (A) and antinuclear (B) new emigrant/transitional B cells are compared between controls (open diamonds), subjects with the PTPN22 "T" risk allele, patients with diverse PID, rheumatoid arthritis (RA), and type 1 diabetes (T1D) (black diamonds). Alteration in either BCR or TLR signaling results in a failure to counterselect developing autoreactive B cells in the bone marrow and results in increased frequencies of polyreactive new emigrant/transitional B cells. IRAK4- and MYD88-deficient new emigrant/transitional B cells were especially enriched in antinuclear clones, as shown in B.

cells including antinuclear B cells, demonstrating that BTK and therefore BCR signaling were essential in regulating the central B cell tolerance checkpoint (Fig. 2).[12] A major role for BCR signaling in the establishment of human B cell tolerance was further demonstrated by the analysis of healthy individuals carrying the *PTPN22* allele encoding an R620W variant associated with the development of many autoimmune diseases including RA, systemic lupus erythematosus (SLE), and T1D.[16–19] Current data indicate that the R620W polymorphism in PTPN22/Lyp leads to decreased BCR signaling, which in turn regulates the establishment of human B cell tolerance.[10,20,21] Indeed, we recently reported that new emigrant/transitional and mature naive B cells from *PTPN22* risk allele carriers contained high frequencies of autoreactive clones

compared to noncarrier donors, revealing defective central and peripheral B cell tolerance checkpoints (Figs. 2 and 3).[10] Hence, a single *PTPN22* risk allele has a dominant effect on altering autoreactive B cell counterselection before any onset of autoimmunity. In addition, similar central and peripheral B cell tolerance defects were also identified in active RA, SLE, and T1D patients, suggesting that these early B cell tolerance defects common to RA, SLE, and T1D may result from specific polymorphisms and precede the onset of these autoimmune diseases (Figs. 2 and 3).[10] These data also further suggest that naive autoreactive B cells produced in RA, SLE, and T1D patients before disease onset may promote the development of autoimmunity, potentially by recognizing and presenting self-antigens to T cells.

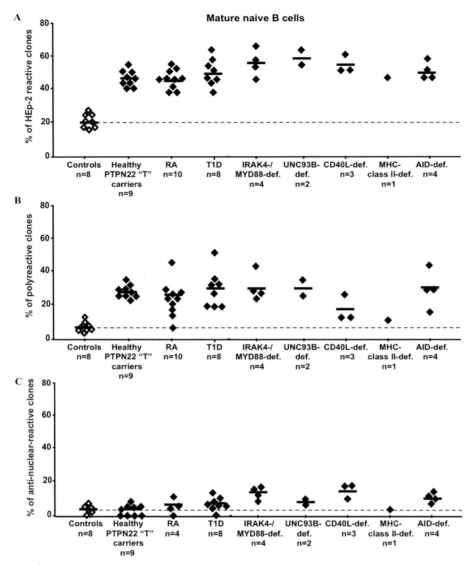

Figure 3. Specific defective peripheral B cell tolerance checkpoint in CD40L- and MHC class II-deficient patients. The frequencies of HEp-2 reactive (A), polyreactive (B), and antinuclear (C) mature naive B cells are compared between controls (open diamonds), subjects with the PTPN22 "T" risk allele, patients with diverse PID, rheumatoid arthritis (RA), and type 1 diabetes (T1D) (black diamonds). Defects in CD40L expression or antigen presentation through MHC class II molecules specifically either interfere with the removal or fail to prevent the accumulation of autoreactive B cells in the periphery. All other subjects who presented central B cell tolerance defects also display large numbers of autoreactive B cells in their mature naive B cell compartment.

Central B cell tolerance is IRAK4/MYD88 dependent

In addition to their BCRs, B cells also express germline-encoded transmembrane receptors called Toll-like receptors (TLRs) that were originally described to bind microbial components but that

are also able to recognize self-antigens.[22] All TLRs except TLR3 as well as transmembrane activator and calcium-modulating cyclophilin ligand interactor (TACI) use IRAK4 and MYD88 to signal.[23–25] In addition, the UNC-93B protein interacts with intracellular TLRs including TLR3, TLR7, TLR8, and TLR9 and seems essential to mediate their functions.[26-30] Additional clues on the regulation of central B cell tolerance came from the analysis of IRAK4-, MYD88-, and UNC-93B–deficient patients. IRAK4-, MYD88-, and UNC-93B–deficient patients showed increased frequencies of polyreactive new emigrant/transitional B cells indicative of a defective central B cell tolerance checkpoint, revealing the importance of the IRAK4/MYD88 pathway in the establishment of central tolerance (Fig. 2A).[30]

In addition, we discovered that ANA clones including those reacting with chromatin were enriched in the new emigrant/transitional B cell compartment when the MYD88/IRAK4 signaling pathway was defective (Fig. 2B).[30] It is tempting to propose that TLR7 and TLR9, which bind nucleic acid containing antigens also recognized by ANAs, are responsible for the MYD88/IRAK4-dependent removal of ANA-expressing clones. However, the proper silencing of ANA-expressing B cells in UNC-93B–deficient patients argues against an involvement of TLR7 and TLR9 in this process, since UNC-93B has been reported to be required for these TLRs to function (Fig. 2B).[27,28,30] Nevertheless, we can hypothesize that TLR7 and TLR9 may mediate the elimination of ANA clones if nucleic acid containing autoantigens bound to antinuclear BCRs may reach these TLRs in the absence of UNC-93B.[28,29,31] Other IRAK4/MYD88-dependent receptors such as TACI[25] may also contribute to the counterselection of B cells expressing ANAs. Altogether, these data suggest that the TLR/BCR coengagement paradigm for B cell activation and proliferation may also apply to the selection of developing B cells in the bone marrow.

Activation-induced cytidine deaminase is essential for central B cell tolerance

Hyper IgM (HIGM) syndromes are PIDs characterized by defects in class switch recombination (CSR) resulting in severely decreased numbers of circulating isotype-switched memory B cells.[32] The genetic basis of HIGM is diverse and is caused by defects in either the CD40L/CD40 pathway essential for B cell activation, germinal center (GC) formation and CSR induction, or the enzymes such as activation-induced cytidine deaminase (AID) required for CSR and somatic hypermutation (SHM).[33-35] Aside from the susceptibility to bacterial infections, HIGM patients are prone to develop autoimmune diseases, suggesting that B cell tolerance is not properly estab-

lished and/or maintained in the absence of CD40L or AID.[36,37] Antibody characteristics and specificity from CD40L-deficient new emigrant/transitional B cells were similar to those from healthy donors suggesting that CD40L, which is not expressed in developing B cells, does not play an important role in the establishment of central B cell tolerance (Fig. 2). In contrast, new emigrant/transitional B cells from autosomal recessive AID-deficient patients express an abnormal immunoglobulin repertoire and a high frequency of polyreactive antibodies, demonstrating that AID is required for the establishment of central B cell tolerance (Fig. 2A).[38] How AID affects central B cell tolerance is currently unknown but because the mechanisms that ensure human central B cell tolerance seem to be mostly controlled by intrinsic B cell factors, AID expression in immature B cells might be relevant to tolerance induction.[8,11,39] Although AID expression was previously believed to be restricted to activated B cells and GCs, we and others have now detected AID transcripts in human and mouse immature B cells, further supporting an earlier role for AID during bone marrow B cell development.[38,40-44] In addition, AID expression is upregulated in mature and immature B cells by BCR, TLR7, TLR9, and TACI triggering.[25,38] Interestingly, all of these receptors have been demonstrated, or are suspected, to be involved in the establishment of early B cell tolerance, potentially further arguing for a relevant intrinsic role for AID in central B cell tolerance (Ref. 38 and data not shown).

Several scenarios could explain how AID might regulate early B cell tolerance. AID might induce DNA lesions that eventually lead to cell death and the elimination of autoreactive clones; AID-deficient B cells may therefore be less sensitive to apoptosis, a mechanism involved in central B cell tolerance, as reported in mice.[44,45] AID deamination of methylated cytidines might also induce DNA demethylation potentially required for the epigenetic regulation of gene expression (and perhaps V(D)J recombination and receptor editing, the most important mechanism for central B cell tolerance[46]). In line with this hypothesis, changes in DNA methylation in individuals carrying a mutated DNA methyltransferase 3B (*DNMT3B*) gene have been reported to interfere with the central counterselection of B cell clones.[47] However, because *AID* gene transcription in human immature B cells is 20–25 times lower than in GC B cells,[38] these low *AID* transcript levels may not be relevant to immature B cell physiology and the removal of developing autoreactive B cells. In this case, early B cell tolerance alteration observed in AID-deficient patients may not result from intrinsic B cell defects but perhaps from a failure to control intestinal microflora.[48] The expansion of autoreactive IgM[+] B cells in AID-deficient patients may then represent a compensatory mechanism to counterbalance the loss of protection by B cells with high affinity in the absence of functional AID. Nonetheless, a major and previously unsuspected role for AID in the removal of developing autoreactive B cells in humans has been reported.[38] Interestingly, a requirement for *AID* expression in central B cell tolerance was also reported in mice,[44] demonstrating a conserved role for AID on tolerance through evolution.

Central B cell tolerance defects correlate with altered receptor editing regulation

Receptor editing is a major central B cell tolerance mechanism by which developing autoreactive B cells can be silenced, especially those that express ANAs.[49,50] Secondary recombination events, first on the kappa locus and then on the lambda locus, provide attempts to edit autoreactive antibodies by substituting light chains until BCR autoreactivity is either abolished or diminished to levels that allow B cell development to proceed.[11,39,50] As a result, upstream variable (V) gene usage combined with downstream joining (J) segments is a signature for secondary recombination events. A first correlation between abnormal regulation of secondary recombination mediating receptor editing and impaired central B cell tolerance in humans was found in XLA patients.[12] The immunoglobulin kappa (Igκ) and lambda chain (Igλ) gene repertoires of new emigrant/transitional B cells from XLA patients were consistent with extensive secondary recombination activity, revealing that BCR signaling play an important role in downregulating such recombination events likely through the termination of *RAG* gene expression.[12,51] Similarly, extensive secondary recombination on both Igκ and Igλ loci was also observed in human Igμ-deficient pro-B cells, further suggesting that IgL gene secondary recombination is a default mechanism in the absence of IgM signaling.[52] Hence, as expected, receptor editing at the pre-B/immature B cell stage likely requires appropriate BCR signaling to be downregulated in order

to properly counterselect autoreactive developing B cells in the bone marrow.[12]

Decreased secondary recombination potentially corresponding to a failure to induce receptor editing may also lead to abnormal central B cell tolerance. Indeed, a subset of common variable immunodeficiency disease (CVID) patients with expanded autoreactive CD21[−/lo] B cell populations (CVID group Ia[53]) suffer from a defective central B cell tolerance checkpoint associated with an Igκ repertoire characterized by a dearth of secondary recombination events.[54,55] Interestingly, new emigrant B cells from untreated active RA patients who also suffer from defective central B cell tolerance[10,56,57] express distinct patterns of Igκ light chain antibody repertoires, some of which altered by defective regulation of secondary recombination, a feature also reported in SLE patient's B cells.[58–60] An alteration in the regulation of secondary recombination events was also reported in IRAK4- and MYD88-deficient patients with defective central B cell tolerance; most ANA-expressing new emigrant/transitional B cells that escaped central tolerance in these patients used kappa chains, demonstrating that editing using lambda chains, which are more efficient in humans at silencing autoreactive antibodies than kappa chains,[61] was not induced in these B cells.[30] In addition, lambda chain usage in IRAK4- and MYD88-deficient B cells did not diminish antibody autoreactivity compared to kappa chain expressing clones, which further suggest defects in receptor editing in these patients. Additional analysis of the Igλ gene repertoire of new emigrant/transitional from IRAK4- and MYD88-deficient patients revealed increased downstream Vλ gene usage combined with upstream Jλ1 usage, the most upstream of all Jλ gene segments, attesting a dearth of secondary recombination on this locus when functional IRAK4/MYD88 complexes could not be expressed.

We conclude that kappa and lambda light chain receptor editing is not efficiently regulated to silence autoreactive and ANA expressing developing B cells in many PID patients who suffer from impaired central B cell tolerance.

Defects in peripheral B cell tolerance

Transgenic mouse models have suggested that CD4[+] T cells may play an important role in the elimination of peripheral autoreactive B cells through MHC class II/T cell receptor; CD40/CD40L and Fas/FasL

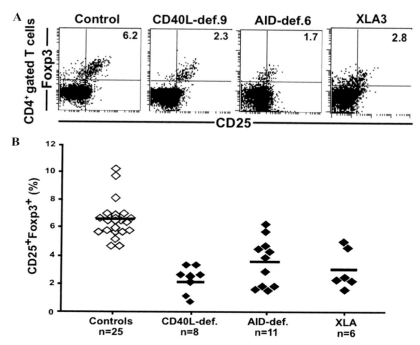

Figure 4. Decreased T_{reg} cell frequency in CD40L-, AID-deficient, and XLA patients. T_{reg} cell frequencies among peripheral CD4+ T cells were assessed by analyzing the proportion of CD25+Foxp3+ cells. Dot plots representative for a healthy control and CD40L-, AID-deficient, and XLA patients are displayed in (A). (B) T_{reg} cell frequencies from all patients were significantly lower than those in healthy controls ($P < 0.0001$ for CD40L-, AID-deficient, and XLA patients).

interactions.[62] To investigate the impact of CD40/CD40L interactions and MHC class II expression on human B cell tolerance, we tested the reactivity of recombinant antibodies isolated from single B cells from CD40L-deficient and MHC class II–deficient patients.[63] We found that although developing autoreactive B cells were properly counterselected in the bone marrow of these patients, mature naive B cells from CD40L- and MHC class II–deficient patients expressed a high proportion of autoreactive antibodies, including ANAs (Figs. 2 and 3).[63] Thus, CD40/CD40L interactions and antigen presentation are essential for peripheral B cell tolerance. In addition, all patients who suffered from a defective central B cell tolerance checkpoint (IRAK4-, MYD88-, UNC-93B-, and AID-deficiencies) also displayed additional selection defects in their periphery, resulting in the accumulation of autoreactive mature naive B cells.[30,38]

The specific defects at the peripheral B cell tolerance checkpoint in CD40L- and MHC class II–deficient patients suggested that a T cell population is involved in the removal of autoreactive B cells in

the periphery.[63] We found that CD40L- and MHC class II–deficient patients displayed decreased T_{reg} cell numbers (Fig. 4).[63] The importance of T_{reg} cells in the establishment and/or the maintenance of peripheral tolerance is demonstrated in mice and humans deficient in Foxp3, who suffer from a severe autoimmune syndrome.[64–66] Similar to CD40L- and MHC class II–deficient patients, individuals with BTK- and AID-deficiency, who suffer from a defective peripheral B cell tolerance checkpoint, also lack isotype-switched memory B cells and display decreased T_{reg} cell frequencies, suggesting a potential involvement for B cells in either the generation or the maintenance of some T_{reg} cells in humans (Fig. 4).[38]

BAFF is a serum cytokine that promotes transitional and mature naive B cell survival. BAFF-deficient mice display profoundly decreased numbers of peripheral B cells.[67] In contrast, mice overexpressing BAFF develop autoimmune disorders similar to SLE and Sjorgren syndrome characterized by the production of autoreactive antibodies, including rheumatoid factor, anti-DNA, and other ANAs.[68] Elevated BAFF concentration

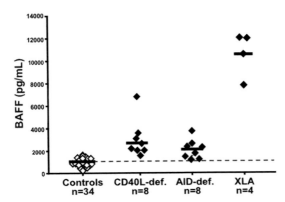

Figure 5. Elevated serum BAFF concentrations in CD40L-, AID-deficient, and XLA patients. BAFF concentrations (pg/mL) in the serum of healthy donor controls (open diamonds), CD40L-, and AID-deficient patients as well as XLA patients (black diamonds) were measured by ELISA. Each diamond represents an individual, and the average is shown with a bar.

inhibits the counterselection of autoreactive new emigrant/transitional B cells that failed to be removed from the B cell population.[69,70] BAFF may also favor the proliferation of some clones by promoting the entry into the cell cycle.[71] Hence, the elevated serum BAFF concentration in CD40L-, MHC class II-, and AID-deficient patients is therefore likely to contribute to the accumulation of autoreactive mature naive B cells in the blood of these patients (Fig. 5).[38,63] We conclude that T_{reg} cells and serum BAFF concentrations may be involved in the regulation of peripheral human B cell tolerance.[38,63]

Perspectives

We have reviewed herein the current data on the establishment of central and peripheral B cell tolerance selecting the naive B cell repertoire. It is obvious that the analysis of additional PID will further increase and refine our understanding on the steps controlling the selection of B cell clones in the mature naive B cell compartment. Several important aspects of early B cell tolerance remain to be investigated: Are TLR7 and TLR9 the receptors responsible for the central removal of antinuclear clones? How does AID deficiency affect central B cell tolerance? and Are T_{reg} cells essential for the removal of autoreactive B cells in the periphery? PID patients deficient for TLR7 or TLR9 have not yet been identified to assess the first question. The mechanisms by which AID deficiency impairs central tolerance may be explored by studying early

B cell tolerance checkpoints in PID patients deficient in molecules acting downstream of AID such as Uracil N-glycosylase (UNG), MSH6, and PMS2, the latter two belonging to the mismatch repair system (MMR) complexes. Finally, the investigation of immune deficiency, polyendocrinopathy, enteropathy, X-linked syndrome (IPEX) patients who carry a mutation in the *FOXP3* gene and suffer from defective T_{reg} cell functions, should determine if T_{reg} cells are involved in the establishment of peripheral B cell tolerance in humans.

Acknowledgments

This work was supported by Grants AI061093, AI071087, AI082713 from NIH-NIAID.

Conflicts of interest

The author declares no conflicts of interest.

References

1. Leslie, D., P. Lipsky & A.L. Notkins. 2001. Autoantibodies as predictors of disease. *J. Clin. Invest.* **108:** 1417–1422.

2. Edwards, J.C.W. *et al.* 2004. Efficacy of B cell-targeted therapy with Rituximab in patients with rheumatoid arthritis. *N. Engl. J. Med.* **350:** 2572–2581.

3. Hauser, S.L. *et al.* 2008. B-cell depletion with rituximab in relapsing-remitting multiple sclerosis. *N. Engl. J. Med.* **358:** 676–688.

4. Pescovitz, M.D. *et al.* 2009. Rituximab, B-lymphocyte depletion, and preservation of beta-cell function. *N. Engl. J. Med.* **361:** 2143–2152.

5. Wardemann, H., *et al.* 2003. Predominant autoantibody production by early human B cell precursors. *Science* **301:** 1374–1377.

6. Meffre, E. *et al.* 2004. Surrogate light chain expressing human peripheral B cells produce self-reactive antibodies. *J. Exp. Med.* **199:** 145–150.

7. Tiller, T. *et al.* 2008. Efficient generation of monoclonal antibodies from single human B cells by single cell RT-PCR and expression vector cloning. *J. Immunol. Methods* **329:** 112–124.

8. Meffre, E. & H. Wardemann. 2008. B-cell tolerance checkpoints in health and autoimmunity. *Curr. Opin. Immunol.* **20:** 632–638.

9. van Zelm, M.C., T. Szczepanski, M. van der Burg & J.J. van Dongen. 2007. Replication history of B lymphocytes reveals homeostatic proliferation and extensive antigen-induced B cell expansion. *J. Exp. Med.* **204:** 645–655.

10. Menard, L. *et al.* 2011. The *PTPN22* allele encoding an R620W variant interferes with the removal of developing autoreactive B cells in humans. *J. Clin. Invest.* **121:** 3635–3644.

11. Goodnow, C.C. 1996. Balancing immunity and tolerance: deleting and tuning lymphocyte repertoires. *Proc. Natl. Acad. Sci. USA* **93:** 2264–2271.

12. Ng, Y.-S., H. Wardemann, J. Chelnis, *et al.* 2004. Bruton's tyrosine kinase (Btk) is essential for human B cell tolerance. *J. Exp. Med.* **200:** 927–934.

13. Grimaldi, C.M., R. Hicks & B. Diamond. 2005. B cell selection and susceptibility to autoimmunity. *J. Immunol.* **174:** 1775–1781.

14. de Weers, M. *et al.* 1994. B-cell antigen receptor stimulation activates the human Bruton's tyrosine kinase, which is deficient in X-linked agammaglobulinemia. *J. Biol. Chem.* **269:** 23857–23860.

15. Kurosaki, T. & S. Tsukada. 2000. BLNK: connecting Syk and Btk to calcium signals. *Immunity* **12:** 1–5.

16. Begovich, A.B. *et al.* 2004. A missense single-nucleotide polymorphism in a gene encoding a protein tyrosine phosphatase (PTPN22) is associated with rheumatoid arthritis. *Am. J. Hum. Genet.* **75:** 330–337.

17. Kyogoku, C. *et al.* 2004. Genetic association of the R620W polymorphism of protein tyrosine phosphatase PTPN22 with human SLE. *Am. J. Hum. Genet.* **75:** 504–507.

18. Bottini, N. *et al.* 2004. A functional variant of lymphoid tyrosine phosphatase is associated with type 1 diabetes. *Nat. Genet.* **36:** 337–338.

19. Michou, L. *et al.* 2007. Linkage proof for PTPN22, a rheumatoid arthritis susceptibility gene and a human autoimmunity gene. *Proc. Natl. Acad. Sci. USA* **104:** 1649–1654.

20. Vang, T. *et al.* 2005. Autoimmune-associated lymphoid tyrosine phosphatase is a gain-of-function variant. *Nat. Genet.* **37:** 1317–1319.

21. Arechiga, A.F. *et al.* 2009. Cutting edge: the PTPN22 allelic variant associated with autoimmunity impairs B cell signaling. *J. Immunol.* **182:** 3343–3347.

22. Marshak-Rothstein, A. 2006. Toll-like receptors in systemic autoimmune disease. *Nat. Rev. Immunol.* **6:** 823–835.

23. Akira, S. & K. Takeda. 2004. Toll-like receptor signaling. *Nat. Rev. Immunol.* **4:** 499–511.

24. Beutler, B. 2004. Inferences, questions and possibilities in Toll-like receptor signalling. *Nature* **430:** 257–263.

25. He, B. *et al.* 2010. The transmembrane activator TACI triggers immunoglobulin class switching by activating B cells through the adaptor MyD88. *Nat. Immunol.* **11:** 836–845.

26. Brinkmann, M.M. *et al.* 2007. The interaction between the ER membrane protein UNC93B and TLR3, 7, and 9 is crucial for TLR signaling. *J. Cell. Biol.* **177:** 265–275.

27. Casrouge, A. *et al.* 2006. Herpes simplex virus encephalitis in human UNC-93B deficiency. *Science* **314:** 308–312.

28. Kim, Y.M., M.M. Brinkmann, M.E. Paquet & H.L. Ploegh. 2008. UNC93B1 delivers nucleotide-sensing toll-like receptors to endolysosomes. *Nature* **452:** 234–238.

29. Tabeta, K. *et al.* 2006. The Unc93b1 mutation 3d disrupts exogenous antigen presentation and signaling via Toll-like receptors 3, 7 and 9. *Nat. Immunol.* **7:** 156–164.

30. Isnardi, I. *et al.* 2008. IRAK-4- and MyD88-dependent pathways are essential for the removal of developing autoreactive B cells in humans. *Immunity* **29:** 746–757.

31. Kim, Y.M., M.M. Brinkmann & H.L. Ploegh. 2007. TLRs bent into shape. *Nat. Immunol.* **8:** 675–677.

32. Gulino, A.V. & L.D. Notarangelo. 2003. Hyper IgM syndromes. *Curr. Opin. Rheumatol.* **15:** 422–429.

33. Lee, W.I. *et al.* 2005. Molecular analysis of a large cohort of patients with the hyper immunoglobulin M (IgM) syndrome. *Blood* **105:** 1881–1890.

34. Muramatsu, M. *et al.* 2000. Class switch recombination and hypermutation require activation-induced cytidine deaminase (AID), a potential RNA editing enzyme [see comments]. *Cell* **102:** 553–563.

35. Revy, P. *et al.* 2000. Activation-induced cytidine deaminase (AID) deficiency causes the autosomal recessive form of the Hyper-IgM syndrome (HIGM2) [see comments]. *Cell* **102:** 565–575.

36. Quartier, P. *et al.* 2004. Clinical, immunologic and genetic analysis of 29 patients with autosomal recessive hyper-IgM syndrome due to activation-induced cytidine deaminase deficiency. *Clin. Immunol.* **110:** 22–29.

37. Durandy, A., S. Peron & A. Fischer 2006. Hyper-IgM syndromes. *Curr. Opin. Rheumatol.* **18:** 369–376.

38. Meyers, G. *et al.* 2011. Activation-induced cytidine deaminase (AID) is required for B-cell tolerance in humans. *Proc. Natl. Acad. Sci. USA* **108:** 11554–11559.

39. Nemazee, D. *et al.* 2000. B-cell-receptor-dependent positive and negative selection in immature B cells. *Curr. Top. Microbiol. Immunol.* **245:** 57–71.

40. Mao, C. *et al.* 2004. T cell-independent somatic hypermutation in murine B cells with an immature phenotype. *Immunity* **20:** 133–144.

41. Han, J.H. *et al.* 2007. Class switch recombination and somatic hypermutation in early mouse B cells are mediated by B cell and Toll-like receptors. *Immunity* **27:** 64–75.

42. Ueda, Y., D. Liao, K. Yang, *et al* 2007. T-independent activation-induced cytidine deaminase expression, class-switch recombination, and antibody production by immature/transitional 1 B cells. *J. Immunol.* **178:** 3593–3601.

43. Kuraoka, M. *et al.* 2009. Activation-induced cytidine deaminase expression and activity in the absence of germinal centers: insights into hyper-IgM syndrome. *J. Immunol.* **183:** 3237–3248.

44. Kuraoka, M. *et al.* 2011. Activation-induced cytidine deaminase mediates central tolerance in B cells. *Proc. Natl. Acad. Sci. USA* **108:** 11560–11565.

45. Zaheen, A. *et al.* 2009. AID constrains germinal center size by rendering B cells susceptible to apoptosis. *Blood* **114:** 547–554.

46. Goodhardt, M. *et al.* 1993. Methylation status of immunoglobulin kappa gene segments correlates with their recombination potential. *Eur. J. Immunol.* **23:** 1789–1795.

47. Blanco-Betancourt, C.E. *et al.* 2004. Defective B-cell-negative selection and terminal differentiation in the ICF syndrome. *Blood* **103:** 2683–2690.

48. Fagarasan, S. *et al.* 2002. Critical roles of activation-induced cytidine deaminase in the homeostasis of gut flora. *Science* **298:** 1424–1427.

49. Halverson, R., R.M. Torres & R. Pelanda. 2004. Receptor editing is the main mechanism of B cell tolerance toward membrane antigens. *Nat. Immunol.* **6:** 645–650.

50. Radic, M.Z. & M. Weigert. 1995. Origins of anti-DNA antibodies and their implications for B-cell tolerance. *Ann. N.Y. Acad. Sci.* **764:** 384–396.

51. Verkoczy, L. *et al.* 2005. A role for nuclear factor kappa B/rel transcription factors in the regulation of the recombinase activator genes. *Immunity* **22:** 519–531.

52. Meffre, E. *et al.* 2001. Immunoglobulin heavy chain expression shapes the B cell receptor repertoire in human B cell development. *J. Clin. Invest.* **108:** 879–886.

53. Warnatz, K. *et al.* 2002. Severe deficiency of switched memory B cells (CD27(+)IgM(−)IgD(−)) in subgroups of patients with common variable immunodeficiency: a new approach to classify a heterogeneous disease. *Blood* **99:** 1544–1551.

54. Isnardi, I. *et al.* 2010. Complement receptor 2/CD21- human naive B cells contain mostly autoreactive unresponsive clones. *Blood* **115:** 5026–5036.

55. Romberg, N., Y.S. Ng, C. Cunningham-Rundles & E. Meffre. 2011. Common variable immunodeficiency patients with increased CD21-/lo B cells suffer from altered receptor editing and defective central B cell tolerance. In press.

56. Samuels, J., Y.-S. Ng, C. Coupillaud, *et al* 2005. Impaired early B cell tolerance in patients with rheumatoid arthritis. *J. Exp. Med.* **201:** 1659–1667.

57. Menard, L., J. Samuels, Y.S. Ng & E. Meffre. 2011. Inflammation-independent defective early B cell tolerance checkpoints in rheumatoid arthritis. *Arthritis Rheum.* **63:** 1237–1245.

58. Bensimon, C., P. Chastagner & M. Zouali. 1994. Human lupus anti-DNA autoantibodies undergo essentially primary V kappa gene rearrangements. *EMBO J.* **13:** 2951–2962.

59. Suzuki, N., T. Harada, S. Mihara & T. Sakane. 1996. Characterization of a germline Vk gene encoding cationic anti-DNA antibody and role of receptor editing for development of the autoantibody in patients with systemic lupus erythematosus. *J. Clin. Invest.* **98:** 1843–1850.

60. Dorner, T., S.J. Foster, N.L. Farner & P.E. Lipsky. 1998. Immunoglobulin kappa chain receptor editing in systemic lupus erythematosus. *J. Clin. Invest.* **102:** 688–694.

61. Wardemann, H., J. Hammersen & M.C. Nussenzweig. 2004. Human autoantibody silencing by immunoglobulin light chains. *J. Exp. Med.* **200:** 191–199.

62. Rathmell, J.C. *et al.* 1995. CD95 (Fas)-dependent elimination of self-reactive B cells upon interaction with CD4+ T cells. *Nature* **376:** 181–184.

63. Hervé, M. *et al.* 2007. CD40 ligand and MHC class II expression are essential for human peripheral B cell tolerance. *J. Exp. Med.* **204:** 1583–1593.

64. Brunkow, M.E. *et al.* 2001. Disruption of a new forkhead/winged-helix protein, scurfin, results in the fatal lymphoproliferative disorder of the scurfy mouse. *Nat. Genet.* **27:** 68–73.

65. Wildin, R.S. *et al.* 2001. X-linked neonatal diabetes mellitus, enteropathy, and endocrinopathy syndrome is the human equivalent of mouse scurfy. *Nat. Genet.* **27:** 18–20.

66. Bennett, C.L. *et al.* 2001. The immune dysregulation, polyendocrinopathy, enteropathy, X-linked syndrome (IPEX) is caused by mutations of FOXP3. *Nat. Genet.* **27:** 20–21.

67. Schiemann, B. *et al.* 2001. An essential role for BAFF in the normal development of B cells through a BCMA-independent pathway. *Science* **293:** 2111–2114.

68. Mackay, F. *et al.* 1999. Mice transgenic for BAFF develop lymphocytic disorders along with autoimmune manifestations. *J. Exp. Med.* **190:** 1697–1710.

69. Lesley, R. *et al.* 2004. Reduced competitiveness of autoantigen-engaged B cells due to increased dependence on BAFF. *Immunity* **20:** 441–453.

70. Thien, M. *et al.* 2004. Excess BAFF rescues self-reactive B cells from peripheral deletion and allows them to enter forbidden follicular and marginal zone niches. *Immunity* **20:** 785–798.

71. Huang, X. *et al.* 2004. Homeostatic cell-cycle control of Blys: induction of cell-cycle entry but not G1/S transition in opposition to p18^{INK4c} and p27^{KIP1}. *Proc. Natl. Acad. Sci. USA* **101:** 17789–17794.

Ann. N.Y. Acad. Sci. ISSN 0077-8923

ANNALS OF THE NEW YORK ACADEMY OF SCIENCES

Issue: *The Year in Human and Medical Genetics: Inborn Errors of Immunity*

Checkpoints of B cell differentiation: visualizing Ig-centric processes

Magdalena A. Berkowska, Mirjam van der Burg, Jacques J.M. van Dongen, and Menno C. van Zelm

Department of Immunology, Erasmus MC, University Medical Center, Rotterdam, the Netherlands

Address for correspondence: M.C. van Zelm, Ph.D., Molecular Immunology Unit, Department of Immunology, Erasmus MC, University Medical Center Rotterdam, Dr. Molewaterplein 50, 3015 GE Rotterdam, the Netherlands. m.vanzelm@erasmusmc.nl

The generation of antibody responses and B cell memory can only take place following multiple steps of differentiation. Key molecular processes during precursor B cell differentiation in bone marrow generate unique antibodies. These antibodies are further optimized via molecular modifications during immune responses in peripheral lymphoid organs. Multiple checkpoints ensure proper differentiation of precursor and mature B lymphocytes. Many of these checkpoints have been found disrupted in patients with a primary immunodeficiency. Based on studies in these patients and in mouse models, new insights have been generated in B cell differentiation and antibody responses. Still, in many patients with impaired antibody formation, it remains unclear how B cells are affected. In this perspective, we present 11 critical processes in B cell differentiation. We discuss how defects in these processes can result in impaired checkpoint selection and how they can be visualized in healthy subjects and patients with immunodeficiency or other immunological disease.

Keywords: B cell; immunoglobulin; selection; repertoire; differentiation; checkpoint

Introduction

B and T lymphocytes have a unique role in the vertebrate immune system, since they seemingly adapt their specificity to the invading pathogen and generate immunological memory. These adaptive capabilities are the result of two independent stages of development (Fig. 1). First, each lymphocyte creates a unique receptor for recognition of pathogens during precursor differentiation in bone marrow (B cell) or thymus (T cell). Together, this results in a large repertoire of antigen receptors with the potential to specifically recognize many different pathogens. Second, the lymphocytes that actually recognize antigen in peripheral lymphoid organs are selected to undergo enormous clonal proliferation, thereby generating huge numbers of daughter cells with the potential to recognize the same pathogen. This clonal expansion generates effector cells for a strong response and long-term memory in the form of memory B and T cells and immunoglobulin (Ig)-producing plasma cells. The host requires a highly dynamic immune system, which maintains a tight balance between the production of a large repertoire of cells with unique receptors and a strong immune response of groups of cells with an antigen-specific, and thereby a more limited (selected), repertoire.

During stepwise B cell differentiation, at least 11 critical processes exist to ensure generation of a selected repertoire (Fig. 1). A developing B cell that is defective in one of these processes will fail to meet subsequent checkpoint requirements and has to be removed from the host's body to prevent disease. The importance of this tightly controlled B cell development is best illustrated by disorders, that is, autoimmune diseases with autoreactive antibodies and B cell malignancies. In these diseases, one or more processes went astray in a developing B cell and the cell was not removed from the repertoire at the subsequent checkpoint. On the other hand, rare inherited disorders that impair immunity (primary immunodeficiencies; PID) often involve an antibody deficiency. In PID

doi: 10.1111/j.1749-6632.2011.06278.x

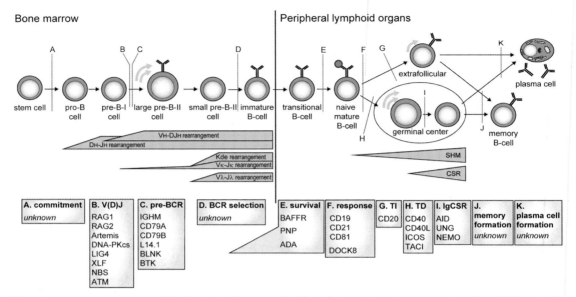

Bone marrow | Peripheral lymphoid organs

Figure 1. Important processes and checkpoints in human B cell differentiation. Schematic representation of B cell differentiation stages in bone marrow and peripheral lymphoid organs. Eleven important processes, of which successful completion is required to meet the subsequent checkpoint, are indicated by letters *A* through *K*. Seven processes have been found impaired due to genetic defects in patients with PID. Thus far, no genetic defects have been found to impair the other four processes that could block B cell differentiation at the accompanying checkpoint: A: B cell commitment; D: B cell antigen receptor (BCR) selection; J: memory B cell formation; K: plasma cell formation.

patients, one or more processes are impaired in all B cells and therefore most or all cells fail to meet the checkpoint requirements, resulting in a differentiation block and removal of most or all cells. Many insights concerning important processes in B cell development and antibody responses have been obtained from studies in animal models. Studies in human subjects are more challenging due to obvious limitations in tissue availability and *in vivo* measurements. Still, many new (technical) developments allow for careful analysis of B cell differentiation checkpoints in human blood and bone marrow.

In this perspective, we present new insights into important checkpoints in B cell differentiation. The main focus will lie on positive selection processes, with limited attention to negative selection against autoreactivity, T cell/B cell interactions, and mucosal Ig responses, which are discussed in accompanying papers.[1–3] We will specifically discuss how these processes and accompanying B cell differentiation checkpoints can be visualized to identify defects in patients with immunological disease.

Critical processes and checkpoints in antigen-independent B cell differentiation

The most defining feature of a B cell is the expression of a surface Ig receptor that can recognize a specific antigenic epitope. One Ig receptor is composed of two identical heavy chains (IgH) and light chains (Igκ or Igλ isotype). In contrast to nearly all other proteins, the constituents of Ig molecules are not encoded by germline DNA. As discovered by Susumu Tonegawa, genetic elements in Ig loci, variable, diversity, and joining genes, need to be rearranged to encode a functional protein through a process named V(D)J recombination.[4,5] To ensure that the total pool of mature B cells consists of cells with unique Ig molecules that together form a large repertoire of antigen specificities, multiple processes need to take place: commitment of multipotent progenitors to the B cell lineage, efficient and ordered recombination of randomly selected V, D, and J genes in the Ig loci, positive selection of functional Ig proteins, and negative selection of autoreactive Igs. Several selection checkpoints ensure that these four processes are successful in consecutive stages of differentiation (Fig. 1; processes A–D). We will here discuss recent insights into these checkpoints and provide suggestions on how to visualize defects in underlying processes.

Commitment of hematopoietic progenitors to the B cell lineage

Hematopoietic stem cells (HSC) in bone marrow are long-lived and self-renewing. They generate multilineage progenitors that are capable of developing into erythroid, myeloid, and lymphoid cells, but do not self-renew (Fig. 2). Thus, every single multilineage progenitor will only differentiate and commit itself to only one of the many specific blood cell types. Extensive studies in mouse models have supported our understanding of their progressive restriction in developmental potential through intermediate steps (reviewed in Refs. 6 and 7). A multilineage progenitor will become restricted to either a lymphoid or myeloid cell fate depending on the levels of transcription factors PU.1 and Ikaros (Fig. 2).[8–11] Myeloid progenitors can develop into

erythrocytes and myeloid cells, including monocytes and granulocytes. The myeloid fate is inhibited by upregulation of E2A and expression of IL-7R, and the resulting lymphoid progenitor can only give rise to NK cells, T cells, and B cells. Upon induction of RAG1, the fate is further specified to the T or B cell lineage, while NK cell potential is lost. These cells can be identified in the mouse based on Ly6D expression.[12] Subsequent expression of EBF1 specifies the B cell fate. These pro-B cells can be identified by intracellular λ5, a component of the surrogate light chain.[12] Still, these cells are not yet fully committed to the B cell lineage and can be directed to the T cell lineage.[13] Only upon expression of Pax5, is the cell fully committed. This pre-B–I cell can be identified based on membrane CD19 expression.

The stepwise processes of restriction, specification, and commitment of HSC to the B cell lineage are extremely difficult to study in humans. Still, several studies have identified differential expression of membrane proteins in progenitor cells prior to commitment to the B cell lineage (Fig. 2B). All early

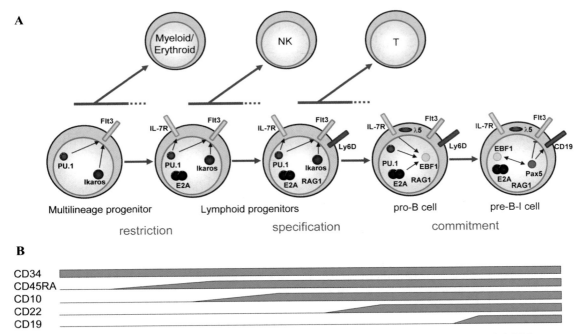

Figure 2. Stepwise control of B cell commitment from hematopoietic stem cells (HSC) in bone marrow. (A) HSC generate multilineage progenitors that have the potential to differentiate into all blood cell lineages. Stepwise, specification and commitment processes take place as a result of tight balances between transcription factors. Ikaros expression and low PU.1 expression levels restrict toward a lymphoid cell fate. Subsequently, E2A and IL-7R signaling specify the B cell program to which the cell becomes committed upon expression of Pax5. (B) Early steps in B cell commitment can be visualized in human bone marrow and neonatal cord blood through differential expression of CD34, CD45RA, CD10, CD22, and CD19.

progenitor cells express CD34. Still, only very recently, long-term repopulating HSC have been purified based on CD49f expression.[14] Multilineage progenitors are negative for CD49f and all lineage markers, and they can still repopulate all blood lineages, but fail to engraft long term.[14] Upon specification to the lymphoid lineage these cells rapidly express CD45RA.[15,16] With further specification to the T/B cell fates CD10 is gradually upregulated,[17] and reaches maximal levels in pro-B cells that coexpress CD22.[17,18] These cells already express RAG proteins and contain D to J gene rearrangements in the Ig heavy chain locus (*IGH*).[18,19] Similar to mice, committed pre-B-I cells can be identified by surface CD19 expression.

Detailed flowcytometric analysis of B cell commitment processes will be relevant to understand and distinguish between conditions that result in a complete absence of precursor B cells in bone marrow. Potential conditions are active infections that cause suppression of the lymphoid compartment, or agammaglobulinemia with a complete absence of precursor B cells in bone marrow (Ref. 20 and unpublished observations, Mirjam van der Burg). Despite our understanding from mouse studies and good candidate genes (e.g., E2A, EBF1, Pax 5), as yet, no genetic defects have been identified in these patients.

V(D)J recombination of Ig loci

In the *IGH* locus, one of each V, D, and J genes are randomly coupled to form a functional exon. Similar rearrangements are initiated between one V and one J gene in the *IGK* and *IGL* loci. The rearrangement process is accompanied by deletion and random insertion of nucleotides (Fig. 3B) at the coupling sides of V, D, and J gene resulting in unique junctions. The combination of V, (D), and J gene segments and the processing of junctional regions create enormous Ig diversity between B cells.

V(D)J recombination is a highly specific process that is only initiated in precursor B cells and precursor T cells in order to generate antigen receptors. Double-stranded DNA breaks are induced by the recombinase activating gene protein products RAG1 and RAG2 that specifically recognize conserved DNA sequences: recombination signal sequence (RSS) (Fig. 3A). The RAG dimers juxtapose the two gene poised to rearrange and nick the DNA of both at the border of the gene and the flanking

RSS.[21–23] The 3'OH at each nick attacks the antiparallel strand to create a DNA hairpin at the gene. Blunt ends remain on the RSS sequences and are directly joined by the nonhomologous end joining (NHEJ) process to create a circular excision product. A protein complex consisting of NBN, MRE11, and RAD50 holds the coding ends together for processing prior to ligation by NHEJ components.[24–27] The proteins Ku70 and Ku80 first bind the coding ends and recruit the catalytic subunit of DNA-dependent protein kinase (DNA-PKcs) and Artemis.[28,29] The protein Artemis nicks the hairpin preferentially at the tip or 1–2 bp 5' of the tip,[30,31] which results in a 3' overhang. Complementary nucleotides can be inserted from the 5' end to generate a blunt end, resulting in the generation, of palindromic (P) nucleotides (Fig. 3B). Furthermore, exonucleases can delete nucleotides, whereas terminal deoxynucleotidyl transferase (TdT) can add random nontemplated (N) nucleotides.[32,33] Finally, the Ku heterodimer recruits a protein complex, including XRCC4, DNA ligase IV, and XLF, that ligates the coding ends.[34–36] The processing of the coding ends before ligation with nucleotide insertions and deletions results in a unique coding joint sequence.

Genetic defects in the RAG proteins and in NHEJ factors greatly impair V(D)J recombination and result in strongly reduced mature B cell (and T cell) numbers. Still, in some patients, incomplete DH to JH gene rearrangements can be found in precursor B cells in bone marrow. The molecular characteristics of DH–JH junctions are highly informative of the impaired phase of the recombination process. The junctional regions in RAG1- or RAG2-deficient patients show normal patterns of nucleotide deletions, additions, and P-nucleotides (Fig. 3C).[27] Apparently, the initiation of the break is impaired, but subsequent processing occurs normally. In contrast, patients with impaired hairpin processing due to Artemis or DNA-PKcs deficiency have junctional regions with longer P-nucleotide stretches due to aberrant hairpin opening (Fig. 3C).[37,38] Finally, patients with defects in ligation of the coding ends due to *LIG4* mutations show increased nucleotide deletion as compared to controls, caused by prolonged exonuclease exposure due to delayed and/or aberrant ligation (Fig. 3C).[39] Thus, while the B cell differentiation defect seems similar, the V(D)J recombination process is impaired in different phases. This can be visualized by molecular analysis of Ig gene rearrangements. While patients with genetic defects in the NBN-encoding gene *NBS* have mature B and T cells with seemingly normal rearrangement patterns,[40] these numbers are decreased due to impaired juxtapositioning of coding ends.[25] These defects in NBN function can best be visualized by fluorescence *in situ* hybridization of precursor B cells with *IGHV* and *IGHC* DNA probes to detect split coding ends.[25]

Pre-B cell antigen receptor (pre-BCR) signaling

Upon the generation of a functional IgH protein, the precursor B cell will express it on the membrane in a complex with signaling proteins CD79A and CD79B and with surrogate light chain proteins VpreB and λ14.1, forming the pre-B cell antigen receptor (pre-BCR); (Figs. 1 and 4). Expression of a functional pre-BCR is an important checkpoint in precursor-B cell differentiation, because downstream signaling pathways are required for further maturation. First, V(D)J recombination at the *IGH*

loci is terminated, followed by induction of proliferation, and subsequently by induction of Ig light chain gene rearrangements (Fig. 4A). The understanding of pre-BCR signaling started upon identification of mutations in the *BTK* gene that were found to underlie X-linked agammaglobulinemia in patients who lacked serum Ig and mature B cells in blood.[41,42] Since then many components and signaling molecules have been identified, some of which are mutated in patients with autosomal recessive agammaglobulinemia (Fig. 1; reviewed in Ref. 43).

The final frontier in the understanding of pre-BCR signaling has been the identification of a potential ligand. Since the pre-BCR signals constitutively, it was suggested that this was induced by its surface expression only, independent of an environmental ligand. However, a series of elegant experiments by Schiff and coworkers have unraveled that the soluble lectin Galectin-1 produced by bone marrow stromal cells can function as a true pre-BCR ligand for human and mouse precursor B cells.[44-46] Galectin-1 can bind to λ14.1 and

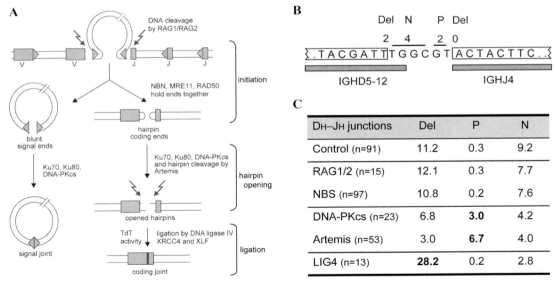

Figure 3. Visualization of Ig repertoire formation processes. (A) Schematic representation of V(D)J recombination. The RAG proteins initiate DNA break formation in two gene at the border of the RSSs. This results in two hairpinned coding ends and two blunt signal ends. The blunt signal ends are directly joined by a complex of Ku70, Ku80, and DNA-PKcs. The coding ends are held together by NBN, MRE1, and RAD50, while Ku70, Ku80, and DNA-PKcs recruit Artemis that cleaves the hairpins. Subsequently, the coding ends are processed by endonucleases and TdT. Finally, a complex of DNA ligase IV, XRCC4, and XLF is required to ligate the ends into a coding joint. (B) Schematic representation of deleted, palindromic (P) and randomly inserted nontemplated (N) nucleotides in a hypothetical *IGHD5–12* to *IGHJ4* gene rearrangement. (C) Junctional region characteristics of *IGHD* to *IGHJ* gene rearrangements in healthy controls and in patients with defects in the initiation, processing, or ligation processes of V(D)J recombination.

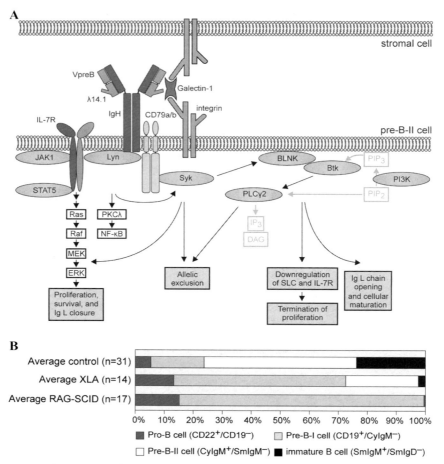

Figure 4. Pre-BCR signaling is required for precursor B cell differentiation. (A) Schematic overview of pre-BCR signaling. Signaling is induced through cross-linking of pre-BCR complexes following binding of λ14.1 to Galectin-1, which is produced by stromal cells and can be presented by integrins. The pre-BCR and the IL-7R signal via Lyn, Syk, Stat5, and the Ras–Raf–MEK–ERK pathway for proliferation. Signaling of the pre-BCR via Syk is also required for allelic exclusion. Furthermore, the pre-BCR signals via BLNK and Btk to limit proliferation and induce Ig light chain rearrangements. (B) BTK-deficient patients have impaired pre-BCR signaling and show a block in differentiation prior to the cytoplasmic Igμ+ pre-B-II cells stage, as compared with healthy controls. This block is partial and clearly differs from V(D)J recombination defects in RAG-deficient patients. Cy, cytoplasmic; Sm, surface membrane.

α4β1, α5β1, and α4β7 integrins, and thereby may function to induce pre-BCR clustering and signaling (Fig. 4A).[45,46]

Defects in pre-BCR signaling lead to a block in differentiation prior to the cytoplasmic Igμ+ pre-B-II cell stage. While the block seemingly occurs at the same differentiation stage as V(D)J recombination defects, most mutations that impair pre-BCR signaling allow development of some Igμ+ pre-B-II cells depending on the affected gene (Fig. 4B).[47] Moreover, pre-BCR signaling defects affect only the B cell lineage.

Control of stepwise Ig gene rearrangements by IL-7 and pre-BCR signaling

One of the major unresolved questions regarding B cell differentiation concerns the highly controlled order in which Ig gene rearrangements are induced. While a common machinery is responsible for V(D)J recombination of three Ig and four T cell receptor (TCR) loci, nearly all precursor B cells rearrange their Ig receptor loci in a strict order: D to J and V to DJ on *IGH*, and only after pre-BCR signaling *IGK* is rearranged prior to *IGL*.

The targeting of recombinase activity to a specific locus (or even clusters of gene segments) is controlled at multiple levels, including DNA methylation,[48] chromatin remodeling,[49] histone acetylation,[50,51] germline transcription[52] and transcription elongation,[53] and large-scale DNA contraction.[54,55] In the *IGH* locus, all mentioned epigenetic changes are first induced in the D, J, and constant regions via the intronic enhancer Eμ. The V regions are likely excluded from these effects through binding of transcription factor CTCF to conserved sites in the V-D region.[56] This allows D to J rearrangements to occur prior to V to DJ rearrangements, which are more tightly controlled. One allele rearranges first and a functional rearrangement prevents V to DJ recombination on the second allele: allelic exclusion (Fig. 4A). While it remains unclear which signals initiate V to DJ rearrangements, this step involves large-scale locus reorganization to position V genes close to the DJ junction and to mediate efficient recombination.[54,57–59] Studies in mouse models have shown that *IGH* locus contraction critically depends on the ubiquitous protein YY1 and on B cell commitment factor Pax5.[60,61] Pax5 seems to mediate contraction by binding to conserved DNA elements in the *IGH* V gene region only in pre-B-I cells, where it acts together with E2A and CTCF that interact with these sequences throughout B cell differentiation.[62]

A role for stromal cell-derived IL-7 in regulation of V to DJ rearrangements in *IGH* via signaling through IL-7R and STAT5 is currently under debate. STAT5 binds to elements in the *IGH* V gene region and distal V to DJ gene rearrangements are severely impaired in STAT5 deficient mouse precursor B cells.[63] However, STAT5 activation is also important for precursor B cell survival and the recombination defects could be rescued by overexpression of the prosurvival gene *BCL2*.[64] In contrast, inhibition of IL-7 signaling was found to induce premature *IGK* rearrangements in pre-B-I cells that lack functional *IGH* gene rearrangements in murine and human B cells.[64,65] Therefore, STAT5 and IL-7 signaling are important for the controlled order of Ig gene rearrangements by suppressing early *IGK* gene rearrangements prior to a functional IgH protein.

The initiation of *IGL* gene rearrangements seemingly coincides with *IGK* rearrangements in small pre-B-II cells.[18] Still, single cell analysis revealed that *IGK* precedes *IGL*: Igκ+ B cells rarely contain *IGL* rearrangements, while Igλ+ B cells are abundant in *IGK* rearrangements.[66,67] Btk-deficient mice have clearly reduced frequencies of Igλ+ B cells.[68] It is well possible that pre-BCR signaling via Btk is important for initiation of *IGL* rearrangements.[68] A potential mechanism is through the upregulation of E2A splice variants E12 and E47. *IGL* gene rearrangements require higher levels of both transcription factors than *IGK* gene rearrangements.[69] It is conceivable that impaired pre-BCR signaling in Btk-deficient mice fails to upregulate E12 and E47 sufficiently for *IGL* rearrangements.

Defects in ordered Ig gene rearrangements could affect B cell numbers and their functionality, because they affect checkpoints in precursor-B cell differentiation. Impaired Ig locus contraction could impair the Ig repertoire diversity. In addition, premature *IGK* gene rearrangements could contain long complementarity determining regions 3 (CDR3) due to increased N-nucleotide additions.[18] These defects are preferentially studied in sorted B cell subsets through molecular analysis of Ig gene rearrangements to visualize V, D, and J gene usage, N-nucleotide additions and in-frame selection. Furthermore, 3D fluorescence *in situ* hybridization or chromosome conformation capture techniques can be used to study Ig locus conformations and long-range interactions.[54,70] The involvement of specific proteins or signaling pathways could be addressed by *in vitro* studies on cultured precursor B cells.[65,71]

Critical processes and checkpoints in antigen-dependent B cell maturation

Following successful antigen-independent differentiation in bone marrow, B cells migrate to peripheral lymphoid organs and recirculate in blood. The cells require external signals for survival by rate-limiting factors, which thereby ensure stable homeostasis of the total B cell pool. Furthermore, only those cells that recognize their cognate antigen initiate further differentiation and generate memory B cells and antibody-producing plasma cells. The maturation pathways differ depending on the anatomic location of the response (e.g., lymph node vs. gut or lung) and the type of antigen (e.g., protein vs. polysaccharide). In this section, we will discuss the survival and maturation processes and the major checkpoints involved.

Survival and maturation of naive B cells

The generation and maintenance of mature B cells critically depend on the membrane expression of a BCR. In its absence, no B cells are generated, while conditional deletion in mature B cells induces cell death.[72,73] BCR-dependent survival signals are provided through a single pathway involving PI3K signaling,[74] a conserved pathway in cellular homeostasis and survival.[75]

Recent bone marrow emigrants are functionally immature, that is, they do not respond to BCR stimulation. These transitional B cells constitute ~5–10% of total B cells in blood of healthy adults and have a characteristic phenotype that includes expression of CD10 and high expression of CD24 and CD38.[76,77] Transitional cells develop into naive mature B cells, a process that is accompanied by homeostatic proliferation of ~two cell cycles.[78] The signals driving maturation and homeostatic proliferation are currently unknown. A good candidate is the cytokine MIF (macrophage migration inhibitory factor). The cytokine functions of MIF were identified several decades ago with respect to monocytes/macrophages.[79,80] More recently, MIF has been shown to induce B cell survival and proliferation through binding to the CD74–CD44 receptor complex and subsequent support of hepatocyte growth factor (HGF)-induced c-MET signaling (Fig. 5A).[81–83] MIF production by dendritic cells in bone marrow is crucial for mature B cell maintenance.[84] It is therefore likely that newly produced B cells circulate, and those that migrate through bone marrow will receive this survival and proliferation signal.

The size of the mature B cell pool is tightly regulated by B cell–activating factor (BAFF). Similar to proliferation-inducing ligand (APRIL), BAFF is a member of the tumor necrosis factor (TNF) family that is implicated in several aspects of B cell survival and Ig isotype switching and production.[85,86] BAFF and APRIL can both bind the BCMA (B cell maturation antigen) and TACI (transmembrane activator and CAML interactor) receptors,[87–91] while BAFF also specifically binds to a third receptor, BAFF-R,[92,93] and APRIL can interact with proteoglycans.[94,95] BAFF-R is quite specifically expressed on B cells and the BAFF–BAFF-R interaction is crucial for survival of naive B cells (Fig. 5B).[85,96] Consequently, genetic ablation of BAFF or BAFF-R in mice and mutations in the human BAFF-R

result in a dramatic reduction of naive mature B cells.[97–99]

Defects in survival and maturation of naive B cells (CD24^{dim}CD38^{dim}IgD$^+$CD27$^-$) can be first identified with flowcytometry of the blood and bone marrow B cell compartments. These would show a reduction in naive mature cells while transitional B cells can still be detected and normal precursor B cell differentiation appears normal. Further insights into the affected processes can be obtained by analysis of surface membrane expression of BAFF-R, CD74, CD44, and serum BAFF and MIF levels. Finally, MIF- or BAFF-induced signaling pathways in B cells can be studied.

Antigen-induced activation and B cell response pathways

Upon binding to its cognate antigen, the BCR induces downstream signaling using the same pathways as the pre-BCR, to initiate target gene transcription (Figs. 4 and 5). In addition, the CD19 complex, consisting of CD19, CD21, CD81, and CD225, is necessary for sufficiently strong signaling of the BCR (Fig. 5B).[100–102] Specifically, signaling molecules are recruited upon phosphorylation of multiple tyrosine residues in the intracellular tail of CD19. Genetic defects in CD19, CD81, and CD21 decrease BCR-mediated signaling and therefore result in impaired B cell responses to antigen.[103–105]

In addition to antigen recognition via the BCR, B cells need a second signal to become activated.[106] Activated T cells can provide such a signal via CD40L that interacts with CD40 on B cells (Fig. 5B). T cell-dependent (TD) B cell responses are characterized by germinal center (GC) formation, extensive B cell proliferation, affinity maturation, and Ig class switch recombination (CSR).[107] Thus, high-affinity memory B cells and Ig-producing plasma cells are formed. Additionally, B cells can respond to T cell-independent (TI) antigens that either activate via the BCR and another (innate) receptor (TI-1) or via extensive cross-linking of the BCR due to the repetitive nature of the antigen (TI-2).[108] TI responses are directed against blood-borne pathogens in the splenic marginal zone and in mucosal tissues (reviewed in Refs. 109,110). B cells express many different pattern recognition receptors, including toll-like receptors (TLRs) and nucleotide oligomerization domain-like receptors (NLRs), that have been implicated in TI responses.[111,112] Furthermore, BAFF and APRIL likely

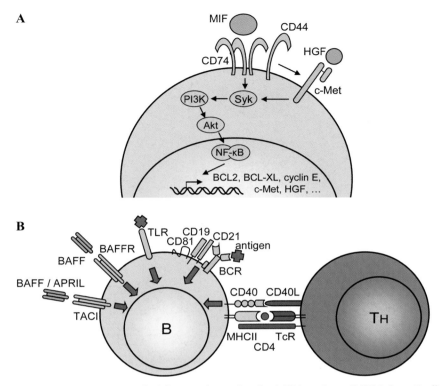

Figure 5. B cell survival and activation signals. (A) Macrophage migration inhibitory factor (MIF) induces B cell survival upon binding to CD74. Subsequent signaling via CD44, Syk, PI3K, and Akt activates NF-κB and induces transcription of survival and proliferation genes. Furthermore, MIF signaling attenuates hepatocyte growth factor (HGF)-induced c-Met signaling, both directly and via transcriptional upregulation of both the *HGF* and *MET* genes. (B) The first B cell activation signal is provided by cognate BCR–antigen interactions and requires the CD19, CD21, CD81 complex for optimal signaling. The second signal can be provided by CD40–CD40L interactions following presentation of antigenic peptides in MHC class II by the B cell to helper T cells. Alternatively, the B cell can receive signals via pattern recognition receptors, such as TLR, or via BAFF–BAFF-R, or BAFF/APRIL–TACI interactions.

support TD and TI responses through binding with TACI and induction of affinity maturation and Ig CSR.[113,114]

It is clear that both the type of antigen and the local tissue environment influence the type of immune response. Therefore, it is to be expected that various types of B cell responses can and need to be generated to provide functional immunity to the diverse pathogens an individual encounters. Importantly, memory B cells derived from these responses recirculate in blood and display unique phenotypes (Fig. 6).[115] Primary GC responses generate CD27$^+$IgM$^+$IgD$^-$ and CD27$^-$IgG$^+$ memory B cells. These cells display similar molecular characteristics with respect to their replication history and somatic hypermutation levels as GC B cells in the childhood tonsil.[115–117] In contrast, IgA- and IgG-class switched CD27$^+$ B cells show an increased replication history and contain high loads of somatic hypermutation (SHM) in their Ig genes, suggestive of secondary TD responses.[78,115]

Besides TD responses, two memory B cell subsets show signs of TI origin: CD27$^+$IgM$^+$IgD$^+$ and CD27$^-$IgA$^+$ show limited proliferation as compared with GC B cells and are present in CD40L-deficient patients. It is debated whether CD27$^+$IgM$^+$IgD$^+$ B cells in healthy adults, are generated from GC responses or independently of T cell help in the splenic marginal zone.[112,118,119] We found reduced replication history and SHM levels in natural effector B cells as compared to CD27$^+$IgM$^+$IgD$^-$ memory B cells.[115] Since

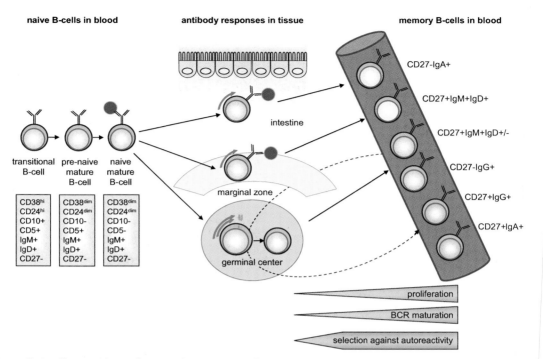

Figure 6. B cell maturation pathways. Naive mature B cells can undergo T cell–independent or T cell–dependent immune responses. TI responses in the gut or splenic marginal zone are characterized by low proliferation and SHM levels as compared with TD responses in GC structures. Secondary responses induce further proliferation and SHM. Despite distinct levels of BCR maturation, all memory B cells display selection against inherently autoreactive IGHV4–34 genes and long IGH-CDR3 regions.

$CD27^+IgM^+IgD^-$ memory B cells highly resemble GC B cells on the molecular level, we concluded that in healthy adults, part of the natural effector B cell compartment is generated outside a GC (Fig. 6). Although the anatomic location of TI CSR toward IgA in human gut remains controversial,[114,120] on the basis of our findings, we can state that $CD27^-IgA^+$ memory B cells resemble IgA^+ cells from the gut lamina propria and seem to be a blood counterpart of this population (Fig. 6).[115]

Importantly, all memory B cell subsets show molecular signs of selection. Their *IGH* gene repertoire is restricted with regard to short IGH-CDR3 regions and reduced *IGHV4–34* gene usage as compared to naive mature B cells.[115,121,122] During an immune response, the proliferating B cells compete for antigen-binding and survival signals, e.g., from Th cells through CD40–CD40L interactions (Fig. 5B).[123] Thus, cells with high affinity receptors survive, while other cells are removed from the repertoire. How selection against long IGH-CDR3 and IGHV4–34, which are both associated with autoreactivity,[124,125] fit into this mechanism

is currently unclear. Still, their frequencies can be important parameters for evaluation of proper antigen selection in patients suspected of having an immunological disease with B cell defects.

Thus, analysis of blood memory B cell subsets can provide information on local and systemic immune responses. Moreover, the end products of TD and TI responses can be independently evaluated through flowcytometric analysis of blood memory B cells and molecular analysis of Ig genes to enable identification of checkpoints in B cell responses.

Terminal differentiation and survival of plasma cells

Plasma cells are derived from activated B cells through a different transcriptional program than memory B cells, mainly involving BLIMP1, XBP-1, and IRF-4 (reviewed in Ref. 126). Furthermore, IL-21, produced by follicular Th cells in the GC, is a potent cytokine involved in induction and maintenance of Ig responses. IL-21 signals through STAT3 to upregulate both BLIMP1 and an inhibitor of plasma cell differentiation, BCL6.[127–129] Still, the duration of IL-21 stimulation and subsequent differential kinetics of STAT3 activation will determine whether plasma cell fate is induced.[130]

Since plasma cells progressively loose membrane BCR expression while maturing, they depend on other mechanisms for survival. Recent studies implicate CD28 for long-term maintenance of plasma cells in bone marrow.[131] The survival signals are provided by the ligands CD80 and CD86 on bone marrow dendritic cells and induce PI3K and NF-κB signaling,[132,133] thereby potentially compensating for the lack of BCR signaling.

While most plasma cells are generated in lymphoid organs and long-lived plasma cells reside in bone marrow, small numbers can be found circulating in blood of healthy adults and have high CD38 and CD27 expression.[134–136] Despite their low numbers in blood (1–5 cells/μL),[137] they display large phenotypic heterogeneity. The total blood plasma cell compartment spans from immature cells that resemble lymph node plasmablasts ($CD20^+sIg^+CD138^-$) to bone marrow plasma cells ($CD20^-sIg^-CD138^+$).[134,137] Moreover, the plasma cells can express one of the various Ig isotypes. Interestingly, the IgA^+ plasma cells are more frequent than IgM^+ or IgG^+.[135,137] These IgA^+ plasma cells display characteristics suggestive of a mucosal origin.[135]

Thus, detailed flowcytometric analysis of blood can provide a lot of information on plasma cell maturation. Such an analysis will not only reveal whether the full maturation pattern is normally present, but also supports dissection of their origin from various maturation pathways. Finally, molecular analysis of Ig-class switched transcripts could provide more insight into normal versus abnormal responses.

Perspectives on PID

Over the past decades, it has become clear that B cell differentiation is a stepwise process involving many important checkpoints. We described here 11 critical processes and accompanying checkpoints in B cell differentiation. In theory, each of these checkpoints can be affected in patients suffering from a PID, and many processes have been found impaired by genetic defects (Fig. 1). More importantly, newly identified key players in each of these processes will be interesting candidate genes affected in patients

in whom currently no molecular diagnosis is established.

Naturally, the defects that result in the most stringent blocks have been characterized first. In recent years, the challenge has therefore been shifted toward patients with milder or atypical phenotypes and later onset of disease. These phenotypes can either be the result of "mild genetic defects" caused by hypomorphic mutations in previously identified PID genes or defects in new candidate genes. To optimize treatment and to preselect proper candidate genes, a good immunological diagnosis is crucial. As illustrated above, much can be learned from understanding the effects of currently identified PID gene mutants, new insights from mouse models and from detailed analysis of B cell differentiation checkpoints in the patient.[138]

Acknowledgments

We thank Mrs. S. de Bruin-Versteeg for assistance in preparing the figures. MAB is supported by a Fellowship from the Ter Meulen Fund–Royal Netherlands Academy of Arts and Sciences. MvdB is supported by a Grant from the foundation "Sophia Kinderziekenhuis Fonds" (SKF; Grant 589). MCvZ is supported by an Erasmus University Rotterdam (EUR)-Fellowship, an Erasmus MC Fellowship, and by Veni Grant 916.110.90 from ZonMW/NWO.

Conflicts of interest

The authors declare no conflicts of interest.

References

1. Meffre, E. 2011. The establishment of early B cell tolerance in humans: Lessons from primary immunodeficiency diseases. *Ann. N.Y. Acad. Sci.* **1246:** 1–10. doi: 10.1111/j.1749-6632.2011.06347.x.
2. Tangye, S. 2011. T cell/B cell interactions in primary immunodeficiencies. *Ann. N.Y. Acad. Sci.* doi: 10.1111/j.1749-6632.2011.06361.x.
3. Cerutti, A., M. Cols, M. Gentile, *et al.* 2011. Regulation of mucosal IgA responses: lessons from primary immunodeficiencies. *Ann. N.Y. Acad. Sci.* doi: 10.1111/j.1749-6632.2011.06266.x.
4. Hozumi, N. & S. Tonegawa. 1976. Evidence for somatic rearrangement of immunoglobulin genes coding for variable and constant regions. *Proc. Natl. Acad. Sci. USA* **73:** 3628–3632.
5. Tonegawa, S. 1983. Somatic generation of antibody diversity. *Nature* **302:** 575–581.
6. Nutt, S.L. & B.L. Kee. 2007. The transcriptional regulation of B cell lineage commitment. *Immunity* **26:** 715–725.

7. Zandi, S., D. Bryder & M. Sigvardsson. 2010. Load and lock: the molecular mechanisms of B-lymphocyte commitment. *Immunol. Rev.* **238:** 47–62.

8. Kondo, M., I.L. Weissman & K. Akashi. 1997. Identification of clonogenic common lymphoid progenitors in mouse bone marrow. *Cell* **91:** 661–672.

9. Akashi, K. *et al.* 2000. A clonogenic common myeloid progenitor that gives rise to all myeloid lineages. *Nature* **404:** 193–197.

10. DeKoter, R.P. & H. Singh. 2000. Regulation of B lymphocyte and macrophage development by graded expression of PU.1. *Science* **288:** 1439–1441.

11. Nichogiannopoulou, A. *et al.* 1999. Defects in hemopoietic stem cell activity in Ikaros mutant mice. *J. Exp. Med.* **190:** 1201–1214.

12. Mansson, R. *et al.* 2008. B-lineage commitment prior to surface expression of B220 and CD19 on hematopoietic progenitor cells. *Blood* **112:** 1048–1055.

13. Rumfelt, L.L. *et al.* 2006. Lineage specification and plasticity in CD19-early B cell precursors. *J. Exp. Med.* **203:** 675–687.

14. Notta, F. *et al.* 2011. Isolation of single human hematopoietic stem cells capable of long-term multilineage engraftment. *Science* **333:** 218–221.

15. Galy, A. *et al.* 1995. Human T, B, natural killer, and dendritic cells arise from a common bone marrow progenitor cell subset. *Immunity* **3:** 459–473.

16. Sanz, E. *et al.* 2010. Ordering human CD34+CD10-CD19+ pre/pro-B-cell and CD19- common lymphoid progenitor stages in two pro-B-cell development pathways. *Proc. Natl. Acad. Sci. USA* **107:** 5925–5930.

17. Ichii, M. *et al.* 2010. The density of CD10 corresponds to commitment and progression in the human B lymphoid lineage. *PLoS One* **5:** e12954.

18. van Zelm, M.C. *et al.* 2005. Ig gene rearrangement steps are initiated in early human precursor B cell subsets and correlate with specific transcription factor expression. *J. Immunol.* **175:** 5912–5922.

19. Bertrand, F.E., 3rd, *et al.* 1997. Ig D(H) gene segment transcription and rearrangement before surface expression of the pan-B-cell marker CD19 in normal human bone marrow. *Blood* **90:** 736–744.

20. Meffre, E. *et al.* 1996. A human non-XLA immunodeficiency disease characterized by blockage of B cell development at an early proB cell stage. *J. Clin. Invest.* **98:** 1519–1526.

21. van Gent, D.C. *et al.* 1997. Stimulation of V(D)J cleavage by high mobility group proteins. *EMBO J.* **16:** 2665–2670.

22. McBlane, J.F. *et al.* 1995. Cleavage at a V(D)J recombination signal requires only RAG1 and RAG2 proteins and occurs in two steps. *Cell* **83:** 387–395.

23. Hiom, K. & M. Gellert. 1997. A stable RAG1-RAG2-DNA complex that is active in V(D)J cleavage. *Cell* **88:** 65–72.

24. Helmink, B.A. *et al.* 2009. MRN complex function in the repair of chromosomal Rag-mediated DNA double-strand breaks. *J. Exp. Med.* **206:** 669–679.

25. van der Burg, M. *et al.* 2010. Loss of juxtaposition of RAG-induced immunoglobulin DNA ends is implicated in the precursor B-cell differentiation defect in NBS patients. *Blood* **115:** 4770–4777.

26. Grawunder, U. & E. Harfst. 2001. How to make ends meet in V(D)J recombination. *Curr. Opin. Immunol.* **13:** 186–194.

27. van Gent, D.C. & M. van der Burg. 2007. Non-homologous end-joining, a sticky affair. *Oncogene* **26:** 7731–7740.

28. Gottlieb, T.M. & S.P. Jackson. 1993. The DNA-dependent protein kinase: requirement for DNA ends and association with Ku antigen. *Cell* **72:** 131–142.

29. Nussenzweig, A. *et al.* 1996. Requirement for Ku80 in growth and immunoglobulin V(D)J recombination. *Nature* **382:** 551–555.

30. Moshous, D. *et al.* 2001. Artemis, a novel DNA double-strand break repair/V(D)J recombination protein, is mutated in human severe combined immune deficiency. *Cell* **105:** 177–186.

31. Schlissel, M.S. 1998. Structure of nonhairpin coding-end DNA breaks in cells undergoing V(D)J recombination. *Mol. Cell. Biol.* **18:** 2029–2037.

32. Benedict, C.L. *et al.* 2000. Terminal deoxynucleotidyl transferase and repertoire development. *Immunol. Rev.* **175:** 150–157.

33. Benedict, C.L., S. Gilfillan & J.F. Kearney. 2001. The long isoform of terminal deoxynucleotidyl transferase enters the nucleus and, rather than catalyzing nontemplated nucleotide addition, modulates the catalytic activity of the short isoform. *J. Exp. Med.* **193:** 89–99.

34. Critchlow, S.E., R.P. Bowater & S.P. Jackson. 1997. Mammalian DNA double-strand break repair protein XRCC4 interacts with DNA ligase IV. *Curr. Biol.* **7:** 588–598.

35. Grawunder, U. *et al.* 1997. Activity of DNA ligase IV stimulated by complex formation with XRCC4 protein in mammalian cells. *Nature* **388:** 492–495.

36. Ahnesorg, P., P. Smith & S.P. Jackson. 2006. XLF interacts with the XRCC4-DNA ligase IV complex to promote DNA nonhomologous end-joining. *Cell* **124:** 301–313.

37. van der Burg, M. *et al.* 2009. A DNA-PKcs mutation in a radiosensitive T-B-SCID patient inhibits Artemis activation and nonhomologous end-joining. *J. Clin. Invest.* **119:** 91–98.

38. van der Burg, M. *et al.* 2007. Defective Artemis nuclease is characterized by coding joints with microhomology in long palindromic-nucleotide stretches. *Eur. J. Immunol.* **37:** 3522–3528.

39. van der Burg, M. *et al.* 2006. A new type of radiosensitive T-B-NK+ severe combined immunodeficiency caused by a LIG4 mutation. *J. Clin. Invest.* **116:** 137–145.

40. Harfst, E. *et al.* 2000. Normal V(D)J recombination in cells from patients with Nijmegen breakage syndrome. *Mol. Immunol.* **37:** 915–929.

41. Tsukada, S. *et al.* 1993. Deficient expression of a B cell cytoplasmic tyrosine kinase in human X-linked agammaglobulinemia. *Cell* **72:** 279–290.

42. Vetrie, D. *et al.* 1993. The gene involved in X-linked agammaglobulinaemia is a member of the src family of protein-tyrosine kinases. *Nature* **361:** 226–233.

43. Conley, M.E. *et al.* 2009. Primary B cell immunodeficiencies: comparisons and contrasts. *Annu. Rev. Immunol.* **27:** 199–227.

44. Gauthier, L. *et al.* 2002. Galectin-1 is a stromal cell ligand of the pre-B cell receptor (BCR) implicated in synapse formation between pre-B and stromal cells and in pre-BCR triggering. *Proc. Natl. Acad. Sci. USA* **99:** 13014–13019.

45. Rossi, B. *et al.* 2006. Clustering of pre-B cell integrins induces galectin-1-dependent pre-B cell receptor relocalization and activation. *J. Immunol.* **177:** 796–803.

46. Espeli, M. *et al.* 2009. Impaired B-cell development at the pre-BII-cell stage in galectin-1-deficient mice due to inefficient pre-BII/stromal cell interactions. *Blood* **113:** 5878–5886.

47. van der Burg, M. *et al.* 2011. Dissection of B-cell development to unravel defects in patients with a primary antibody deficiency. *Adv. Exp. Med. Biol.* **697:** 183–196.

48. Mostoslavsky, R. *et al.* 1998. Kappa chain monoallelic demethylation and the establishment of allelic exclusion. *Genes Dev.* **12:** 1801–1811.

49. Maes, J. *et al.* 2001. Chromatin remodeling at the Ig loci prior to V(D)J recombination. *J. Immunol.* **167:** 866–874.

50. McBlane, F. & J. Boyes. 2000. Stimulation of V(D)J recombination by histone acetylation. *Curr. Biol.* **10:** 483–486.

51. Chowdhury, D. & R. Sen. 2001. Stepwise activation of the immunoglobulin mu heavy chain gene locus. *EMBO J.* **20:** 6394–6403.

52. Yancopoulos, G.D. & F.W. Alt. 1985. Developmentally controlled and tissue-specific expression of unrearranged VH gene segments. *Cell* **40:** 271–281.

53. Abarrategui, I. & M.S. Krangel. 2006. Regulation of T cell receptor-alpha gene recombination by transcription. *Nat. Immunol.* **7:** 1109–1115.

54. Jhunjhunwala, S. *et al.* 2008. The 3D structure of the immunoglobulin heavy-chain locus: implications for long-range genomic interactions. *Cell* **133:** 265–279.

55. Jhunjhunwala, S. *et al.* 2009. Chromatin architecture and the generation of antigen receptor diversity. *Cell* **138:** 435–448.

56. Featherstone, K. *et al.* 2010. The mouse immunoglobulin heavy chain V-D intergenic sequence contains insulators that may regulate ordered V(D)J recombination. *J. Biol. Chem.* **285:** 9327–9338.

57. Kosak, S.T. *et al.* 2002. Subnuclear compartmentalization of immunoglobulin loci during lymphocyte development. *Science* **296:** 158–162.

58. Roldan, E. *et al.* 2005. Locus 'decontraction' and centromeric recruitment contribute to allelic exclusion of the immunoglobulin heavy-chain gene. *Nat. Immunol.* **6:** 31–41.

59. Sayegh, C. *et al.* 2005. Visualization of looping involving the immunoglobulin heavy-chain locus in developing B cells. *Genes Dev.* **19:** 322–327.

60. Fuxa, M. *et al.* 2004. Pax5 induces V-to-DJ rearrangements and locus contraction of the immunoglobulin heavy-chain gene. *Genes Dev.* **18:** 411–422.

61. Liu, H. *et al.* 2007. Yin Yang 1 is a critical regulator of B-cell development. *Genes Dev.* **21:** 1179–1189.

62. Ebert, A. *et al.* 2011. The distal V(H) gene cluster of the Igh locus contains distinct regulatory elements with Pax5 transcription factor-dependent activity in pro-B cells. *Immunity* **34:** 175–187.

63. Bertolino, E. *et al.* 2005. Regulation of interleukin 7-dependent immunoglobulin heavy-chain variable gene rearrangements by transcription factor STAT5. *Nat. Immunol.* **6:** 836–843.

64. Malin, S. *et al.* 2010. Role of STAT5 in controlling cell survival and immunoglobulin gene recombination during pro-B cell development. *Nat. Immunol.* **11:** 171–179.

65. Nodland, S.E. *et al.* 2011. IL-7R expression and IL-7 signaling confer a distinct phenotype on developing human B-lineage cells. *Blood* **118:** 2116–2127.

66. Engel, H., A. Rolink & S. Weiss. 1999. B cells are programmed to activate kappa and lambda for rearrangement at consecutive developmental stages. *Eur. J. Immunol.* **29:** 2167–2176.

67. van der Burg, M. *et al.* 2001. Ordered recombination of immunoglobulin light chain genes occurs at the IGK locus but seems less strict at the IGL locus. *Blood* **97:** 1001–1008.

68. Dingjan, G.M. *et al.* 2001. Bruton's tyrosine kinase regulates the activation of gene rearrangements at the lambda light chain locus in precursor B cells in the mouse. *J. Exp. Med.* **193:** 1169–1178.

69. Beck, K. *et al.* 2009. Distinct roles for E12 and E47 in B cell specification and the sequential rearrangement of immunoglobulin light chain loci. *J. Exp. Med.* **206:** 2271–2284.

70. Degner, S.C. *et al.* CCCTC-binding factor (CTCF) and cohesin influence the genomic architecture of the Igh locus and antisense transcription in pro-B cells. *Proc. Natl. Acad. Sci. USA* **108:** 9566–9571.

71. Johnson, S.E. *et al.* 2005. Murine and human IL-7 activate STAT5 and induce proliferation of normal human pro-B cells. *J. Immunol.* **175:** 7325–7331.

72. Lam, K.P., R. Kuhn & K. Rajewsky. 1997. In vivo ablation of surface immunoglobulin on mature B cells by inducible gene targeting results in rapid cell death. *Cell* **90:** 1073–1083.

73. Torres, R.M. *et al.* 1996. Aberrant B cell development and immune response in mice with a compromised BCR complex. *Science* **272:** 1804–1808.

74. Srinivasan, L. *et al.* 2009. PI3 kinase signals BCR-dependent mature B cell survival. *Cell* **139:** 573–586.

75. Engelman, J.A., J. Luo & L.C. Cantley. 2006. The evolution of phosphatidylinositol 3-kinases as regulators of growth and metabolism. *Nat. Rev. Genet.* **7:** 606–619.

76. Cuss, A.K. *et al.* 2006. Expansion of functionally immature transitional B cells is associated with human immunodeficient states characterized by impaired humoral immunity. *J. Immunol.* **176:** 1506–1516.

77. Sims, G.P. *et al.* 2005. Identification and characterization of circulating human transitional B cells. *Blood* **105:** 4390–4398.

78. van Zelm, M.C. *et al.* 2007. Replication history of B lymphocytes reveals homeostatic proliferation and extensive antigen-induced B cell expansion. *J. Exp. Med.* **204:** 645–655.

79. Calandra, T. *et al.* 1994. The macrophage is an important and previously unrecognized source of macrophage migration inhibitory factor. *J. Exp. Med.* **179:** 1895–1902.

80. George, M. & J.H. Vaughan. 1962. In vitro cell migration as a model for delayed hypersensitivity. *Proc. Soc. Exp. Biol. Med.* **111:** 514–521.

81. Gore, Y. *et al.* 2008. Macrophage migration inhibitory factor induces B cell survival by activation of a CD74-CD44 receptor complex. *J. Biol. Chem.* **283:** 2784–2792.

82. Matza, D. *et al.* 2002. Invariant chain induces B cell maturation in a process that is independent of its chaperonic activity. *Proc. Natl. Acad. Sci. USA* **99:** 3018–3023.

83. Shachar, I. & R.A. Flavell. 1996. Requirement for invariant chain in B cell maturation and function. *Science* **274:** 106–108.

84. Sapoznikov, A. *et al.* 2008. Perivascular clusters of dendritic cells provide critical survival signals to B cells in bone marrow niches. *Nat. Immunol.* **9:** 388–395.

85. Mackay, F. *et al.* 2003. BAFF and APRIL: a tutorial on B cell survival. *Annu. Rev. Immunol.* **21:** 231–264.

86. Dillon, S.R. *et al.* 2006. An APRIL to remember: novel TNF ligands as therapeutic targets. *Nat. Rev. Drug Discov.* **5:** 235–246.

87. Gross, J.A. *et al.* 2000. TACI and BCMA are receptors for a TNF homologue implicated in B-cell autoimmune disease. *Nature* **404:** 995–999.

88. Marsters, S.A. *et al.* 2000. Interaction of the TNF homologues BLyS and APRIL with the TNF receptor homologues BCMA and TACI. *Curr. Biol.* **10:** 785–788.

89. Thompson, J.S. *et al.* 2000. BAFF binds to the tumor necrosis factor receptor-like molecule B cell maturation antigen and is important for maintaining the peripheral B cell population. *J. Exp. Med.* **192:** 129–135.

90. Wu, Y. *et al.* 2000. Tumor necrosis factor (TNF) receptor superfamily member TACI is a high affinity receptor for TNF family members APRIL and BLyS. *J. Biol. Chem.* **275:** 35478–35485.

91. Yu, G. *et al.* 2000. APRIL and TALL-I and receptors BCMA and TACI: system for regulating humoral immunity. *Nat. Immunol.* **1:** 252–256.

92. Thompson, J.S. *et al.* 2001. BAFF-R, a newly identified TNF receptor that specifically interacts with BAFF. *Science* **293:** 2108–2111.

93. Yan, M. *et al.* 2001. Identification of a novel receptor for B lymphocyte stimulator that is mutated in a mouse strain with severe B cell deficiency. *Curr. Biol.* **11:** 1547–1552.

94. Hendriks, J. *et al.* 2005. Heparan sulfate proteoglycan binding promotes APRIL-induced tumor cell proliferation. *Cell. Death Differ.* **12:** 637–648.

95. Ingold, K. *et al.* 2005. Identification of proteoglycans as the APRIL-specific binding partners. *J. Exp. Med.* **201:** 1375–1383.

96. Schneider, P. 2005. The role of APRIL and BAFF in lymphocyte activation. *Curr. Opin. Immunol.* **17:** 282–289.

97. Gross, J.A. *et al.* 2001. TACI-Ig neutralizes molecules critical for B cell development and autoimmune disease. Impaired B cell maturation in mice lacking BLyS. *Immunity* **15:** 289–302.

98. Schiemann, B. *et al.* 2001. An essential role for BAFF in the normal development of B cells through a BCMA-independent pathway. *Science* **293:** 2111–2114.

99. Warnatz, K. *et al.* 2009. B-cell activating factor receptor deficiency is associated with an adult-onset antibody deficiency syndrome in humans. *Proc. Natl. Acad. Sci. USA* **106:** 13945–13950.

100. Carter, R.H. & D.T. Fearon. 1992. CD19: lowering the threshold for antigen receptor stimulation of B lymphocytes. *Science* **256:** 105–107.

101. van Noesel, C.J., A.C. Lankester & R.A. van Lier. 1993. Dual antigen recognition by B cells. *Immunol. Today* **14:** 8–11.

102. Fearon, D.T. & M.C. Carroll. 2000. Regulation of B lymphocyte responses to foreign and self-antigens by the CD19/CD21 complex. *Annu. Rev. Immunol.* **18:** 393–422.

103. Kimmig, L.M. *et al.* 2008. Further insights into human CD21 deficiency. *Clin. Exp. Immunol.* **154:** 221–221 (abstract).

104. van Zelm, M.C. *et al.* 2006. An antibody-deficiency syndrome due to mutations in the CD19 gene. *N. Engl. J. Med.* **354:** 1901–1912.

105. van Zelm, M.C. *et al.* 2010. CD81 gene defect in humans disrupts CD19 complex formation and leads to antibody deficiency. *J. Clin. Invest.* **120:** 1265–1274.

106. Bretscher, P. & M. Cohn. 1970. A theory of self-nonself discrimination. *Science* **169:** 1042–1049.

107. MacLennan, I.C. 1994. Germinal centers. *Annu. Rev. Immunol.* **12:** 117–139.

108. Mond, J.J. *et al.* 1995. T cell independent antigens. *Curr. Opin. Immunol.* **7:** 349–354.

109. Cerutti, A. 2008. The regulation of IgA class switching. *Nat. Rev. Immunol.* **8:** 421–434.

110. Weill, J.C., S. Weller & C.A. Reynaud. 2009. Human marginal zone B cells. *Annu. Rev. Immunol.* **27:** 267–285.

111. Delgado, M.F. *et al.* 2009. Lack of antibody affinity maturation due to poor Toll-like receptor stimulation leads to enhanced respiratory syncytial virus disease. *Nat. Med.* **15:** 34–41.

112. Weller, S. *et al.* 2001. CD40-CD40L independent Ig gene hypermutation suggests a second B cell diversification pathway in humans. *Proc. Natl. Acad. Sci. USA* **98:** 1166–1170.

113. He, B. *et al.* 2010. The transmembrane activator TACI triggers immunoglobulin class switching by activating B cells through the adaptor MyD88. *Nat. Immunol.* **11:** 836–845.

114. He, B. *et al.* 2007. Intestinal bacteria trigger T cell-independent immunoglobulin A(2) class switching by inducing epithelial-cell secretion of the cytokine APRIL. *Immunity* **26:** 812–826.

115. Berkowska, M.A. *et al.* 2011. Human memory B cells originate from three distinct germinal center-dependent and -independent maturation pathways. *Blood* **118:** 2150–2158.

116. Fecteau, J.F., G. Cote & S. Neron. 2006. A new memory CD27-IgG+ B cell population in peripheral blood expressing VH genes with low frequency of somatic mutation. *J. Immunol.* **177:** 3728–3736.

117. Wei, C. *et al.* 2007. A new population of cells lacking expression of CD27 represents a notable component of the B cell memory compartment in systemic lupus erythematosus. *J. Immunol.* **178:** 6624–6633.

118. Weller, S. *et al.* 2004. Human blood IgM "memory" B cells are circulating splenic marginal zone B cells harboring a prediversified immunoglobulin repertoire. *Blood* **104:** 3647–3654.

119. Agematsu, K. *et al.* 1998. Absence of IgD-CD27(+) memory B cell population in X-linked hyper-IgM syndrome. *J. Clin. Invest.* **102:** 853–860.

120. Boursier, L. *et al.* 2005. Human intestinal IgA response is generated in the organized gut-associated lymphoid tissue

but not in the lamina propria. *Gastroenterology* **128:** 1879–1889.

121. Pugh-Bernard, A.E. *et al.* 2001. Regulation of inherently autoreactive VH4–34 B cells in the maintenance of human B cell tolerance. *J. Clin. Invest.* **108:** 1061–1070.

122. Wu, Y.C. *et al.* 2010. High-throughput immunoglobulin repertoire analysis distinguishes between human IgM memory and switched memory B-cell populations. *Blood* **116:** 1070–1078.

123. Rajewsky, K. 1996. Clonal selection and learning in the antibody system. *Nature* **381:** 751–758.

124. Potter, K.N. *et al.* 2002. Evidence for involvement of a hydrophobic patch in framework region 1 of human V4–34-encoded Igs in recognition of the red blood cell I antigen. *J. Immunol.* **169:** 3777–3782.

125. Wardemann, H. *et al.* 2003. Predominant autoantibody production by early human B cell precursors. *Science* **301:** 1374–1377.

126. Schmidlin, H., S.A. Diehl & B. Blom. 2009. New insights into the regulation of human B-cell differentiation. *Trends Immunol.* **30:** 277–285.

127. Avery, D.T. *et al.* 2010. B cell-intrinsic signaling through IL-21 receptor and STAT3 is required for establishing long-lived antibody responses in humans. *J. Exp. Med.* **207:** 155–171.

128. Ettinger, R. *et al.* 2005. IL-21 induces differentiation of human naive and memory B cells into antibody-secreting plasma cells. *J. Immunol.* **175:** 7867–7879.

129. Ozaki, K. *et al.* 2004. Regulation of B cell differentiation and plasma cell generation by IL-21, a novel inducer of Blimp-1 and Bcl-6. *J. Immunol.* **173:** 5361–5371.

130. Diehl, S.A. *et al.* 2008. STAT3-mediated up-regulation of BLIMP1 is coordinated with BCL6 down-regulation to control human plasma cell differentiation. *J. Immunol.* **180:** 4805–4815.

131. Rozanski, C.H. *et al.* 2011. Sustained antibody responses depend on CD28 function in bone marrow-resident plasma cells. *J. Exp. Med.* **208:** 1435–1446.

132. Bahlis, N.J. *et al.* 2007. CD28-mediated regulation of multiple myeloma cell proliferation and survival. *Blood* **109:** 5002–5010.

133. Tu, Y., A. Gardner & A. Lichtenstein. 2000. The phosphatidylinositol 3-kinase/AKT kinase pathway in multiple myeloma plasma cells: roles in cytokine-dependent survival and proliferative responses. *Cancer Res.* **60:** 6763–6770.

134. Caraux, A. *et al.* 2010. Circulating human B and plasma cells. Age-associated changes in counts and detailed characterization of circulating normal CD138- and CD138+ plasma cells. *Haematologica* **95:** 1016–1020.

135. Mei, H.E. *et al.* 2009. Blood-borne human plasma cells in steady state are derived from mucosal immune responses. *Blood* **113:** 2461–2469.

136. Odendahl, M. *et al.* 2005. Generation of migratory antigen-specific plasma blasts and mobilization of resident plasma cells in a secondary immune response. *Blood* **105:** 1614–1621.

137. Perez-Andres, M. *et al.* 2010. Human peripheral blood B-cell compartments: a crossroad in B-cell traffic. *Cytometry B Clin. Cytom.* **78**(Suppl 1): S47–S60.

138. Driessen, G.J. *et al.* 2011. B-cell replication history and somatic hypermutation status identify distinct pathophysiological backgrounds in common variable immunodeficiency. *Blood* [Epub ahead of print] PMID: 22042693. doi:10.1182/blood-2011-06-361881.

Ann. N.Y. Acad. Sci. ISSN 0077-8923

ANNALS OF THE NEW YORK ACADEMY OF SCIENCES

Issue: *The Year in Human and Medical Genetics: Inborn Errors of Immunity*

DOCK8 deficiency

Helen C. Su, Huie Jing, and Qian Zhang

Laboratory of Host Defenses, National Institute of Allergy and Infectious Diseases, National Institutes of Health, Bethesda, Maryland

Address for correspondence: Helen Su, Building 10CRC, Room 5W3940, 10CRC Center Dr., MSC 1456, Bethesda, MD 20892-1456. hsu@niaid.nih.gov

The discovery that loss-of-function mutations in the gene *DOCK8* are responsible for most forms of autosomal recessive hyper-IgE syndrome and some forms of combined immunodeficiency without elevated serum IgE has led to studies into the immunopathogenesis of this disease. In this review, we relate the clinical features of this disease to studies using patients' cells and a mouse model of Dock8 deficiency, which have revealed how DOCK8 regulates T and B cell numbers and functions. The results of these studies help to explain how the absence of DOCK8 contributes to patients' susceptibility to viral, fungal, and bacterial infections. However, unanswered questions remain regarding how the absence of DOCK8 also leads to high IgE and allergic disease, predisposition for malignancy, and unusual clinical features, such as CNS abnormalities and autoimmunity, observed in some patients.

Keywords: DOCK8; hyper-IgE syndrome; combined immunodeficiency; lymphopenia

Introduction

DOCK8 deficiency is an autosomal recessive primary immunodeficiency (PID) disease caused by loss-of-function mutations in the *DOCK8* gene.[1,2] The gene encodes for a member of the DOCK180 family of atypical guanine nucleotide exchange factors that activate Rho-family GTPases such as RAC and CDC42.[3–5] The Rho-family GTPases have important roles in diverse cell functions including cell division, survival, adhesion, migration, activation, and differentiation. DOCK8 itself is highly expressed within the immune system. Thus, not surprisingly, patients with DOCK8 deficiency present with multiple abnormalities of the immune system, including defective T cell function and impaired production of antigen-specific antibodies. These lead to persistent viral infections of the skin, mucocutaneous candidiasis, recurrent sinopulmonary infections, atopic dermatitis, and other allergic disease, malignancies, and sometimes autoimmunity. This review will focus on the different aspects of disease and what is currently understood about immunopathological mechanisms contributing to their clinical manifestations.

Disease classification

The hyper-IgE syndromes are characterized by eczema, skin abscesses caused by *Staphylococcus aureus* infections, recurrent pneumonias, and elevated serum IgE.[6] Most forms of hyper-IgE syndrome are due to autosomal dominant *STAT3* mutations (called Job's syndrome).[7–9] Job's syndrome also features pneumatoceles, scoliosis or pathological fractures, and delayed exfoliation of primary teeth, which are not characteristic of autosomal recessive hyper-IgE syndrome.[10] In one patient with autosomal recessive hyper-IgE syndrome, who additionally had an unusual susceptibility to mycobacterial and viral skin infections, *TYK2* loss-of-function mutations were found.[11] However, no additional hyper-IgE syndrome patients with *TYK2* mutations have since been identified.[12] Instead, it now appears that *DOCK8* mutations account for most cases of autosomal recessive hyper-IgE syndrome.

The classification of DOCK8 deficiency as predominantly an autosomal recessive hyper-IgE syndrome may, however, reflect an ascertainment bias. This is suggested by our identification of several patients with DOCK8 deficiency whose serum IgE was

doi: 10.1111/j.1749-6632.2011.06295.x

either borderline high, or even normal on repeated testing.[1] A similar situation exists for *TYK2* deficiency, as a second patient with *TYK2* mutations was recently identified who, unlike the first patient, had normal serum IgE.[13] Furthermore, either normal or elevated serum IgE can be seen in several other immunodeficiencies, including the Wiskott–Aldrich syndrome, leaky SCID/Omenn's syndrome, atypical complete DiGeorge syndrome, IPEX syndrome, and Comèl–Netherton syndrome.[14] Because T lymphopenia and/or lymphocyte dysfunction are central to these disorders, the variably dysregulated serum IgE most likely is a consequence of T cell dysregulation.

The situation seems to be similar for DOCK8 deficiency, which is characterized by lymphopenia, especially of CD4$^+$ T cells.[1,2,15] Depending upon the patient, lymphopenia may also affect, in decreasing order, CD8$^+$ T cells, NK cells, and/or B cells. Furthermore, within the CD8$^+$ T cell compartment, both naive and memory phenotype subsets are often decreased, while cells having an "exhausted" phenotype are increased.[16] Although it is not known whether homeostatic proliferation in the periphery is also impaired, when stimulated *in vitro* through their antigen receptors DOCK8-deficient T cells expand poorly from peripheral blood mononuclear cells.[1,2,16] Their poor expansion results from poor cell division, particularly of the CD8$^+$ T cells, and appears to progress with age. The lymphopenia may also result in part from decreased thymic output, as supported by recent findings of decreased T cell receptor excision circles (TRECs) in three young patients.[17] Additionally, patients show functional abnormalities including decreased production of antiviral cytokines, such as IFN-γ and TNF-α, by CD8$^+$ T cells that otherwise do not have impaired cytotoxicity, and poor antibody function (see below).[1] Thus, a variety of mechanisms seems to contribute to the infectious susceptibility of DOCK8-deficient patients, particularly to viral infections, and may also contribute to other clinical features (discussed below).

Similar to the patients, Dock8-deficient mice, which were generated by *N*-ethyl-*N*-nitrosourea (ENU) mutagenesis, also show decreased T cell numbers in the spleen, lymph nodes, and blood.[15,16,18] The decreased numbers, especially in the naive T cell compartment, may reflect in part decreased thymic output of CD4$^+$ T cells, as well

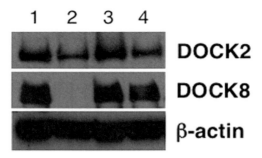

Figure 1. DOCK2 expression in DOCK8 deficiency. Lysates were prepared from EBV-transformed human B cells derived from a DOCK8-deficient patient (lane 2) and healthy controls (lanes 1, 3, 4). Lanes were each loaded with 30 μg of protein. Immunoblotting for DOCK2, DOCK8, or β-actin proteins was performed, as described.[1] Anti-DOCK2 antibodies were from Abcam (Cambridge, UK).

as decreased T cell survival.[15,16] Nonetheless, unlike DOCK8-deficient patients, T cells from Dock8-deficient mice showed only mild defects in activation, cell division, and cytokine production, and the mice were not reported to have high serum IgE.[15,16,18] Although more work is needed to characterize the T cell responses in the mice, particularly during allergic challenges, the reported findings are consistent with observations that all patients have lymphopenia and/or lymphocyte dysfunction, but not all have high serum IgE. Intriguingly, the findings in the Dock8-deficient mice resemble those in Dock2-deficient mice, whose abnormalities include T cell lymphopenia, decreased thymic output, poor T cell proliferation, but variable IgE levels.[19–23] No DOCK2-deficient humans have yet been identified, although the mouse studies predict a phenotype that probably overlaps with DOCK8 deficiency. Nevertheless, these two related DOCK180 family members appear to exert nonredundant functions in the immune system, as DOCK8-deficient patients express normal levels of DOCK2 protein in Epstein–Barr virus (EBV)–transformed B cells (Fig. 1) and *Herpesvirus saimiri*-transformed T cells (Jing and Su, data not shown). Our results also suggest that DOCK8 does not act through DOCK2 by stabilizing DOCK2 protein in lymphocytes.

Overall, despite some differences, both patient and mouse observations support the classification of DOCK8 deficiency as a form of combined immunodeficiency that encompasses autosomal recessive hyper-IgE syndrome, but also includes cases that are not hyper-IgE syndrome.

Viral infections

A distinctive feature of DOCK8 deficiency that helps to distinguish it from other disorders is the difficulty controlling viral infections of the skin.[1,2] Offending pathogens are typically herpes simplex virus (HSV), human papillomavirus (HPV), molluscum contagiosum virus (MCV), and varicella-zoster virus (VZV). Eczema herpeticum, chronic ulcerating orolabial or anogenital HSV infections, or HSV keratitis often occur. Florid verrucous and flat warts, macular lesions resembling those seen in epidermodysplasia verruciformis, and anogenital warts are common. Extensive and sometimes confluent MCV skin lesions are also observed, as well as severe primary varicella or outbreaks of herpes zoster.

In comparison to the skin viral infections, DOCK8-deficient patients generally do not have difficulty controlling systemic viral infections. Low-level cytomegalovirus (CMV) or EBV viremia is rarely detected in some patients.[2] Although asymptomatic, these may become problematic upon further immunosuppression, such as when used during hematopoietic cell transplantation (HCT).[24] Several cases of progressive multifocal leukoencephalopathy (PML) due to JC virus have also been observed, although no cases of HSV or VZV encephalitis have been reported.[2]

To understand better patients' viral susceptibility, Dock8-deficient mice have recently been studied during experimental infections with either vaccinia virus or influenza. The mice recovered normally from acute infection and did not display any clinically worse disease. Their clinical course was consistent with their acute T cell responses, which were almost comparable to those from normal mice. However, antigen-specific CD8+ T cell numbers and responses were decreased at later times and following rechallenge, supporting a defect in CD8+ T cell memory.[15,16]

Although a defect in T cell memory can help to explain the chronic persistence of the viral infections in the DOCK8-deficient patients, their lack of problems with systemic viral infections suggests additional defects in local antiviral immunity within the skin. In this regard, immunoblotting demonstrated that nonimmune cell types contained within skin, such as fibroblasts, keratinocytes, and endothelial cells, do not normally express DOCK8 protein

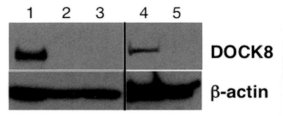

Figure 2. DOCK8 expression in keratinocytes, fibroblasts, and endothelial cells. Lysates were prepared from primary human keratinocytes (lane 2), fibroblasts (lane 3), endothelial cells (lane 5), and T cells (lanes 1 and 4), derived from healthy controls. The left and right blots were loaded with 50 or 40 μg of protein per lane, respectively, and immunoblotting for DOCK8 or β-actin proteins was performed, as described.[1]

(Fig. 2). Thus, DOCK8-expressing immune cells contained within the skin seem to be important for control of the viral skin infections, as underscored by the ability of HCT to cure this aspect of disease in DOCK8-deficient patients (see below). Besides impaired production of antiviral cytokines by DOCK8-deficient T cells[1] and poor antiviral CD8+ T cell memory responses,[15,16] disease could also reflect a requirement for DOCK8 in production of antiviral type I interferons from plasmacytoid dendritic cells (similar to what has been shown for Dock2-deficient mice),[25] and/or defects of these immune cells in migrating to the skin to exert their antiviral functions. This latter possibility is particularly intriguing, as Dock2-deficient mice, which resemble Dock8-deficient mice, have lymphocyte chemotaxis abnormalities.[19–21] Moreover, other diseases such as the Wiskott–Aldrich syndrome or the WHIM (warts, hypogammaglobulinemia, infections, myelokathexis) syndrome, which involve cytoskeletal or chemokine abnormalities that affect immune cell trafficking, display a similar predilection for chronic viral infections and, in the former case, eczema of the skin.[26,27] Thus, further studies may provide insight into unique aspects of local immunity and host defense within the skin.

Fungal infections

Although less problematic, fungal infections are almost equally prevalent as viral infections in DOCK8 deficiency.[2] Patients tend to present with mucocutaneous candidiasis, and more rarely *Pneumocystis jirovecii*, Histoplasmosis, or Cryptococcal meningitis. Filamentous mold infections have not been reported. The predilection for *Candida* infections probably reflects this organism's ubiquitous presence and normal coexistence as a commensal in healthy people.

The fungal susceptibility in DOCK8-deficient patients can be explained by decreased numbers of T helper type 17 (Th17) CD4[+] T cells.[28–31] Th17 cells are important for directing protective neutrophil responses against fungi and extracellular bacteria. Their importance has recently been demonstrated in patients with impaired IL-17 functions, who have chronic mucocutaneous candidiasis, *Staphylococcus aureus* folliculitis, and respiratory tract infections.[32] Patients with Job's syndrome due to autosomal dominant *STAT3* mutations also have mucocutaneous candidiasis due to severely decreased Th17 cell numbers.[29,33–35] Production of chemokines and antimicrobial peptides by keratinocytes or bronchial epithelial cells, but not other cell types, in turn, depends upon the synergistic actions of IL-17 and proinflammatory cytokines.[36] Thus, the systemic defect in Th17 cells could thereby predispose to *Candida* and *Staphyloccocus* infections of the skin.

When compared to Job's syndrome patients, the numbers of Th17 cells in DOCK8-deficient patients seem to be variably decreased (Fig. 3A).[28,30] Furthermore, naive T cells from DOCK8-deficient patients can be differentiated *in vitro* to express RORγt but not IL-17, whereas naive T cells from Job's syndrome patients are blocked in their ability to differentiate into either RORγt- or IL-17-expressing cells.[28] Thus, the loss of these DOCK8-deficient T cells occurs at a later step of Th17 differentiation or survival after RORγt expression. One possibility is that the defect in Th17 generation could reflect a global impairment in T cell differentiation into, or survival of, different effector subpopulations. This possibility was raised by observations of impaired production of IL-2 (Fig. 3B) and IFN-γ by *ex vivo* CD4[+] T cells,[15] suggesting a defect also in generating Th1 cells. However, a global impairment seems unlikely given that Th2 cells are concomitantly increased in DOCK8-deficient patients.[15] The molecular details of how DOCK8 expression might normally contribute to the generation of Th17 cells are presently unknown. Although *STAT3* could normally have other transcriptional targets involved in early Th17 differentiation, one possibility is that it also promoted DOCK8 transcription. However,

microarray analysis and chromatin immunoprecipitation of CD4[+] T cells from *Stat3*-deficient mice, differentiated under Th17 conditions, did not support this explanation.[37] Thus, a clear explanation for the effects of DOCK8 deficiency on Th17 cells for antifungal immunity is lacking.

Sinopulmonary infections

Patients with DOCK8 deficiency have recurrent sinus, lung, and middle ear infections, which often require multiple sinus surgeries or placement of myringotomy tubes, and sometimes lead to complications such as mastoiditis or bronchiectasis.[1,2] A variety of organisms are responsible, mostly Gram-positive and Gram-negative bacteria, such as *Streptococcus pneumoniae* and *Haemophilus influenzae*, but also fungi, such as *Pneumocystis jirovecii*, and viruses such as respiratory adenovirus. Additionally, some patients have recurrent or persistent gastrointestinal infections due to *Salmonella* enteritis, Giardiasis, or viruses such as norovirus.

The recurrent sinopulmonary as well as gastrointestinal infections are consistent with humoral immune abnormalities, which have been well characterized in Dock8-deficient mice generated by ENU mutagenesis.[18] Screening of these mice revealed defective production of long-lasting, mature, T cell-dependent antibody responses upon primary or secondary challenge. The mice lack marginal zone B cells in the spleen and display atrophic germinal centers. Following antigenic challenge, Dock8-deficient B cells, adoptively transferred into normal mice, undergo somatic hypermutation but fail to select out mature, high affinity, isotype-switched cells. Moreover, their B cells form abnormally organized immune synapses. Thus, the absence of Dock8 confers a defect intrinsic to B cells, although whether defective T cell help contributes to defective antibody responses was not examined. Recapitulating the abnormal B cell function in the mice, humans with DOCK8 deficiency have variably defective specific antibodies against T cell-independent (i.e., pneumococcal polysaccharide) and T cell-dependent vaccines.[1] Furthermore, in two patients who had been immunized and rechallenged with the T cell-dependent neoantigen bacteriophage φX174, both the primary and secondary antibody responses were impaired, and there was also no isotype switching.[1] In light of these observations, administration of intravenous

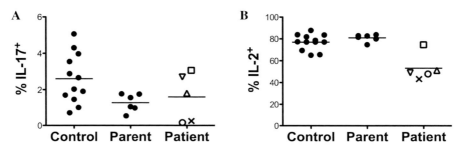

Figure 3. IL-17 or IL-2 expression in DOCK8-deficient CD4[+] T cells. Intracellular flow cytometric analysis for (A) IL-17 or (B) IL-2 expression in purified T cells from DOCK8-deficient parents and their patients, as well as healthy controls, was performed as described.[1] Additional antibodies used were PE anti-IL-17A (eBioscience) or PE anti-IL-2 (BD Biosciences). Shown are the percent positive of gated CD8[−]CD45RO[+] T cells, with each symbol designating an individual study subject and horizontal bars designating the means.

immunoglobulin, not surprisingly, decreases the frequency of sinopulmonary infections in some patients.

Despite many similarities, the antibody responses in DOCK8-deficient humans and mice differ in several aspects.[1] Unlike the mice, whose levels of total serum immunoglobulins are normal, patients often have high serum IgG and almost all have high IgE. Serum IgA can be high or low, whereas IgM is usually low. This puzzling pattern could suggest accelerated isotype switching, as well as differential effects on memory B cells or plasma cells. In further contrast to the mice, germinal centers were present and well formed in one patient who had lymph node available for histopathologic analysis (A. Freeman, unpublished data). Whether these apparent species differences reflect the repeated antigenic challenges that humans encounter in the natural environment is unknown. More work is needed to clarify the pathophysiologic mechanisms leading to the humoral immune abnormalities in DOCK8-deficient humans.

Atopic disease

In DOCK8-deficient patients, atopic dermatitis begins during infancy, before other symptoms such as viral skin infections develop. Patients have frequent infections of the skin, including abscesses, caused by *Staphyloccoccus aureus* and, rarely, *Acinetobacter baumanii*, and sensitization to *Staphylococcus aureus* further exacerbates the atopic dermatitis. During evaluation, patients are usually found to have high serum IgE and eosinophilia, which are also characteristic of Job's syndrome.

However, unlike Job's syndrome patients, patients with DOCK8 deficiency develop other manifestations of atopic disease.[1] Most patients have severe allergies to multiple foods or aeroallergens, including anaphylaxis, and a subset also develops eosinophilic esophagitis. Asthma is also common. These allergic manifestations reflect increased numbers of Th2 CD4[+] T cells, which express IL-4 or IL-13 to promote allergic disease, in the patients.[15]

Although Dock8-deficient mice were not reported in their original description to have high serum IgE, eosinophilia, or allergic disease, the absence of these findings could reflect genetic background differences and/or lack of environmental exposure to allergens.[18] Dock8-deficient mice do produce increased numbers of IL-4–expressing cells, despite similar numbers of GATA3-expressing cells, when their naive CD4[+] T cells are differentiated *in vitro* under Th2-polarizing conditions.[15] Dock2-deficient mice were also not initially appreciated as having allergic disease. However, when backcrossed onto an allergy-prone BALB/c genetic background, Dock2-deficient mice spontaneously developed blepharitis, with eosinophilic and mast cell infiltration into skin, elevated total serum IgE, and skewing towards Th2 CD4[+] T cell responses that promote allergic disease.[23] The exaggerated IL-4 signaling results from a failure to internalize and degrade the IL-4 receptor alpha chain by disrupting normal microtubular function for lysosomal trafficking. Whether a similar mechanism operates in DOCK8 deficiency has not yet been determined. Interestingly, after HCT of one patient, who achieved full donor T cell reconstitution but had mixed chimerism in other immune cells, eczema resolved while food allergies, although lessened, persisted.[38] These observations suggest that DOCK8-deficient T cells play an important role in allergic disease, but that other immune cell types in which DOCK8 might be normally expressed, including mast cells and eosinophils, could also contribute to disease. More work is needed to clarify a potential role of DOCK8 in T helper cell differentiation, as well as mast cell and eosinophil functions.

Malignancies

Similar to many other PIDs, DOCK8 deficiency is associated with an increased likelihood of developing cancer, with ~20% of patients going on to develop at least one cancer and ~10% of patients dying from cancer.[39] The most common malignancy seen in these patients is squamous cell carcinomas, to which the chronic HPV infections of the skin contribute. Because most patients develop significant disease before becoming sexually active, whether they would otherwise go on to develop cervical cancer from genitally acquired high-risk HPV types is unknown, although cervical intraepithelial dysplasia has been observed. The second most common malignancy following squamous cell carcinoma is lymphoma. Both EBV[−] diffuse large B cell lymphoma and EBV[+] Burkitt lymphoma have been observed. Lymphomas tend to be extranodal and have included primary CNS lymphoma as well as cutaneous T cell leukemia/lymphoma. Unusual cancers that have been sporadically reported in DOCK8-deficient patients include microcystic adenoma and leiomyoma.[1,40]

In addition to direct oncogenic effects of certain viruses, the increased incidence of cancers in DOCK8-deficient patients could reflect impaired tumor surveillance resulting from defective CD8 T cell functions.[1] Whether NK cell functions are also defective and contribute to the increased cancers is unknown. Furthermore, the over- or underexpression of other related DOCK180 family members has been shown to influence invasiveness or migration of cancers.[31,41–47] Because many cancers originating in the normal population acquire deletions or other abnormalities in DOCK8 expression, these observations suggest the possibility that DOCK8 might have a tumor suppressor function, which needs further evaluation.

Autoimmune disease

Autoimmune diseases can be seen in PIDs characterized by partial T cell deficiency, including DOCK8 deficiency. Several patients have developed autoimmune hemolytic anemia.[2] Furthermore, although a significant proportion of CNS abnormalities result from documented or suspected CNS infection, CNS vasculitis has been reported in some patients.[2] Whether the CNS vasculitis in some DOCK8-deficient patients reflects an infectious, autoimmune, and/or autoinflammatory process is unclear. Interestingly, vascular abnormalities are also found in Job's syndrome, which have been proposed to result from abnormal *STAT3* activity in vascular tissues during development or tissue remodeling.[48,49] However, the possibility that the pathogenesis of vascular abnormalities in both Job's syndrome and DOCK8 deficiency results from the hypereosinophilia common to both disorders has not yet been investigated.

Hematopoietic cell transplantation

To date, the outcomes after HCT of five patients, who were retrospectively confirmed as having DOCK8 deficiency, have been reported in the literature.[24,38,50,51] After myeloablative, reduced-intensity conditioning, patients received fully matched, related, or unrelated donor bone marrow or CD34[+] peripheral blood stem cells. They achieved nearly 100% donor chimerism in their T cells, but only after transient worsening of viral infections including MCV. With the exception of one patient who had congenital asplenia and died of *Klebsiella pneumoniae* sepsis, after T cell reconstitution the remaining four patients were cured of infectious complications for (at the time when reported) as long as six years after transplantation. Interestingly, in one patient who had mixed chimerism (98% T cells, 35% B cells, 53% mononuclear cells, 6% granulocytes), the eczema and viral infections of the skin, as well as recurrent sinopulmonary infections, resolved concurrently with restoration of lymphocyte numbers and function, including the ability to generate specific antibodies.[38] This patient continued to have food allergies, although she was less severely affected than prior to HCT, whereas allergies completely resolved in another patient after HCT.[24]

Together, these results suggest that the lack of DOCK8 expression within lymphocytes, primarily T cells, drives most of the infectious susceptibility and skin problems in the patients. Because Dock8-deficient bone marrow cells are at a competitive disadvantage for reconstituting the T cell compartment after adoptive transfer in mice, reduced-intensity conditioning regimens should be adequate for curative HCT therapy in patients, which indeed seems to be the case.[15,16,18] Outcomes will presumably be improved in patients undergoing HCT early in disease, before they develop chronic infections and deterioration of end-organ function that could contribute to complications. Whether HCT will prevent the future occurrence of malignancies remains to be seen.

Conclusions

DOCK8 deficiency in humans causes a form of combined immunodeficiency characterized by prominent lymphopenia and lymphocyte dysfunction, and is often accompanied by high serum IgE. This disease presents with a diverse constellation of signs and symptoms, which include problems with cutaneous viral, *Candida*, and bacterial infections, atopic disease, and malignancies. The infectious susceptibility can be a consequence of lymphopenia resulting from defective T cell proliferation, impaired generation of Th17 cells, impaired T cell production of antiviral cytokines, poor CD8$^+$ T cell memory, and defective affinity maturation with poor persistence of antibody responses. However, many unanswered questions remain about the pathogenesis of this disease. For example, it is unknown what role, if any, DOCK8 plays in the functions of other immune cell types, such as NK cells, dendritic cells, eosinophils, and mast cells. Furthermore, how DOCK8 deficiency leads to the development of high serum IgE and allergic disease or other infrequently observed manifestations, such as CNS abnormalities or autoimmune disease, has not yet been experimentally addressed. Investigation into these and other questions will help elucidate the normal function of DOCK8 in regulating immune responses for health and disease.

Acknowledgments

We thank Dr. Yu Zhang for her bioinformatics analysis of the NCBI published dataset GSE26553, Dr. Manfred Boehm (NHLBI, NIH) for endothelial cells, and Dr. Alexandra Freeman for many helpful discussions. Patients, their parents, and healthy controls were studied after written informed consent was obtained for enrollment in an NIAID IRB-approved protocol. This work was supported by the Intramural Research Program of the National Institutes of Health, the National Institute of Allergy and Infectious Diseases.

Conflicts of interest

The authors declare no conflicts of interest.

References

1. Zhang, Q. *et al.* 2009. Combined immunodeficiency associated with DOCK8 mutations. *N. Engl. J. Med.* **361:** 2046–2055.
2. Engelhardt, K.R. *et al.* 2009. Large deletions and point mutations involving the dedicator of cytokinesis 8 (DOCK8) in the autosomal-recessive form of hyper-IgE syndrome. *J. Allergy Clin. Immunol.* **124:** 1289–1302.e1284.
3. Ruusala, A. & P. Aspenstrom. 2004. Isolation and characterisation of DOCK8, a member of the DOCK180-related regulators of cell morphology. *FEBS Lett.* **572:** 159–166.
4. Cote, J.F. & K. Vuori. 2002. Identification of an evolutionarily conserved superfamily of DOCK180-related proteins with guanine nucleotide exchange activity. *J. Cell. Sci.* **115:** 4901–4913.
5. Tybulewicz, V.L. & R.B. Henderson. 2009. Rho family GTPases and their regulators in lymphocytes. *Nat. Rev. Immunol.* **9:** 630–644.
6. Freeman, A.F. & S.M. Holland. 2010. Clinical manifestations of hyper IgE syndromes. *Dis. Markers* **29:** 123–130.
7. Minegishi, Y. *et al.* 2007. Dominant-negative mutations in the DNA-binding domain of STAT3 cause hyper-IgE syndrome. *Nature* **448:** 1058–1062.
8. Holland, S.M. *et al.* 2007. STAT3 mutations in the hyper-IgE syndrome. *N. Engl. J. Med.* **357:** 1608–1619.
9. Woellner, C. *et al.* 2010. Mutations in STAT3 and diagnostic guidelines for hyper-IgE syndrome. *J. Allergy Clin. Immunol.* **125:** 424–432.
10. Renner, E.D. *et al.* 2004. Autosomal recessive hyperimmunoglobulin E syndrome: a distinct disease entity. *J. Pediatr.* **144:** 93–99.
11. Minegishi, Y. *et al.* 2006. Human tyrosine kinase 2 deficiency reveals its requisite roles in multiple cytokine signals involved in innate and acquired immunity. *Immunity* **25:** 745–755.
12. Woellner, C. *et al.* 2007. The hyper IgE syndrome and mutations in TYK2. *Immunity* **26:** 535; author reply 536.
13. Grant, A.V. *et al.* 2011. Accounting for genetic heterogeneity in homozygosity mapping: application to Mendelian susceptibility to mycobacterial disease. *J. Med. Genet.* **48:** 567–571.
14. Ozcan, E., L.D. Notarangelo & R.S. Geha. 2008. Primary immune deficiencies with aberrant IgE production. *J. Allergy Clin. Immunol.* **122:** 1054–1062; quiz 1063–1054.
15. Lambe, T. *et al.* 2011. DOCK8 is essential for T-cell survival and the maintenance of CD8(+) T-cell memory. *Eur. J. Immunol.* [Epub ahead of print] doi: 10.1002/eji.201141759.
16. Randall, K.L. *et al.* 2011. DOCK8 deficiency cripples CD8 T cells in humans and mice. *J. Exp. Med.* **208:** 2305–2320.

17. Dasouki, M. *et al.* 2011. Deficient T Cell Receptor Excision Circles (TRECs) in autosomal recessive hyper IgE syndrome caused by DOCK8 mutation: implications for pathogenesis and potential detection by newborn screening. *Clin. Immunol.* **141:** 128–132.

18. Randall, K.l. *et al.* 2009. Dock8 mutations cripple B cell immunological synapses, germinal centers and long-lived antibody production. *Nat. Immunol.* **10:** 1283–1291.

19. Fukui, Y. *et al.* 2001. Haematopoietic cell-specific CDM family protein DOCK2 is essential for lymphocyte migration. *Nature* **412:** 826–831.

20. Nombela-Arrieta, C. *et al.* 2004. Differential requirements for DOCK2 and phosphoinositide-3-kinase gamma during T and B lymphocyte homing. *Immunity* **21:** 429–441.

21. Nombela-Arrieta, C. *et al.* 2007. A central role for DOCK2 during interstitial lymphocyte motility and sphingosine-1-phosphate-mediated egress. *J. Exp. Med.* **204:** 497–510.

22. Sanui, T. *et al.* 2003. DOCK2 is essential for antigen-induced translocation of TCR and lipid rafts, but not PKC-theta and LFA-1, in T cells. *Immunity* **19:** 119–129.

23. Tanaka, Y. *et al.* 2007. T helper type 2 differentiation and intracellular trafficking of the interleukin 4 receptor-alpha subunit controlled by the Rac activator Dock2. *Nat. Immunol.* **8:** 1067–1075.

24. Barlogis, V. *et al.* 2011. Successful allogeneic hematopoietic stem cell transplantation for DOCK8 deficiency. *J. Allergy Clin. Immunol.* **128:** 420–422.e2.

25. Gotoh, K. *et al.* 2010. Selective control of type I IFN induction by the Rac activator DOCK2 during TLR-mediated plasmacytoid dendritic cell activation. *J. Exp. Med.* **207:** 721–730.

26. Blundell, M.P. *et al.* 2010. The Wiskott–Aldrich syndrome: the actin cytoskeleton and immune cell function. *Dis. Markers* **29:** 157–175.

27. Bachelerie, F. 2010. CXCL12/CXCR4-axis dysfunctions: markers of the rare immunodeficiency disorder WHIM syndrome. *Dis. Markers* **29:** 189–198.

28. Al Khatib, S. *et al.* 2009. Defects along the T(H)17 differentiation pathway underlie genetically distinct forms of the hyper IgE syndrome. *J. Allergy Clin. Immunol.* **124:** 342–348, 348.e341–345.

29. Milner, J.D. *et al.* 2008. Impaired T(H)17 cell differentiation in subjects with autosomal dominant hyper-IgE syndrome. *Nature* **452:** 773–776.

30. Schimke, L.F. *et al.* 2010. Diagnostic approach to the hyper-IgE syndromes: immunologic and clinical key findings to differentiate hyper-IgE syndromes from atopic dermatitis. *J. Allergy Clin. Immunol.* **126:** 611–617.e611.

31. Zhang, Q. *et al.* 2010. Genetic, clinical, and laboratory markers for DOCK8 immunodeficiency syndrome. *Dis. Markers* **29:** 131–139.

32. Puel, A. *et al.* 2011. Chronic mucocutaneous candidiasis in humans with inborn errors of interleukin-17 immunity. *Science* **332:** 65–68.

33. Ma, C.S. *et al.* 2008. Deficiency of Th17 cells in hyper IgE syndrome due to mutations in STAT3. *J. Exp. Med.* **205:** 1551–1557.

34. de Beaucoudrey, L. *et al.* 2008. Mutations in STAT3 and IL12RB1 impair the development of human IL-17-producing T cells. *J. Exp. Med.* **205:** 1543–1550.

35. Renner, E.D. *et al.* 2008. Novel signal transducer and activator of transcription 3 (STAT3) mutations, reduced T(H)17 cell numbers, and variably defective STAT3 phosphorylation in hyper-IgE syndrome. *J. Allergy Clin. Immunol.* **122:** 181–187.

36. Minegishi, Y. *et al.* 2009. Molecular explanation for the contradiction between systemic Th17 defect and localized bacterial infection in hyper-IgE syndrome. *J. Exp. Med.* **206:** 1291–1301.

37. Yang, X.P. *et al.* 2011. Opposing regulation of the locus encoding IL-17 through direct, reciprocal actions of STAT3 and STAT5. *Nat. Immunol.* **12:** 247–254.

38. Bittner, T.C. *et al.* 2010. Successful long-term correction of autosomal recessive hyper-IgE syndrome due to DOCK8 deficiency by hematopoietic stem cell transplantation. *Klin. Padiatr.* **222:** 351–355.

39. Su, H.C. 2010. Dedicator of cytokinesis 8 (DOCK8) deficiency. *Curr. Opin. Allergy Clin. Immunol.* **10:** 515–520.

40. Lei, J.Y. *et al.* 2000. Microcystic adnexal carcinoma associated with primary immunodeficiency, recurrent diffuse herpes simplex virus infection, and cutaneous T-cell lymphoma. *Am. J. Dermatopathol.* **22:** 524–529.

41. Sato, M. *et al.* 2005. Identification of chromosome arm 9p as the most frequent target of homozygous deletions in lung cancer. *Genes Chromosomes Cancer* **44:** 405–414.

42. Takahashi, K. *et al.* 2006. Homozygous deletion and reduced expression of the DOCK8 gene in human lung cancer. *Int. J. Oncol.* **28:** 321–328.

43. Heidenblad, M. *et al.* 2004. Genome-wide array-based comparative genomic hybridization reveals multiple amplification targets and novel homozygous deletions in pancreatic carcinoma cell lines. *Cancer Res.* **64:** 3052–3059.

44. Kang, J.U. *et al.* 2010. Frequent silence of chromosome 9p, homozygous DOCK8, DMRT1 and DMRT3 deletion at 9p24.3 in squamous cell carcinoma of the lung. *Int. J. Oncol.* **37:** 327–335.

45. Takada, H. *et al.* 2006. Genomic loss and epigenetic silencing of very-low-density lipoprotein receptor involved in gastric carcinogenesis. *Oncogene* **25:** 6554–6562.

46. Idbaih, A. *et al.* 2008. Genomic changes in progression of low-grade gliomas. *J. Neurooncol.* **90:** 133–140.

47. Saelee, P. *et al.* 2009. Novel PNLIPRP3 and DOCK8 gene expression and prognostic implications of DNA loss on chromosome 10q25.3 in hepatocellular carcinoma. *Asian Pac. J. Cancer Prev.* **10:** 501–506.

48. Yavuz, H. & R. Chee. 2010. A review on the vascular features of the hyperimmunoglobulin E syndrome. *Clin. Exp. Immunol.* **159:** 238–244.

49. Freeman, A.F. *et al.* 2011. Coronary artery abnormalities in hyper-IgE syndrome. *J. Clin. Immunol.* **31:** 338–345.

50. Gatz, S.A. *et al.* 2011. Curative treatment of autosomal-recessive hyper-IgE syndrome by hematopoietic cell transplantation. *Bone Marrow Transplant* **46:** 552–556.

51. McDonald, D.R. *et al.* 2010. Successful engraftment of donor marrow after allogeneic hematopoietic cell transplantation in autosomal-recessive hyper-IgE syndrome caused by dedicator of cytokinesis 8 deficiency. *J. Allergy Clin. Immunol.* **126:** 1304–1305.e3.

Ann. N.Y. Acad. Sci. ISSN 0077-8923

ANNALS OF THE NEW YORK ACADEMY OF SCIENCES
Issue: *The Year in Human and Medical Genetics: Inborn Errors of Immunity*

Molecular mechanisms of the immunological abnormalities in hyper-IgE syndrome

Yoshiyuki Minegishi and Masako Saito

Department of Immune Regulation, Tokyo Medical and Dental University, Tokyo, Japan

Address for correspondence: Yoshiyuki Minegishi, 1-5-45 Yushima, Bunkyo-ku, Tokyo 113-8519, Japan. yminegishi.mbch@tmd.ac.jp

Hyper-IgE syndrome (HIES) is a primary immunodeficiency characterized by atopic dermatitis associated with extremely high serum IgE levels and susceptibility to staphylococcal skin abscesses and pneumonia. Recent studies have identified dominant negative mutations in the signal transducer and activator of transcription 3 gene (*STAT3*) as a major molecular cause of classical hyper-IgE syndrome, but the molecular mechanisms underlying this syndrome remain unclear. We recently showed that the impaired development of interleukin 17 (IL-17)–producing T helper cells (Th17 cells) due to defective IL-6 and IL-23 signaling in T cells, and the impaired generation of induced regulatory T (iT_{reg}) cells from defective IL-10 signaling in dendritic cells, may account for the immunological abnormalities of hyper-IgE syndrome. These findings open up possibilities for exploring new approaches to the treatment of HIES patients.

Keywords: Th17 cell; iTreg cell; staphylococcal infection; atopic dermatitis; STAT3

Introduction

Hyper-IgE syndrome (HIES) is a complex primary immunodeficiency disorder (PID) characterized by recurrent staphylococcal skin abscesses and pneumonia, atopic dermatitis, and extremely high serum IgE levels.[1,2] Recent studies have demonstrated the multisystem nature of HIES,[3] the signs of which are not restricted to the immune system, extend to skeletal and lung parenchymal abnormalities, such as osteoporosis, fracture with minor trauma, scoliosis, hyperextensive joints, retention of primary teeth, bronchiectasis, and pneumatocele. Dominant-negative mutations in *STAT3* have been identified as a major molecular cause of the multisystem HIES.[4,5] However, our understanding of the molecular mechanism underlying this syndrome remains limited. In this review, we focus on the molecular mechanisms underlying immunological manifestations of HIES due to dominant negative mutations in *STAT3*.

STAT3

STAT3 plays a critical role in signal transduction for many cytokines and growth factors, including those of the γc family (IL-2, IL-4, IL-7, IL-9, IL-15, IL-21), the gp130 family (IL-6, IL-11, IL-27, IL-31), the IL-10 family (IL-10, IL-19, IL-20, IL-22, IL-24, IL-26, IL-28, IL-29), and receptor-type tyrosine kinases (M-CSF, Flt-3, PDGF, EGF, FGF, GH, IGF) (Table 1).[6] STAT3 functions as a transcription factor, binding to promoter regions and initiating transcription of its target genes. STAT3 mediates signaling for about 40 cytokines and growth factors. It is, therefore, not straightforward to determine which pathway, in which cell type is critical for the signs of HIES. Studies of a null mutation of the *STAT3* gene in mice demonstrated that STAT3 was essential for embryo survival close to the time of implantation (E6.5–E7.5).[7] Other studies of mice with a tissue-specific deletion of *STAT3* demonstrated the critical role of STAT3 in cell survival, proliferation, migration, apoptosis, and inflammation in diverse cells including keratinocytes, hepatocytes, thymic epithelial cells, respiratory epithelial cells, neurons, lymphocytes, and macrophages.[8] The multisystem signs in HIES patients probably reflect the diverse functions *in vivo* of STAT3 in humans.

Th17 cells

Th17 cells—a subset of helper T cells producing cytokines including IL-17A, IL-17F, and IL-22—

doi: 10.1111/j.1749-6632.2011.06280.x

Ann. N.Y. Acad. Sci. 1246 (2011) 34–40 © 2011 New York Academy of Sciences.

Table 1. Ligands, receptors, and Jak family kinases upstream of STAT3

	Ligands		Receptors		Jak family kinases		
γc family	IL-2	γc	IL-2Ra	IL-2Rb	Jak1	Jak3	
	IL-4	γc	IL-4Ra		Jak1	Jak3	
	IL-7	γc	IL-7Ra		Jak1	Jak3	
	IL-9	γc	IL-9Ra		Jak1	Jak3	
	IL-15	γc	IL-15Ra	IL-2Rb	Jak1	Jak3	
	IL-21	γc	IL-21R		Jak1	Jak3	
IFNs	IFN-α	IFNAR1	IFNAR2		Jak1	Tyk2	
	IFN-β	IFNAR1	IFNAR2		Jak1	Tyk2	
	IFN-γ	IFNGR1	IFNGR2		Jak1	Jak2	
IL-12/23	IL-12	IL-12Rb1	IL-12Rb2		Jak2	Tyk2	
	IL-23	IL-12Rb1	IL-23R		Jak2	Tyk2	
gp130 family	IL-6	gp130	IL-6Ra		Jak1	Jak2	Tyk2
	IL-11	gp130	IL-11Ra		Jak1	Jak2	Tyk2
	IL-27	gp130	IL-27Ra		Jak1	Jak3	
	IL-31	gp130	IL-31Ra		Jak1	Jak3	
	LIF	gp130	LIFR		Jak1	Jak3	
	OSM	gp130	OSMRb		Jak1	Jak3	
	CNTF	gp130	CNTFR		Jak1	Jak3	
	CT-1	gp130	CT-1R		Jak1	Jak3	
IL-10 family	IL-10	IL-10R2	IL-10R1		Jak1	Tyk2	
	IL-19	IL-20R1	IL-20R2		Jak1	Jak2	
	IL-20	IL-20R1	IL-20R2		Jak1	Jak2	
	IL-22	IL-10R2	IL-22R		Jak1	Tyk2	
	IL-24	IL-20R1	IL-20R2		Jak1	Jak2	
	IL-26	IL-10R2	IL-20R1		Jak1	Jak2	
	IL-28	IL-10R2	IL-28R1		Jak1	Tyk2	
	IL-29	IL-10R2	IL-28R1		Jak1	Tyk2	
Receptor type	M-CSF	M-CSFR			–		
	Flt3L	Flt3			–		
	PDGF	PDGFR			–		
	EGF	EGFR			–		
	FGF	FGFR			–		
	GH	GHR			–		
	IGF	IGFR			–		
Others	IL-5	βc	IL-5Ra		Jak1	Jak2	
	G-CSF	G-CSFR			Jak1	Jak2	Tyk2
	Leptin	LEPR			Jak2		
	PAF	PAFR			Jak2		

have been extensively studied as inducers of autoimmune disorders.[9–13] Recent studies have also indicated that Th17 cells play a key role in host defense against extracellular bacteria and fungi.[14,15] Interestingly, most staphylococcal and Candida infections occurring in patients with HIES are confined to the skin and lung, whereas in patients with chronic granulomatous disease—another human primary immunodeficiency—staphylococcal infections are frequently systemic.[16] These clinical observations suggest that Th17 cytokines play an important role in host defense on the

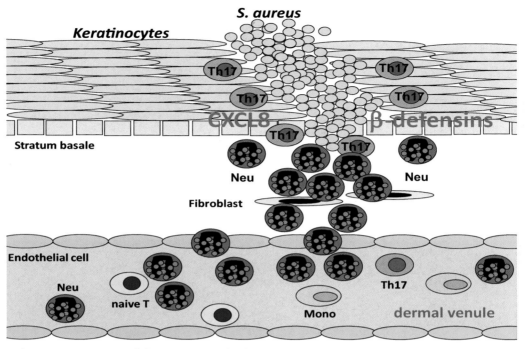

Figure 1. Protection against *Staphylococcus aureus* at the skin. The production of Th17 cytokines is severely decreased in HIES patients, which is required for the production of antimicrobial peptides, including β-defensin 2 and β-defensin 3, and neutrophil-recruiting chemokines, including CXCL8 (IL-8) from keratinocytes. The lack of antimicrobial peptides and neutrophil-recruiting chemokines may result in the susceptibility to staphylococcal infection in the skin.

surface of the body, particularly in the skin and airways.

Many reports have indicated that the production of Th17 cytokines, including IL-17A, IL-17F, and IL-22, by activated T cells from HIES patients is much lower than those from control individuals, whereas the production of other proinflammatory cytokines, including IFN-γ, IL-1β, and TNF-α, is unaffected.[17–21] Such findings raise the questions of why and how systemic Th17 cell defects lead to staphylococcal infections restricted to the skin and lungs.

Insight into these questions was provided by the experimental observation that while supernatant from activated T cells from normal subjects induce keratinocyte and bronchial epithelial cell production of neutrophil-recruiting chemokines and β-defensins, supernatant from activated T cells from STAT3-deficient patients does not.[21] Human primary keratinocytes and bronchial epithelial cells do not produce sufficiently large amounts of neutrophil-recruiting chemokines and β-defensins in response to Th17 cytokines or classical proin-

flammatory cytokines.[21] Further support for these findings was provided by the demonstration *in vitro* that neutralization of Th17 cytokines decreases the production of the chemokines and defensins.[21] In contrast to those data, primary dermal fibroblasts and endothelial cells were found to respond equally well to T cell supernatants from HIES patients and controls. Thus, keratinocytes and bronchial epithelial cells respond differently from other types of cells (e.g., fibroblasts and endothelial cells) to Th17 cytokines, with Th17 cytokines playing a more important role in the production of chemokines and β-defensins in epithelial cells. One interpretation of this observation is that epithelial cells are always exposed to external stimuli and therefore have developed a system that is unresponsive to a single stimulation (such as Th17 cytokines) yet are responsive to combinations of stimulations. By contrast, internal cells, including fibroblasts and endothelial cells, must respond to single stimuli more rapidly because such first signals are often indicative of pathogen invasion, which requires an immediate response.

These previously published data[21] strongly indicate that Th17 cytokines play a crucial role in human host defense against *Staphylococcus aureus*, particularly at the surface barriers of the body (Fig. 1). Systemic T cell defects are converted into local defects, because only keratinocytes and bronchial epithelial cells require cytokines produced by Th17 cells in order to secrete neutrophil-recruiting chemokines and antimicrobial peptides. These findings provide at least a partial explanation for the restriction of staphylococcal infections to the skin and lungs of HIES patients and highlight the physiological role of Th17 cytokines in protection against extracellular pathogens in humans.[21]

Induced regulatory T cells

One of the potential mechanisms of atopic dermatitis development in HIES is an acceleration of Th2 cell activity.[22–24] Effector Th2 cells are considered to be the major cell type that responds to allergens and produces Th2 cytokines, including IL-4, IL-5, IL-9, and IL-13. These Th2 cytokines induce changes in blood vessels, upregulate adhesion molecules, and recruit eosinophils. Th2 cytokines also induce class switching to IgE.[25] Recently identified cytokines such as IL-25, IL-31, and IL-33 also participate in Th2 cell-mediated inflammatory diseases.[26–28] In addition to Th2 cells, Th1 cells play a role in the pathogenesis of atopic dermatitis—contributing at a later time point—by inducing the apoptosis of epithelial cells.[29]

Another potential mechanism by which atopic dermatitis may develop in HIES patients is by impairment of regulatory T (T_{reg}) cell activity; T_{reg} cells are key mediators of peripheral tolerance that suppress effector Th2 cells. The transcription factor Foxp3 is an important regulator of the development, function, and survival of T_{reg} cells, as clearly demonstrated by primary immunodeficiency in which patients lack FOXP3 gene expression and present with severe autoimmune and atopic phenotypes. Mutations in the human FOXP3 gene (*FOXP3*) result in immune dysregulation, polyendocrinopathy, enteropathy, and X-linked (IPEX) syndrome.[30,31] Foxp3 deficiency in mice also leads to atopic phenotypes.[32,33]

There are at least two types of Foxp3+ T_{reg} cells: natural T_{reg} (nT_{reg}) cells and induced T_{reg} (iT_{reg}) cells. Natural T_{reg} cells develop in the thymus, whereas iT_{reg} cells develop in the periphery. TGF-β

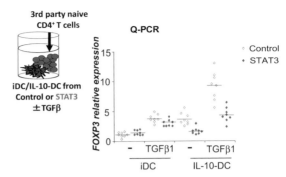

Figure 2. Q-PCR analysis of relative *FOXP3* mRNA expression (FOXP3/HPRT) after the co-culture of third-party allogeneic naive CD4+ T cells from a control subject with untreated immature DCs (iDCs) or IL-10-DCs from eight controls and eight *STAT3* patients in the absence or presence of exogenous TGF-β1. IL-10-DCs upregulate *FOXP3* expression as efficiently as TGF-β1 and the combination of IL-10-DCs and TGF-β synergistically upregulates the expression of *FOXP3*.

plays a crucial role in the induction of iT_{reg} cells; its expression in the presence of TCR stimulation converts naive Foxp3−CD4+ T cells into Foxp3+ iT_{reg} cells.[34–37] In addition to soluble factors, dendritic cells play a key role in the induction of T_{reg} cells.[38,39]

It has been shown that dendritic cells of patients with HIES display defective IL-10 signaling, which results in impaired suppression of cytokine production and T cell proliferation. In addition, dendritic cells from HIES patients are defective in generating Foxp3+ iT_{reg} cells by IL-10 treatment.[40] Defective generation of iT_{reg} cells in response to IL-10 has also been observed in the other form of HIES that results from TYK2 deficiency.[41]

In terms of the molecular mechanisms involved, IL-10 normally upregulates the expression of PD-L1 and ILT-4 on the surface of dendritic cells, and both of these molecules are required for the induction of Foxp3+ iT_{reg} cells.[40] In addition, IL-10–treated dendritic cells induce iT_{reg} cells as efficiently as does TGF-β, and the combination of IL-10-treated dendritic cells and TGF-β synergistically induces iT_{reg} cells (Fig. 2). Both of these IL-10–mediated pathways are likely defective in HIES patients. IL-10 signaling in dendritic cells is crucial for generating iT_{reg} cells *in vivo* and thus for maintaining an appropriate Th2–T_{reg} cell balance to prevent hyper-IgE syndrome.

Many studies have suggested that IL-10 is one of the key regulators of atopic dermatitis. The exposure of the skin to allergens induces allergen-specific unresponsiveness due to the production of IL-10[42,43] that modulates Langerhans cells and dermal dendritic cells to induce allergen-specific tolerance. A defect in IL-10–mediated tolerance to innocuous environmental antigens may thus be one of the mechanisms underlying the atopic dermatitis in hyper-IgE syndrome. Indeed, in humans it has been shown that low IL-10 is involved in the molecular pathogenesis of atopic disorders; the frequency of allergen-specific, IL-10–secreting T cells is significantly higher in nonatopic individuals than in atopic patients;[44] and IL-10 levels are inversely correlated with the severity of human allergic diseases.[45,46] Also, effective allergen-specific immunotherapies increase IL-10 synthesis by T cells.[47,48]

In rodent studies, mice lacking IL-10 or the IL-10 receptor spontaneously develop inflammation in the large intestine,[49–51] and mice with T_{reg} cell-specific IL-10 deficiency also display inflammation of body surfaces that are in contact with the environment, such as the colon, lungs, and skin.[52] In humans, mutations in the genes encoding IL-10 or IL-10 receptor subunits have been found in patients with early-onset enterocolitis.[53]

HIES patients, however, do not display a marked increase in the frequency of enterocolitis despite the impairment of IL-10 signaling, which may reflect partial IL-10 signaling. In addition to this IL-10 signaling defect, patients with STAT3 mutations have defective Th17 cell development. Thus, the combination of Th17 cell deficiency and an IL-10 signaling defect may prevent the development of enterocolitis but induce atopic dermatitis in HIES patients.[54]

Naive CD4$^+$ T cells educated by IL-10–treated dendritic cells have antigen-specific iT_{reg} activity.[55] A previous study showed that the generation of FOXP3$^+$ iT_{reg} cells by IL-10–treated dendritic cells is impaired in HIES patients.[40] Because T_{reg} cells mediate peripheral tolerance and play a central role in determining several immune diseases, including autoimmunity, chronic infections, tumors, and allergies,[56] FOXP3$^+$ T_{reg} cells are likely involved in protecting humans against allergic diseases, as patients with IPEX syndrome suffer from allergic symptoms. Consistent with this, peripheral blood mononuclear cells (PBMCs) from atopic patients proliferate more extensively and produce more Th2 cytokines in response to allergen than do PBMCs from nonatopic healthy individuals.[57] However, patients with atopic dermatitis have normal numbers of T_{reg} cells in the periphery—likely nT_{reg} cells—with normal suppressive activity.[58] Such results suggest that iT_{reg} cells may be more important than nT_{reg} cells for controlling atopic dermatitis. Indeed, a recent study in two mouse strains—one capable of generating iT_{reg} cells but not nT_{reg} cells and the other unable to generate either iT_{reg} or nT_{reg} cells—suggested that iT_{reg} cells control allergic inflammation in response to innocuous environmental allergens, whereas nT_{reg} cells do not.[59]

Therapeutic implications

Some patients with HIES are doing well with conventional treatments, but the other patients suffer from severe clinical manifestations, such as early-onset pneumonia and subsequent pneumatocele formation, which is further complicated by multidrug-resistant *Pseudomonas* and *Aspergillus* infections. A significant number of patients in their twenties die of pulmonary hemorrhage due to fungal vascular invasion and brain metastasis of fungal disease.[60] At present, it is not clear that this diversity of clinical courses is caused by environmental or genetic factors. Previous studies suggested that the molecular mechanisms underlying the immunological manifestations of HIES, including staphylococcal pneumonia are likely to be caused by T cell defects, and that these defects could be corrected by stem cell transplantation. Future studies need to identify a subgroup of HIES patients with poor prognosis, which will provide an opportunity to improve clinical outcome by early stem cell transplantation before the onset of severe infections and parenchymal lung sequelae. Furthermore, stem cell transplantation might be beneficial for some HIES patients even after the episodes of pneumonia and parenchymal lung complications.

Acknowledgments

This work is supported by grants-in-aid from the Japanese Ministry of Education, Culture, Sports, Science and Technology (22021015, 22390205); JST; CREST; and Research on Intractable Diseases from the Ministry of Health, Labor and Welfare.

Conflicts of interest

The authors declare no conflicts of interest.

References

1. Grimbacher, B., S.M. Holland & J.M. Puck. 2005. Hyper-IgE syndromes. *Immunol. Rev.* **203:** 244–250.

2. Minegishi, Y. 2009. Hyper-IgE syndrome. *Curr. Opin. Immunol.* **21:** 487–492.

3. Grimbacher, B., S.M. Holland, J.I. Gallin, *et al.* 1999. Hyper-IgE syndrome with recurrent infections—an autosomal dominant multisystem disorder. *N. Engl. J. Med.* **340:** 692–702.

4. Holland, S.M., F.R. DeLeo, H.Z. Elloumi, *et al.* 2007. STAT3 mutations in the hyper-IgE syndrome. *N. Engl. J. Med.* **357:** 1608–1619.

5. Minegishi, Y., M. Saito, S. Tsuchiya, *et al.* 2007. Dominant-negative mutations in the DNA-binding domain of STAT3 cause hyper-IgE syndrome. *Nature* **448:** 1058–1062.

6. Levy, D.E. & C.K. Lee. 2002. What does STAT3 do? *J. Clin. Invest.* **109:** 1143–1148.

7. Takeda, K., K. Noguchi, W. Shi, *et al.* 1997. Targeted disruption of the mouse STAT3 gene leads to early embryonic lethality. *Proc. Natl. Acad. Sci. USA* **94:** 3801–3804.

8. Akira, S. 2000. Roles of STAT3 defined by tissue-specific gene targeting. *Oncogene* **19:** 2607–2611.

9. Bettelli, E., T. Korn & V.K. Kuchroo. 2007. Th17: the third member of the effector T cell trilogy. *Curr. Opin. Immunol.* **19:** 652–657.

10. Korn, T., M. Oukka, V. Kuchroo & E. Bettelli. 2007. Th17 cells: effector T cells with inflammatory properties. *Semin. Immunol.* **19:** 362–371.

11. Diveu, C., M.J. McGeachy & D.J. Cua. 2008. Cytokines that regulate autoimmunity. *Curr. Opin. Immunol.* **20:** 663–668.

12. Dong, C. 2008. TH17 cells in development: an updated view of their molecular identity and genetic programming. *Nat. Rev. Immunol.* **8:** 337–348.

13. Ouyang, W., J.K. Kolls & Y. Zheng. 2008. The biological functions of T helper 17 cell effector cytokines in inflammation. *Immunity* **28:** 454–467.

14. Aujla, S.J., P.J. Dubin & J.K. Kolls. 2007. Th17 cells and mucosal host defense. *Semin. Immunol.* **19:** 377–382.

15. Iwakura, Y., S. Nakae, S. Saijo & H. Ishigame. 2008. The roles of IL-17A in inflammatory immune responses and host defense against pathogens. *Immunol. Rev.* **226:** 57–79.

16. Winkelstein, J.A., M.C. Marino, R.B. Johnston, Jr., *et al.* 2000. Chronic granulomatous disease. Report on a national registry of 368 patients. *Medicine* **79:** 155–169.

17. de Beaucoudrey, L., A. Puel, O. Filipe-Santos, *et al.* 2008. Mutations in STAT3 and IL12RB1 impair the development of human IL-17-producing T cells. *J. Exp. Med.* **205:** 1543–1550.

18. Ma, C.S., G.Y. Chew, N. Simpson, *et al.* 2008. Deficiency of Th17 cells in hyper IgE syndrome due to mutations in STAT3. *J. Exp. Med.* **205:** 1551–1557.

19. Milner, J.D., J.M. Brenchley, A. Laurence, *et al.* 2008. Impaired T(H)17 cell differentiation in subjects with autosomal dominant hyper-IgE syndrome. *Nature* **452:** 773–776.

20. Renner, E.D., S. Rylaarsdam, S. Anover-Sombke, *et al.* 2008. Novel signal transducer and activator of transcription 3 (STAT3) mutations, reduced T(H)17 cell numbers, and variably defective STAT3 phosphorylation in hyper-IgE syndrome. *J. Allergy Clin. Immunol.* **122:** 181–187.

21. Minegishi, Y., M. Saito, M. Nagasawa, *et al.* 2009. Molecular explanation for the contradiction between systemic Th17 defect and localized bacterial infection in hyper-IgE syndrome. *J. Exp. Med.* **206:** 1291–1301.

22. Akdis, C.A. & M. Akdis. 2009. Mechanisms and treatment of allergic disease in the big picture of regulatory T cells. *J. Allergy Clin. Immunol.* **123:** 735–746.

23. Umetsu, D.T. & R.H. DeKruyff. 2006. The regulation of allergy and asthma. *Immunol. Rev.* **212:** 238–255.

24. Lloyd, C.M. & C.M. Hawrylowicz. 2009. Regulatory T cells in asthma. *Immunity* **31:** 438–49.

25. Hammad, H. & B.N. Lambrecht. 2008. Dendritic cells and epithelial cells: linking innate and adaptive immunity in asthma. *Nat. Rev. Immunol.* **8:** 193–204.

26. Dillon, S.R., C. Sprecher, A. Hammond, *et al.* 2004. Interleukin 31, a cytokine produced by activated T cells, induces dermatitis in mice. *Nat. Immunol.* **5:** 752–760.

27. Kakkar, R. & R.T. Lee. 2008. The IL-33/ST2 pathway: therapeutic target and novel biomarker. *Nat. Rev. Drug Discov.* **7:** 827–840.

28. Wang, Y.H., P. Angkasekwinai, N. Lu, *et al.* 2007. IL-25 augments type 2 immune responses by enhancing the expansion and functions of TSLP-DC-activated Th2 memory cells. *J. Exp. Med.* **204:** 1837–1847.

29. Trautmann, A., M. Akdis, D. Kleemann, *et al.* 2000. T cell-mediated Fas-induced keratinocyte apoptosis plays a key pathogenetic role in eczematous dermatitis. *J. Clin. Invest.* **106:** 25–35.

30. Wildin, R.S., F. Ramsdell, J. Peake, *et al.* 2001. X-linked neonatal diabetes mellitus, enteropathy and endocrinopathy syndrome is the human equivalent of mouse scurfy. *Nat. Genet.* **27:** 18–20.

31. Bennett, C.L., J. Christie, F. Ramsdell, *et al.* 2001. The immune dysregulation, polyendocrinopathy, enteropathy, X-linked syndrome (IPEX) is caused by mutations of FOXP3. *Nat. Genet.* **27:** 20–21.

32. Fontenot, J.D., M.A. Gavin & A.Y. Rudensky. 2003. Foxp3 programs the development and function of $CD4^+CD25^+$ regulatory T cells. *Nat. Immunol.* **4:** 330–336.

33. Lin, W., N. Truong, W.J. Grossman, *et al.* 2005. Allergic dysregulation and hyperimmunoglobulinemia E in Foxp3 mutant mice. *J. Allergy Clin. Immunol.* **116:** 1106–1115.

34. Chen, W., W. Jin, N. Hardegen, *et al.* 2003. Conversion of peripheral $CD4^+CD25-$ naive T cells to $CD4^+CD25^+$ regulatory T cells by TGF-beta induction of transcription factor Foxp3. *J. Exp. Med.* **198:** 1875–1886.

35. Coombes, J.L., K.R. Siddiqui, C.V. Arancibia-Carcamo, *et al.* 2007. A functionally specialized population of mucosal $CD103^+$ DCs induces $Foxp3^+$ regulatory T cells via a TGF-beta and retinoic acid-dependent mechanism. *J. Exp. Med.* **204:** 1757–1764.

36. Zheng, S.G., J. Wang, P. Wang, *et al.* 2007. IL-2 is essential for TGF-beta to convert naive $CD4^+CD25^-$ cells to $CD25^+Foxp3^+$ regulatory T cells and for expansion of these cells. *J. Immunol.* **178:** 2018–2027.

37. Rubtsov, Y.P. & A.Y. Rudensky. 2007. TGFbeta signalling in control of T-cell-mediated self-reactivity. *Nat. Rev. Immunol.* **7:** 443–453.

38. Steinman, R.M., D. Hawiger & M.C. Nussenzweig. 2003. Tolerogenic dendritic cells. *Annu. Rev. Immunol.* **21:** 685–711.

39. Rutella, S., S. Danese & G. Leone. 2006. Tolerogenic dendritic cells: cytokine modulation comes of age. *Blood* **108:** 1435–1440.

40. Saito, M., M. Nagasawa, H. Takada, *et al.* 2011. Defective IL-10 signaling in hyper-IgE syndrome results in impaired generation of tolerogenic dendritic cells and induced regulatory T cells. *J. Exp. Med.* **208:** 235–249.

41. Minegishi, Y., M. Saito, T. Morio, *et al.* 2006 Human TYK2 deficiency reveals requisite roles of TYK2 in multiple cytokine signals involved in innate and acquired immunity. *Immunity* **25:** 745–755.

42. Enk, A.H. & S.I. Katz. 1992. Early molecular events in the induction phase of contact sensitivity. *Proc. Natl. Acad. Sci. USA* **89:** 1398–1402.

43. Enk, A.H., V.L. Angeloni, M.C. Udey & S.I. Katz. 1993. Inhibition of Langerhans cell antigen-presenting function by IL-10. A role for IL-10 in induction of tolerance. *J. Immunol.* **151:** 2390–2398.

44. Akdis, M., J. Verhagen, A. Taylor, *et al.* 2004. Immune responses in healthy and allergic individuals are characterized by a fine balance between allergen-specific T regulatory 1 and T helper 2 cells. *J. Exp. Med.* **199:** 1567–1575.

45. Borish, L., A. Aarons, J. Rumbyrt, *et al.* 1996. Interleukin-10 regulation in normal subjects and patients with asthma. *J. Allergy Clin. Immunol.* **97:** 1288–1296.

46. Lim, S., E. Crawley, P. Woo & P.J. Barnes. 1998. Haplotype associated with low interleukin-10 production in patients with severe asthma. *Lancet* **352:** 113.

47. Francis, J.N., S.J. Till & S.R. Durham. 2003. Induction of IL-10+CD4+CD25+ T cells by grass pollen immunotherapy. *J. Allergy Clin. Immunol.* **111:** 1255–1261.

48. Vissers, J.L., B.C. van Esch, G.A. Hofman, *et al.* 2004. Allergen immunotherapy induces a suppressive memory response mediated by IL-10 in a mouse asthma model. *J. Allergy Clin. Immunol.* **113:** 1204–1210.

49. Kuhn, R., J. Lohler, D. Rennick, *et al.* 1993. Interleukin-10-deficient mice develop chronic enterocolitis. *Cell* **75:** 263–274.

50. Davidson, N.J., M.W. Leach, M.M. Fort, *et al.* 1996. T helper cell 1-type CD4+ T cells, but not B cells, mediate colitis in interleukin 10-deficient mice. *J. Exp. Med.* **184:** 241–251.

51. Spencer, S.D., F. Di Marco, J. Hooley, *et al.* 1998. The orphan receptor CRF2-4 is an essential subunit of the interleukin 10 receptor. *J. Exp. Med.* **187:** 571–578.

52. Rubtsov, Y.P., J.P. Rasmussen, E.Y. Chi, *et al.* 2008. Regulatory T cell-derived interleukin-10 limits inflammation at environmental interfaces. *Immunity* **28:** 546–558.

53. Glocker, E.O., A. Hennigs, M. Nabavi, *et al.* 2009. A homozygous CARD9 mutation in a family with susceptibility to fungal infections. *N. Engl. J. Med.* **361:** 1727–1735.

54. Brand, S. 2009. Crohn's disease: Th1, Th17 or both? The change of a paradigm: new immunological and genetic insights implicate Th17 cells in the pathogenesis of Crohn's disease. *Gut* **58:** 1152–1167.

55. Steinbrink, K., E. Graulich, S. Kubsch, *et al.* 2002. CD4(+) and CD8(+) anergic T cells induced by interleukin-10-treated human dendritic cells display antigen-specific suppressor activity. *Blood* **99:** 2468–2476.

56. Hawrylowicz, C.M. & A. O'Garra. 2005. Potential role of interleukin-10-secreting regulatory T cells in allergy and asthma. *Nat. Rev. Immunol.* **5:** 271–283.

57. Ling, E.M., T. Smith, X.D. Nguyen, *et al.* 2004. Relation of CD4+CD25+ regulatory T-cell suppression of allergen-driven T-cell activation to atopic status and expression of allergic disease. *Lancet* **363:** 608–615.

58. Ou, L.S., E. Goleva, C. Hall & D.Y. Leung. 2004. T regulatory cells in atopic dermatitis and subversion of their activity by superantigens. *J. Allergy Clin. Immunol.* **113:** 756–763.

59. Curotto de Lafaille, M.A., N. Kutchukhidze, S. Shen, *et al.* 2008. Adaptive Foxp3+ regulatory T cell-dependent and – independent control of allergic inflammation. *Immunity* **29:** 114–126.

60. Freeman, A.F., D.E. Kleiner, H. Nadiminti, *et al.* 2007. Causes of death in hyper-IgE syndrome. *J. Allergy Clin. Immunol.* **119:** 1234–1240.

Ann. N.Y. Acad. Sci. ISSN 0077-8923

ANNALS OF THE NEW YORK ACADEMY OF SCIENCES

Issue: *The Year in Human and Medical Genetics: Inborn Errors of Immunity*

Perspectives on common variable immune deficiency

Joon H. Park, Elena S. Resnick, and Charlotte Cunningham-Rundles

Department of Medicine and the Immunology Institute, Mount Sinai School of Medicine, New York, New York

Address for correspondence: Charlotte Cunningham-Rundles, M.D., Ph.D., Departments of Medicine and Pediatrics, The Immunology Institute, Mount Sinai School of Medicine, 1425 Madison Avenue, New York, NY 10029. Charlotte.Cunningham-Rundles@mssm.edu

Common variable immunodeficiency (CVID) is considered to be a collection of genetic immune defects with complex inheritance patterns. While the main phenotype is loss of B cell function, the majority of the genetic mechanisms leading to CVID remain elusive. In the past two decades there have been increasing efforts to unravel the genetic defects in CVID. Here, we provide an overview of our current understanding of the genetic basis of these defects, as revealed over time by earlier linkage studies in large cohorts, analysis of families with recessive inheritance, targeted gene approaches, and genome-wide association studies using single nucleotide polymorphism arrays and copy number variation, and whole genome studies.

Keywords: common variable immunodeficiency; hypogammaglobulinemia; IgA deficiency; genome-wide association studies; single nucleotide polymorphism; copy number variations; recessive genes

Introduction

The programmed development and maintenance of B cells capable of producing, in great abundance for an indefinite period of time, virtually unlimited numbers of antibody specificities is one of the most enigmatic features of biology. Each step in this complex process requires a sequence of transcription factors, cell surface interactions, migratory stimuli, cytokines, and the appropriate niche locations to sponsor these events. Even when formed and functional, new B cells are subjected to continual counterselection to exclude self-reactivity and, finally, to equip emerging clones with a high degree of specificity for previously selected antigens. B cells have several fates, a prominent one being the maturation into long-lived plasma cells that are generated first in lymphoid organs and ultimately in the bone marrow, where they can survive for many years. Another fate of the appropriately activated B cell is differentiation into memory B cells, a CD40L-dependent fate that ensures continued capability to produce antibodies, even after the passage of long periods of time. The final products of selected B cells—serum immune globulins—represent about 20% of serum

protein, but this does not include the extensive production of IgA, the most abundantly produced Ig, as at least 80% of IgA-secreting B cells reside in the gastrointestinal mucosa.

Considering the extensive biological effort manifest in B cell biology, it may be surprising to consider that an equally extensive network of genetic influences—some working singly, others as collective influences—must support the many stages of B cell biology. The study of B cells with single gene defects has elucidated some of the most essential components of B cell biology, especially for the early events of B cell survival and activation. However, the most common of these events—common variable immunodeficiency (CVID)—is for the most part not yet well understood, thus providing a still open field for exploration.

Patients with CVID have a marked reduction in serum levels of IgG (usually < 3 g/L) and usually IgA (< 0.05 g/L), with reductions in serum IgM in about half of all cases.[1–6] With the loss of antibody, patients have a high incidence of infectious disease, but also paradoxically these same patients are also prone to both inflammatory and autoimmune disorders. CVID affects approximately 1/25,000 Caucasians,

doi: 10.1111/j.1749-6632.2011.06338.x

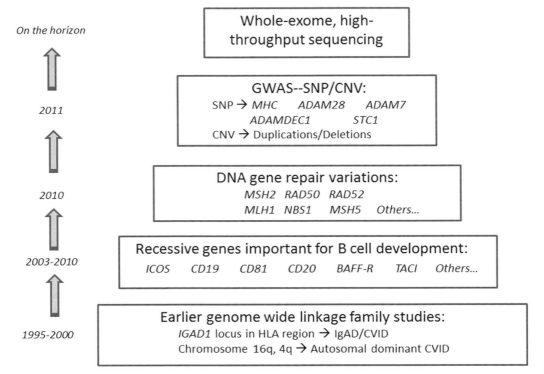

Figure 1. Genetics of CVID. This figure summarizes the evolution of various attempts at deciphering the genetics of CVID. The numbers on the left indicate the year of publication for each phase of the discovery.

but the frequency among Americans of African descent is estimated to be 20-fold lower.[7] CVID has been recognized for more than six decades,[8] and while it is considered to be a genetic immune disease, family members of CVID patients are usually normal, suggesting more complex inheritance for most subjects. As the hallmark of CVID is loss of humoral immunity, the World Health Organization classifies this immune defect among the B cell defects; however, variably impaired T cell, monocyte, and dendritic cell functions have been long described, suggesting that this syndrome bears some resemblance to combined immune defects.

In the past two decades, there have been a number of attempts to unravel the genetic defects in CVID. These have included earlier and more modern genome-wide studies, index families with multiply affected members, families with inheritance of recessive genes important in B cell development, and targeted gene approaches. Here, we review these and describe some of the newly emerging themes in this field (see Fig. 1).

Earlier genome-wide linkage and family studies

While CVID is not commonly found in more than one member of a family, for about 10% of subjects other first-degree relatives may be either hypogammaglobulinemic or may have selective IgA deficiency (IgAD).[9,10] A number of earlier studies concentrated on these families, which revealed several putative susceptibility loci. Concentrating first on families with selective IgA deficiency, Vořechovský *et al.* examined 101 multiple-case families, containing a total of 554 informative family members, with IgA deficiency and CVID and identified susceptibility loci within the HLA region on chromosome 6p.[11] Linkage analysis of this cohort indicated a putative susceptibility locus termed *IGAD1*. Of the 110 haplotypes shared by 258 affected family members, a single haplotype accounted for the majority of *IGAD1* contributions to the development of IgAD/CVID in this cohort. For unclear reasons, in this data set affected mothers transmitting the phenotype to their offspring were overrepresented compared to affected males, although this was not apparent in multiple-case families with a predominance of affected mothers (however, it should be noted that previous work suggested that the offspring of IgA-deficient mothers may not develop IgA due to transplacental transmission of anti-IgA antibodies).[12] Subsequent work also suggested that selected *HLA-DQ/DR* haplotypes conferred either protection or susceptibility to IgAD and CVID.[13] The strong influence of the MHC region was more recently noted in several other cohorts; in one, the majority of patients inherited HLA *DQ2, *DR7, *DR3 (17), *B8, and/or *B44. B44 was present in almost half, and was the most common susceptibility allele.[14] A strong influence of the MHC region was again recently noted in whole-genome studies, described in detail below.[15]

Reinvestigating the same cohort as Vořechovský *et al.* but restricting the focus to families in which at least one case of CVID was known, another study suggested linkage of autosomal dominant CVID to chromosome 16q.[16] A candidate gene considered here was *WWOX* (WW-domain containing oxidoreductase), but no mutations were found. As described below, a large heterozygous deletion in this same region was later noted for one subject in whole-genome studies, suggesting the need for additional studies of this region.[15]

Further studies examined another extended family with autosomal inheritance pattern of immune deficiency. In this family, six cases of CVID—five of IgAD and three of dysgammaglobulinemia—over five generations were found.[17] Linkage analysis performed on this family identified an area of interest on chromosome 4. Further genotype analysis of nine markers on chromosome 4q was used to find similar markers in 32 additional families, suggesting the existence of a disease-causing gene for autosomal-dominant CVID/IgAD in this region. The authors suggested several candidate genes, including *DAPP1*, a B cell signaling molecule, mutation of which leads to IgG3 deficiency in mice, and *BANK1*, which plays a role in B cell response to antigens,[18] but these have also not been validated.

Recessive genes important for B cell development

Some of the most incisive advances in CVID have more recently emerged from studies of families with a consanguineous background, demonstrating that mutations in single genes important in B cell biology can lead to the CVID phenotype.

Inducible costimulator

The inducible costimulator (ICOS) is a cell surface receptor structurally and functionally closely related to CD28[19] and expressed on activated T cells. Functionally, ICOS is important for the production of IL-10, a cytokine implicated in the generation of B cell memory and plasma cells.[20–23] Grimbacher *et al.* described a homozygous deletion of ICOS gene (*ICOS*) inherited as an autosomal recessive trait in four CVID related patients.[24] As interaction of ICOS with its unique ligand ICOS-L plays an important role in T cell help for late B cell differentiation, class-switching, memory B cell generation, and the numbers of memory and switched memory B cells were substantially reduced in the patients with *ICOS* deletion, as were serum immunoglobulin concentrations. Thus, ICOS deficiency resulted in defective T cell help for late B cell differentiation, suggesting an explanation for the clinical phenotype of CVID in these subjects. Extending this work, Salzer *et al.* identified other individuals in the same kindred, all of whom carried the identical large genomic deletion of *ICOS*.[25] Later, Takahashi *et al.* reported an in-depth analysis of T cell function in two siblings with ICOS deficiency.[26] While the brother displayed mild skin infections and impaired immunoglobulin class switching, the sister exhibited more severe manifestations, including immunodeficiency, inflammatory bowel disease, interstitial pneumonitis, rheumatoid arthritis, and psoriasis. Their work demonstrated an extensive T cell dysfunction, decreased memory T cell compartment, and an imbalance between effector and regulatory cells that may underlie immunodeficiency and/or autoimmunity observed in the sister. While mutations of the ICOS-L gene (*ICOSLG*) could theoretically lead to a similar CVID phenotype, subjects bearing such a mutation have not been identified.

CD19 deficiency

Four surface proteins (CD19, CD21, CD81, and CD225) on the surface of mature B cells form a complex that signals in conjunction with the B cell antigen receptor, thereby decreasing the threshold for activation by antigen.[27] Of these, CD19 appears early and remains on B cells during differentiation until maturation into plasma cells. In 2006, van Zelm *et al.* reported four patients from two unrelated families who had hypogammaglobulinemia and mutation of the *CD19* gene.[28] One patient, from Turkey, had an insertional mutation in both alleles of *CD19* leading to a frame shift, while three other patients, adult hypogammaglobulinemic siblings from Colombia, were homozygous for deletion resulting in a premature stop codon in the intracellular domain. In these patients, CD27[+] memory B cells were decreased, and the response of the patients' B cells to *in vitro* stimulation through the B cell receptor was impaired, as was antibody response to rabies vaccination. The patients were on immunoglobulin replacement, but antibody deficiency was documented *de novo*. Another case of CD19 deficiency was described a year later in a Japanese patient with CVID.[29] This patient, who had a very similar clinical phenotype as other patients with CD19 deficiency, had a compound heterozygous mutation in *CD19*, both of which were novel mutations. More recently in 2011, two additional patients with CD19 deficiency from two different families were reported.[30] One of these patients was a girl of Moroccan descent born to consanguineous parents who demonstrated selective IgG1 deficiency, conserved antibody response against protein antigens on vaccination, and, interestingly, glomerulonephritis consistent with a diagnosis of IgA nephropathy.

CD81 deficiency

As CD81 forms a part of CD19 complex, it may not be surprising that mutations of CD81 could mimic the defects of *CD19*. This was demonstrated by van Zelm *et al.*, who reported the first case in a six-year-old girl born to consanguineous parents.[31] Similar to the CD19-deficient patients reported earlier, she had hypogammaglobulinemia, decreased memory B cell numbers, impaired specific antibody responses, and an absence of CD19-expressing B cells. The sequence analysis demonstrated normal *CD19* alleles but a homozygous splice site *CD81* mutation resulting in a complete lack of CD19 protein expression. The requirement of intact *CD81* for *CD19* expression and function was also validated in CD81-knockout mice, which demonstrated that *CD19* expression is reduced on mature B cells and antibody production in response to T cell-dependent antigens is impaired.[32-34]

CD20 deficiency

CD20, one of the first B cell–specific differentiation antigens identified,[35] belongs to the membrane-spanning 4-domains (MS4A) family of molecules[36] and is expressed on pre-B and mature B cells but is lost upon differentiation into plasma cells.[37] While CD20 is likely involved in the regulation of B cell activation and proliferation,[38,39] its precise role in B cell physiology has remained elusive. In 2010, Kuijpers *et al.* reported a young Turkish patient, born to a consanguineous marriage, with CD20 deficiency due to a homozygous mutation in a splice junction of the CD20 gene (*MS4A1*) resulting in nonfunctional mRNA species.[40] The clinical features of this patient overlapped with CVID, namely, persistent hypogammaglobulinemia, recurrent bronchopneumonia, reduction in memory B cells, and markedly reduced ability to respond to pneumococcal polysaccharides. Additional cases of mutations in the CD20 gene remain to be found.

BAFF-R deficiency

B cell activating factor receptor (BAFF-R), a member of the TNF receptor superfamily, is encoded by three exons of the *TNFRSF13C* gene located on chromosome 22q13.[41,42] BAFF, also called BLyS, is a ligand of BAFF-R, and studies have demonstrated the importance of BAFF/BAFF-R interaction in B cell survival. Mice deficient in either BAFF or BAFF-R are characterized by a block of B cell development at the transitional stage.[43-48] Initial attempts to identify potential mutations in *BAFF-R* led to sequencing of the *BAFF-R* gene in patients with CVID who had very low B cell numbers. These demonstrated three novel variants present at the heterozygous state leading to amino acid substitutions.[49] These variants, however, were found to be polymorphic variants as they had no effect on the expression of the *BAFF-R* gene both at the mRNA and protein level. A few years later, Warnatz *et al.* identified two adult siblings (but one with CVID), born to a consanguineous marriage, carrying a homozygous deletion in the *BAFF-R* gene, resulting in undetectable BAFF-R expression.[50] One sibling had low serum immunoglobulins (IgG and IgM, but normal IgA) and poor antibody responses to protein vaccines and pneumococcal polysaccharides. The other, who was clinically well, had only a slightly reduced serum IgG and IgM, but preserved antibody production to tetanus, showing some discordance. The authors concluded that deletion of the *BAFF-R* gene causes a characteristic immunological phenotype, but it does not necessarily lead to a clinically manifest immunodeficiency state.

Transmembrane activator and calcium-modulating cyclophilin ligand interactor mutations

Transmembrane activator and calcium-modulating cyclophilin ligand interactor (TACI) is expressed on mature B cells and binds its ligands BAFF and APRIL (a proliferation-inducing ligand). The activation of TACI leads to T cell-dependent and T cell-independent responses and isotype switch.[51–53] TACI is encoded by *TNFRSF13B*, and knockout mice (*TNFRSF13B*[−/−]) develop a lymphoproliferative disorder, autoimmunity, and splenomegaly, suggesting, in addition to its role in B cell activation, an inhibitory role of TACI in signaling.[54–56] Using a candidate gene approach, Salzer *et al.* reported the mutations in *TNFRSF13B* encoding TACI in 13 individuals with CVID.[57] They demonstrated homozygosity for several coding variants (C104R, A181E, and S144X); in addition, heterozygous coding variants (C104R, A181E, S194X, and R202H) were identified. At the same time, Castigli *et al.* noted similar findings, and demonstrated dominant inheritance in other cohorts.[58] In general, mutations in *TNFRSF13B* are found in about 8% of CVID patients.[59,60] The extracellular mutation, C104R, and a transmembrane, A181E, constitute a majority of mutations identified, with heterozygosity occurring far more common than homozygosity. C104R leads to a disruption of a region important for binding the ligands, BAFF, and APRIL; the transmembrane mutations are presumed to lead to impaired BAFF and APRIL signaling. While TACI mutations are significantly associated with the CVID phenotype,[60] and in these subjects with both autoimmunity and lymphoid hyperplasia, some of the same mutations can be found in clinically healthy relatives, suggesting the role of other factors.[59] Even homozygous mutations in C104R did not lead to hypogammaglobulinemia in one of the three siblings of a family in which both parents bore one heterozygous mutation.[61] Thus mutations in *TNFRSF13B*, while biologically of great interest, are not diagnostic for CVID or predictive of the development of this immune defect, suggesting that routine testing for *TNFRSF13B* mutations is not recommended for these purposes.

Other targeted gene approaches

Along with family studies, there have been a number of attempts to extend an understanding of CVID by investigating if mutations in selected genes important in B cell development could be identified. Seeking mutations or polymorphisms in IL-10,[62,63] IL-10 receptor, IL-21, and IL-21 receptor,[64] all cytokines important for B cell maturation, has not proven fruitful thus far. The chemokine receptor gene *CXCR4*, mutated in WHIM (warts, hypogammaglobulinemia, infections, myelokathexis) syndrome, has also been investigated as alternative phenotypes, not including warts, that could lead to forms of CVID, but was not found mutated in one large group of subjects (Cunningham-Rundles, unpublished data).

Single nucleotide polymorphisms and copy number studies

Extensive genome-wide association studies (GWAS) using single nucleotide polymorphism (SNP) arrays have recently enabled high-throughput genotyping of genomic DNA and investigation of copy number variations (CNVs). A 2010 GWAS study of IgAD patients from Sweden and Iceland identified associations with variants in *IFIH1* and *CLEC16A*, both known to be associated with autoimmune disease, as well as associations with class II alleles in the HLA region.[65] The first GWAS SNP and CNV study on CVID patients collected from four medical centers investigated 610,000 SNPs of 363 CVID subjects compared to 3,031 controls.[15] Again, a strong association with the MHC region was revealed, and associations with the disintegrin and metalloproteinases 28 (*ADAM28*), *ADAM7, ADAMDEC1*, and stanniocalcin-1 (*STC1*) were suggested. Recent studies have noted that CVID is characterized by fairly stereotypic phenotypic patterns associated with selected inflammatory/autoimmune medical complications.[1,2,6,66–69] Thus, the CVID subjects were classified by these phenotypes, including cancers, lymphoma, lymphadenopathy, nodular regenerative hyperplasia of the liver, lymphoid interstitial pneumonitis (LIP), bronchiectasis, biopsy-proved granuloma, gastrointestinal enteropathy, malabsorption, splenectomy, cytopenias, organ-specific autoimmunity, low IgM

(<50 mg/dL), low IgA (<10 mg/dL), low B cell number (CD19$^+$ cells <1%), and young age at symptom onset (<10 years).[15] SNP analysis revealed genes associated with particular phenotypes, including mitogen-activated protein kinase kinase kinase 7-interacting protein 3 (*MAP3K7IP3*), significantly associated with low IgA. Genes significantly associated with lymphoma included *PFTK1*, *HAVCR1*, and *KIAA0834*. The gene *CACNA1C* (calcium channel, voltage-dependent, L-type, alpha 1C subunit) was found associated with gastrointestinal enteropathy.[15]

In addition to SNP investigation, CNV analyses uncovered several novel genes that were significantly associated with CVID. Of these, 84 CNV deletions and 98 duplications were identified in one or more patients, but were not found in any of the 2,766 control subjects. Some of these also overlapped with the GWAS part of the study. Five deletions and 11 duplications were found to be recurrent in the patient group and were significantly increased in CVID cases compared with controls; 15 regions were unique to CVID cases. Specifically, a significant number of subjects had duplications in *ORC4L*, which is essential for initiation of DNA replication in immune cells and has previously been associated with B cell lymphoproliferative disorders.[70] Examination of the overall CNV burden of both large (100 kb) and rare (<1%) CNVs revealed that deletions were significantly enriched in CVID cases, and all but five of the 182 CNVs, exclusive to the CVID cohort, were intraexonic.[15] These findings suggest that CNVs may represent alterations in genes that could disrupt normal genetic and/or cellular function in individual subjects with CVID.

DNA gene repair in CVID

In the process of class switch recombination and somatic hypermutation, a developing B cell undergoes multiple rounds of DNA double-stranded breaks, which must be repaired or the damage will lead to apoptosis. However, B cells have evolved numerous signaling pathways that lead to repair and permit proliferation of intact B cells.[71,72] While a number of DNA repair defects have been characterized, it is interesting that a number of them, such as defects of RAG1 or RAG2, Artemis, *Cernunnos*, ligase 4, and Nijmegen breakage syndrome, lead to a loss of B cells, and in some cases loss of T cells. Under normal circumstances, B cells undergo class switch

recombination to produce a functionally diverse antibody repertoire. This process is catalyzed by activation-induced cytidine deaminase (AID) and uracil-DNA glycosylase (UNG); mutations in these account for two of the versions of the hyper-IgM syndrome.[73–75] With inappropriate DNA repair, a predisposition to radiation damage and cancer are plausible outcomes. As CVID subjects have an increased propensity to cancer (lymphoma in particular)[76,77] and appear to have increased cellular radio sensitivity,[78–80] it is plausible that DNA gene repair variations could also account for some forms of CVID. In this vein, and returning to the MHC theme previously observed in CVID, Sekine *et al.* examined genetic variations in MSH5, a member of the mutS family of proteins involved in DNA mismatch repair and encoded in the MHC region. Several unique alleles of MSH5 were shown to have genetic associations with both CVID and IgAD.[81] More recently, Offer *et al.* surveyed 27 candidate DNA metabolism genes and found that other markers in several mismatch repair proteins were associated with IgAD/CVID.[82] Resequencing was used to investigate these genes, and four rare, nonsynonymous alleles were found associated with IgAD/CVID: two in MutL homolog 1 (*MLH1*), one in *RAD50*, a protein involved in DNA double-strand break repair, and one in Nijmegen breakage syndrome 1 (*NBN*). A premature RAD50 stop codon identified in one conferred an increased sensitivity to ionizing radiation.[82]

Conclusions

CVID is a complex, multifocal disease, the genetic origins of which are beginning to be at least partially understood. Further large cohort studies using whole-exome sequencing and other high-throughput methods, along with international studies with subjects from diverse genetic backgrounds, will be needed in the future to illuminate the many causes of this disease and possibly therapeutic targets.

Acknowledgments

This work was supported by the National Institutes of Health, AI 101093, AI-467320, AI-48693, NIAID Contract 03-22, and the David S. Gottesman Immunology Chair.

Conflicts of interest

The authors declare no conflicts of interest.

References

1. Cunningham-Rundles, C. & C. Bodian. 1999. Common variable immunodeficiency: clinical and immunological features of 248 patients. *Clin. Immunol.* **92:** 34–48.
2. Chapel, H., M. Lucas, M. Lee, *et al.* 2008. Common variable immunodeficiency disorders: division into distinct clinical phenotypes. *Blood* **112:** 277–286.
3. Conley, M.E., A.K. Dobbs, D.M. Farmer, *et al.* 2009. Primary B cell immunodeficiencies: comparisons and contrasts. *Annu. Rev. Immunol.* **27:** 199–227.
4. Cunningham-Rundles, C. 2001. Common variable immunodeficiency. *Curr. Allergy Asthma Rep.* **1:** 421–429.
5. Notarangelo, L.D., A. Fischer, R.S. Geha, *et al.* 2009. Primary immunodeficiencies: 2009 update. *J. Allergy Clin. Immunol.* **124:** 1161–1178.
6. Chapel, H. & C. Cunningham-Rundles. 2009. Update in understanding common variable immunodeficiency disorders (CVIDs) and the management of patients with these conditions. *Br. J. Haematol.* **145:** 709–727.
7. Schroeder, H.W., Jr., H.W. Schroeder, 3rd & S.M. Sheikh. 2004. The complex genetics of common variable immunodeficiency. *J. Investig. Med.* **52:** 90–103.
8. Sanford, J.P., C.B. Favour & M.S. Tribeman. 1954. Absence of serum gamma globulins in an adult. *N. Engl. J. Med.* **250:** 1027–1029.
9. Vorechovsky, I., H. Zetterquist, R. Paganelli, *et al.* 1995. Family and linkage study of selective IgA deficiency and common variable immunodeficiency. *Clin. Immunol. Immunopathol.* **77:** 185–192.
10. Burrows, P.D. & M.D. Cooper. 1997. IgA deficiency. *Adv. Immunol.* **65:** 245–276.
11. Vorechovsky, I., M. Cullen, M. Carrington, *et al.* 2000. Fine mapping of IGAD1 in IgA deficiency and common variable immunodeficiency: identification and characterization of haplotypes shared by affected members of 101 multiple-case families. *J. Immunol.* **164:** 4408–4416.
12. Petty, R.E., D.D. Sherry & J. Johannson. 1985. Anti-IgA antibodies in pregnancy. *N. Engl. J. Med.* **313:** 1620–1625.
13. Kralovicova, J., L. Hammarstrom, A. Plebani, *et al.* 2003. Fine-scale mapping at IGAD1 and genome-wide genetic linkage analysis implicate HLA-DQ/DR as a major susceptibility locus in selective IgA deficiency and common variable immunodeficiency. *J. Immunol.* **170:** 2765–2775.
14. Waldrep, M.L., Y. Zhuang & H.W. Schroeder, Jr. 2009. Analysis of TACI mutations in CVID & RESPI patients who have inherited HLA B*44 or HLA*B8. *BMC Med. Genet.* **10:** 100.
15. Orange, J.S., J.T. Glessner, E. Resnick, *et al.* 2011. Genome-wide association identifies diverse causes of common variable immunodeficiency. *J. Allergy Clin. Immunol.* **127:** 1360–1367 e1366.
16. Schaffer, A.A., J. Pfannstiel, A.D. Webster, *et al.* 2006. Analysis of families with common variable immunodeficiency (CVID) and IgA deficiency suggests linkage of CVID to chromosome 16q. *Hum. Genet.* **118:** 725–729.
17. Nijenhuis, T., I. Klasen, C.M. Weemaes, *et al.* 2001. Common variable immunodeficiency (CVID) in a family: an autosomal dominant mode of inheritance. *Neth. J. Med.* **59:** 134–139.
18. Finck, A., J.W. Van der Meer, A.A. Schaffer, *et al.* 2006. Linkage of autosomal-dominant common variable immunodeficiency to chromosome 4q. *Eur. J. Hum. Genet.* **14:** 867–875.
19. Hutloff, A., A.M. Dittrich, K.C. Beier, *et al.* 1999. ICOS is an inducible T-cell co-stimulator structurally and functionally related to CD28. *Nature* **397:** 263–266.
20. Choe, J. & Y.S. Choi. 1998. IL-10 interrupts memory B cell expansion in the germinal center by inducing differentiation into plasma cells. *Eur. J. Immunol.* **28:** 508–515.
21. Kindler, V. & R.H. Zubler. 1997. Memory, but not naive, peripheral blood B lymphocytes differentiate into Ig-secreting cells after CD40 ligation and costimulation with IL-4 and the differentiation factors IL-2, IL-10, and IL-3. *J. Immunol.* **159:** 2085–2090.
22. Rousset, F., E. Garcia, T. Defrance, *et al.* 1992. Interleukin 10 is a potent growth and differentiation factor for activated human B lymphocytes. *Proc. Natl. Acad. Sci. USA* **89:** 1890–1893.
23. Witsch, E.J., M. Peiser, A. Hutloff, *et al.* 2002. ICOS and CD28 reversely regulate IL-10 on re-activation of human effector T cells with mature dendritic cells. *Eur. J. Immunol.* **32:** 2680–2686.
24. Grimbacher, B., A. Hutloff, M. Schlesier, *et al.* 2003. Homozygous loss of ICOS is associated with adult-onset common variable immunodeficiency. *Nat. Immunol.* **4:** 261–268.
25. Salzer, U., A. Maul-Pavicic, C. Cunningham-Rundles, *et al.* 2004. ICOS deficiency in patients with common variable immunodeficiency. *Clin. Immunol.* **113:** 234–240.
26. Takahashi, N., K. Matsumoto, H. Saito, *et al.* 2009. Impaired CD4 and CD8 effector function and decreased memory T cell populations in ICOS-deficient patients. *J. Immunol.* **182:** 5515–5527.
27. Carter, R.H. & D.T. Fearon. 1992. CD19: lowering the threshold for antigen receptor stimulation of B lymphocytes. *Science* **256:** 105–107.
28. van Zelm, M.C., I. Reisli, M. van der Burg, *et al.* 2006. An antibody-deficiency syndrome due to mutations in the CD19 gene. *N. Engl. J. Med.* **354:** 1901–1912.
29. Kanegane, H., K. Agematsu, T. Futatani, *et al.* 2007. Novel mutations in a Japanese patient with CD19 deficiency. *Genes Immun.* **8:** 663–670.
30. Vince, N., D. Boutboul, G. Mouillot, *et al.* 2011. Defects in the CD19 complex predispose to glomerulonephritis, as well as IgG1 subclass deficiency. *J. Allergy Clin. Immunol.* **127:** 538–541 e531–535.
31. van Zelm, M.C., J. Smet, B. Adams, *et al.* 2010. CD81 gene defect in humans disrupts CD19 complex formation and leads to antibody deficiency. *J. Clin. Invest.* **120:** 1265–1274.
32. Maecker, H.T. & S. Levy. 1997. Normal lymphocyte development but delayed humoral immune response in CD81-null mice. *J. Exp. Med.* **185:** 1505–1510.
33. Miyazaki, T., U. Muller & K.S. Campbell. 1997. Normal development but differentially altered proliferative responses of lymphocytes in mice lacking CD81. *EMBO J.* **16:** 4217–4225.

34. Tsitsikov, E.N., J.C. Gutierrez-Ramos & R.S. Geha. 1997. Impaired CD19 expression and signaling, enhanced antibody response to type II T independent antigen and reduction of B-1 cells in CD81-deficient mice. *Proc. Natl. Acad. Sci. USA* **94:** 10844–10849.

35. Stashenko, P., L.M. Nadler, R. Hardy & S.F. Schlossman. 1980. Characterization of a human B lymphocyte-specific antigen. *J. Immunol.* **125:** 1678–1685.

36. Liang, Y., T.R. Buckley, L. Tu, *et al.* 2001. Structural organization of the human MS4A gene cluster on Chromosome 11q12. *Immunogenetics* **53:** 357–368.

37. Tedder, T.F. & P. Engel. 1994. CD20: a regulator of cell-cycle progression of B lymphocytes. *Immunol. Today* **15:** 450–454.

38. Tedder, T.F., A.W. Boyd, A.S. Freedman, *et al.* 1985. The B cell surface molecule B1 is functionally linked with B cell activation and differentiation. *J. Immunol.* **135:** 973–979.

39. Tedder, T.F., A. Forsgren, A.W. Boyd, *et al.* 1986. Antibodies reactive with the B1 molecule inhibit cell cycle progression but not activation of human B lymphocytes. *Eur. J. Immunol.* **16:** 881–887.

40. Kuijpers, T.W., R.J. Bende, P.A. Baars, *et al.* 2010. CD20 deficiency in humans results in impaired T cell-independent antibody responses. *J. Clin. Invest.* **120:** 214–222.

41. Mackay, F., P. Schneider, P. Rennert & J. Browning. 2003. BAFF AND APRIL: a tutorial on B cell survival. *Annu. Rev. Immunol.* **21:** 231–264.

42. Ng, L.G., A.P. Sutherland, R. Newton, *et al.* 2004. B cell-activating factor belonging to the TNF family (BAFF)-R is the principal BAFF receptor facilitating BAFF costimulation of circulating T and B cells. *J. Immunol.* **173:** 807–817.

43. Batten, M., J. Groom, T.G. Cachero, *et al.* 2000. BAFF mediates survival of peripheral immature B lymphocytes. *J. Exp. Med.* **192:** 1453–1466.

44. Gross, J.A., S.R. Dillon, S. Mudri, *et al.* 2001. TACI-Ig neutralizes molecules critical for B cell development and autoimmune disease. Impaired B cell maturation in mice lacking BLyS. *Immunity* **15:** 289–302.

45. Sasaki, Y., S. Casola, J.L. Kutok, *et al.* 2004. TNF family member B cell-activating factor (BAFF) receptor-dependent and -independent roles for BAFF in B cell physiology. *J. Immunol.* **173:** 2245–2252.

46. Schiemann, B., J.L. Gommerman, K. Vora, *et al.* 2001. An essential role for BAFF in the normal development of B cells through a BCMA-independent pathway. *Science* **293:** 2111–2114.

47. Shulga-Morskaya, S., M. Dobles, M.E. Walsh, *et al.* 2004. B cell-activating factor belonging to the TNF family acts through separate receptors to support B cell survival and T cell-independent antibody formation. *J. Immunol.* **173:** 2331–2341.

48. Yan, M., J.R. Brady, B. Chan, *et al.* 2001. Identification of a novel receptor for B lymphocyte stimulator that is mutated in a mouse strain with severe B cell deficiency. *Curr. Biol.* **11:** 1547–1552.

49. Losi, C.G., A. Silini, C. Fiorini, *et al.* 2005. Mutational analysis of human BAFF receptor TNFRSF13C (BAFF-R) in patients with common variable immunodeficiency. *J. Clin. Immunol.* **25:** 496–502.

50. Warnatz, K., U. Salzer, M. Rizzi, *et al.* 2009. B-cell activating factor receptor deficiency is associated with an adult-onset antibody deficiency syndrome in humans. *Proc. Natl. Acad. Sci. USA* **106:** 13945–13950.

51. Castigli, E., S.A. Wilson, S. Scott, *et al.* 2005. TACI and BAFF-R mediate isotype switching in B cells. *J. Exp. Med.* **201:** 35–39.

52. Litinskiy, M.B., B. Nardelli, D.M. Hilbert, *et al.* 2002. DCs induce CD40-independent immunoglobulin class switching through BLyS and APRIL. *Nat. Immunol.* **3:** 822–829.

53. Sakurai, D., Y. Kanno, H. Hase, *et al.* 2007. TACI attenuates antibody production costimulated by BAFF-R and CD40. *Eur. J. Immunol.* **37:** 110–118.

54. Seshasayee, D., P. Valdez, M. Yan, *et al.* 2003. Loss of TACI causes fatal lymphoproliferation and autoimmunity, establishing TACI as an inhibitory BLyS receptor. *Immunity.* **18:** 279–288.

55. von Bulow, G.U., J.M. van Deursen & R.J. Bram. 2001. Regulation of the T-independent humoral response by TACI. *Immunity* **14:** 573–582.

56. Yan, M., H. Wang, B. Chan, *et al.* 2001. Activation and accumulation of B cells in TACI-deficient mice. *Nat. Immunol.* **2:** 638–643.

57. Salzer, U., H.M. Chapel, A.D. Webster, *et al.* 2005. Mutations in TNFRSF13B encoding TACI are associated with common variable immunodeficiency in humans. *Nat. Genet.* **37:** 820–828.

58. Castigli, E., S.A. Wilson, L. Garibyan, *et al.* 2005. TACI is mutant in common variable immunodeficiency and IgA deficiency. *Nat. Genet.* **37:** 829–834.

59. Zhang, L., L. Radigan, U. Salzer, *et al.* 2007. Transmembrane activator and calcium-modulating cyclophilin ligand interactor mutations in common variable immunodeficiency: clinical and immunologic outcomes in heterozygotes. *J. Allergy Clin. Immunol.* **120:** 1178–1185.

60. Pan-Hammarstrom, Q., U. Salzer, L. Du, *et al.* 2007. Reexamining the role of TACI coding variants in common variable immunodeficiency and selective IgA deficiency. *Nat. Genet.* **39:** 429–430.

61. Martinez-Pomar, N., D. Detkova, J.I. Arostegui, *et al.* 2009. Role of TNFRSF13B variants in patients with common variable immunodeficiency. *Blood* **114:** 2846–2848.

62. Rezaei, N., A. Aghamohammadi, M. Mahmoudi, *et al.* Association of IL-4 and IL-10 gene promoter polymorphisms with common variable immunodeficiency. *Immunobiology*, **215:** 81–87.

63. Fritsch, A., U. Junker, H. Vogelsang & L. Jager. 1994. On interleukins 4, 6 and 10 and their interrelationship with immunoglobulins G and M in common variable immunodeficiency. *Cell Biol. Int.* **18:** 1067–1075.

64. Borte, S., Q. Pan-Hammarstrom, C. Liu, *et al.* 2009. Interleukin-21 restores immunoglobulin production ex vivo in patients with common variable immunodeficiency and selective IgA deficiency. *Blood* **114:** 4089–4098.

65. Ferreira, R.C., Q. Pan-Hammarstrom, R.R. Graham, *et al.* 2010. Association of IFIH1 and other autoimmunity risk alleles with selective IgA deficiency. *Nat. Genet.* **42:** 777–780.

66. Cunningham-Rundles, C. 1989. Clinical and immunologic analyses of 103 patients with common variable immunodeficiency. *J. Clin. Immunol.* **9:** 22–33.

67. Hermaszewski, R.A. & A.D. Webster. 1993. Primary hypogammaglobulinaemia: a survey of clinical manifestations and complications. *Q. J. Med.* **86:** 31–42.

68. Kainulainen, L., J. Nikoskelainen & O. Ruuskanen. 2001. Diagnostic findings in 95 Finnish patients with common variable immunodeficiency. *J. Clin. Immunol.* **21:** 145–149.

69. Quinti, I., A. Soresina, G. Spadaro, *et al.* 2007. Long-term follow-up and outcome of a large cohort of patients with common variable immunodeficiency. *J. Clin. Immunol.* **27:** 308–316.

70. Radojkovic, M., S. Ristic, A. Divac, *et al.* 2009. Novel ORC4L gene mutation in B-cell lymphoproliferative disorders. *Am. J. Med. Sci.* **338:** 527–529.

71. Loizou, J.I., R. Sancho, N. Kanu, *et al.* 2011. ATMIN is required for maintenance of genomic stability and suppression of B cell lymphoma. *Cancer Cell* **19:** 587–600.

72. Nussenzweig, A. & M.C. Nussenzweig. 2011. Origin of chromosomal translocations in lymphoid cancer. *Cell* **141:** 27–38.

73. Durandy, A., S. Peron & A. Fischer. 2006. Hyper-IgM syndromes. *Curr. Opin. Rheumatol.* **18:** 369–376.

74. Imai, K., G. Slupphaug, W.I. Lee, *et al.* 2003. Human uracil-DNA glycosylase deficiency associated with profoundly impaired immunoglobulin class-switch recombination. *Nat. Immunol.* **4:** 1023–1028.

75. Revy, P., T. Muto, Y. Levy, *et al.* 2000. Activation-induced cytidine deaminase (AID) deficiency causes the autosomal recessive form of the Hyper-IgM syndrome (HIGM2). *Cell* **102:** 565–575.

76. Cunningham-Rundles, C. 2010. How I treat common variable immune deficiency. *Blood* **116:** 7–15.

77. Cunningham-Rundles, C., D.L. Cooper, T.P. Duffy & J. Strauchen. 2002. Lymphomas of mucosal-associated lymphoid tissue in common variable immunodeficiency. *Am. J. Hematol.* **69:** 171–178.

78. Aghamohammadi, A., M. Moin, A. Kouhi, *et al.* 2008. Chromosomal radiosensitivity in patients with common variable immunodeficiency. *Immunobiology* **213:** 447–454.

79. Palanduz, S., A. Palanduz, I. Yalcin, *et al.* 1998. *In vitro* chromosomal radiosensitivity in common variable immune deficiency. *Clin. Immunol. Immunopathol.* **86:** 180–182.

80. Vorechovsky, I., D. Scott, M.R. Haeney & D.A. Webster. 1993. Chromosomal radiosensitivity in common variable immune deficiency. *Mutat. Res.* **290:** 255–264.

81. Sekine, H., R.C. Ferreira, Q. Pan-Hammarstrom, *et al.* 2007. Role for Msh5 in the regulation of Ig class switch recombination. *Proc. Natl. Acad. Sci. USA* **104:** 7193–7198.

82. Offer, S.M., Q. Pan-Hammarstrom, L. Hammarstrom & R.S. Harris. 2010. Unique DNA repair gene variations and potential associations with the primary antibody deficiency syndromes IgAD and CVID. *PLoS One* **5:** e12260.

Ann. N.Y. Acad. Sci. ISSN 0077-8923

ANNALS OF THE NEW YORK ACADEMY OF SCIENCES

Issue: *The Year in Human and Medical Genetics: Inborn Errors of Immunity*

DNA repair: the link between primary immunodeficiency and cancer

Noel FCC de Miranda, Andrea Björkman, and Qiang Pan-Hammarström

Division of Clinical Immunology, Department of Laboratory Medicine, Karolinska Institutet at Karolinska University Hospital Huddinge, Stockholm, Sweden

Address for correspondence: Qiang Pan-Hammarström, Division of Clinical Immunology, Department of Laboratory Medicine, Karolinska Institutet at Karolinska University Hospital Huddinge, SE-14186, Stockholm, Sweden. Qiang. Pan-Hammarstrom@ki.se

The adaptive component of the immune system depends greatly on the generation of genetic diversity provided by lymphocyte-specific genomic rearrangements. V(D)J recombination, class switch recombination (CSR), and somatic hypermutation (SHM) constitute complex and vulnerable processes that are orchestrated by a multitude of DNA repair pathways. When inherited defects in certain DNA repair proteins are present, lymphocyte development can be compromised and, consequently, patients can develop primary immunodeficiencies (PIDs). PID patients often have a strong predisposition for cancer development as a result of genomic instability generated from defective DNA repair mechanisms. Tumors of lymphoid origin are one of the most common PID-associated cancers, likely due to DNA lesions resulting from defective V(D)J, CSR, and SHM. In this review, we describe PID syndromes that confer an increased risk for cancer development. Furthermore, we discuss the role of the affected proteins in tumorigenesis/lymphomagenesis.

Keywords: primary immunodeficiency; cancer; DNA repair; V(D)J recombination; class switch recombination; genomic instability

Introduction

Genetic diversity—the basis of evolution—is partly provided by sexual reproduction and meiotic recombination during gametes formation.[1] Fallible DNA repair mechanisms provide an additional source of diversity by allowing the establishment of mutations during DNA replication.[2] Nevertheless, a delicate balance between the generation of genetic variation and fidelity of DNA replication is paramount to guaranteeing cellular viability and normal ontogenesis.[3]

The immune system depends greatly on genetic diversity. Humans have experienced what can be referred to as an "evolutionary arms race" with a myriad of pathogens, where the capacity to deal with infection has been crucial for human survival.[4] B and T lymphocytes constitute the cellular component of the adaptive immune system, which is characterized by its specificity and immunological memory.[5] Lymphocytes are capable of recognizing

a multitude of antigens, due to somatic recombination of their antigen-binding receptors. The B and T cell receptor (*BCR* and *TCR*, respectively) loci are modified by complex (and therefore vulnerable to mutation) genetic rearrangements carried out by multiple DNA repair and damage response protein complexes.[6]

Variations in DNA repair genes might compromise the balance between the replication fidelity of DNA and tolerance for a limited degree of genetic variation. Ultimately, cellular viability is endangered and malignant transformation of cells can occur.[7] Additionally, defects in some DNA repair proteins greatly affect lymphocyte development due to their crucial role in the generation of B and T cell receptors.[8] Primary immunodeficiencies (PIDs) associated with defects in DNA repair develop in an autosomal recessive setting and generally associate with other phenotypes such as cellular radiosensitivity, developmental defects, and predisposition to cancer.[9] All of the above are primed by the

doi: 10.1111/j.1749-6632.2011.06322.x

inability of cells to deal with DNA lesions created during lymphocyte development or caused by environmental insults.[10] Accordingly, these diseases are frequently referred to as *genomic instability syndromes*.[11] This review connects the mechanisms of lymphocyte development and malignant transformation in the context of DNA repair deficiencies. We describe DNA repair disorders that simultaneously predispose for the development of PID and cancer, and discuss the role of the affected DNA repair genes in tumorigenesis.

Genetics of lymphocyte development

In order for B and T lymphocytes to express a great variety of antigen-binding receptors, the *BCR* and *TCR* genes undergo a number of lymphocyte-specific genetic rearrangements. V(D)J recombination refers to the combinatorial joining of the variable (*V*), diversity (*D*), and joining (*J*) *BCR* and *TCR* gene segments.[12] Immunoglobulin (*Ig*) loci are further modified by class switch recombination (CSR), which replaces the heavy chain constant (C_H) region from C_μ to C_γ, C_α, or C_ε and results in the production of IgG, IgA, or IgE antibodies, respectively.[13] Finally, the affinity between antibodies and antigens is fine-tuned by the introduction of point mutations in the V region of Igs by the process of somatic hypermutation (SHM).[14]

V(D)J recombination is initiated by the binding of the lymphocyte-specific factors RAG1 and RAG2 to defined recombination signal sequences situated at the ends of all V, D, and J gene segments; this leads to the creation of double strand breaks (DSBs).[15,16] These DSB lesions activate DNA damage response proteins (e.g., ATM, 53BP1, and NBN), which in turn recruit members of the nonhomologous end-joining (NHEJ) pathway responsible for resolving the newly formed DSBs.[17] NHEJ is performed by a plethora of proteins, of which seven are considered indispensable: Ku70 and Ku80, XRCC4, DNA ligase 4, Artemis, DNA-PKcs, and Cernunnos, where deficiencies in any of the latter may result in immunodeficiency.[6]

CSR and SHM are B cell-specific processes initiated by activation-induced cytidine deaminase (AID).[18] AID converts cytosines into uracils, creating U/G mismatches that are recognized and processed by proteins from the base excision repair (BER) pathway (UNG, APE1) and mismatch repair (MMR) pathway (MSH2/MSH6, MLH1/PMS2, and

EXO1).[19] During CSR, the BER and MMR proteins produce DSBs in switch regions situated upstream of each *Ig* C_H gene. Like in V(D)J recombination, these breaks are also repaired by NHEJ, leading to the replacement of C_μ positioned downstream of the *Ig* V region.[19,20] In the context of SHM, the processing of mismatches instead results in point mutations.[14]

Another DSB repair pathway, considered imprecise and associated with chromosomal instability, is the alternative-end-joining (alt-EJ) pathway. The alt-EJ pathway is activated when one or a few of the classical NHEJ components are missing. However, this is still under debate, as alt-EJ probably involves numerous pathways depending on the missing NHEJ factor.[17] Alt-EJ usually makes use of longer sequence microhomologies, as well as insertions and deletions, compared to the classical NHEJ pathway.[19,21] Several proteins have been suggested to participate in alt-EJ, such as the MRN complex (NBN, Rad50, and MRE11), CtIP, DNA ligase 1 and 3, PARP1, and XRCC1.[19,20] In antibody diversification processes, it is thought that alt-EJ occurs during normal CSR and that it becomes dominant when NHEJ is impaired,[22-25] whereas the RAG enzymes are believed to inhibit the use of alt-EJ during V(D)J recombination, even when NHEJ factors are missing.[26]

PIDs deriving from DNA repair defects

The crucial role of DNA repair during lymphocyte development explains the PID phenotype of patients carrying defects in certain DNA repair genes. Since V(D)J recombination, CSR, and SHM share several DNA repair proteins or pathways, deficiencies of the latter might affect more than one process (Fig. 1). Thus, ATM, DNA ligase 4, Cernunnos, DNA-PKcs, or Artemis deficiencies affect V(D)J recombination and CSR, whereas some patients lacking MMR proteins or NBN display impaired CSR and SHM.[9,27] Proteins with important functions during V(D)J recombination would theoretically give the most serious immunodeficiency, since it affects both B and T cell development. Hence, patients with mutated *RAG1* or *RAG2* suffer from severe combined immunodeficiency (SCID), which is characterized by a complete lack of B and T cells and is often lethal during the first year of life unless it is treated by hematopoietic stem cell transplantation.[28,29] Another form of SCID with additional radiosensitivity,

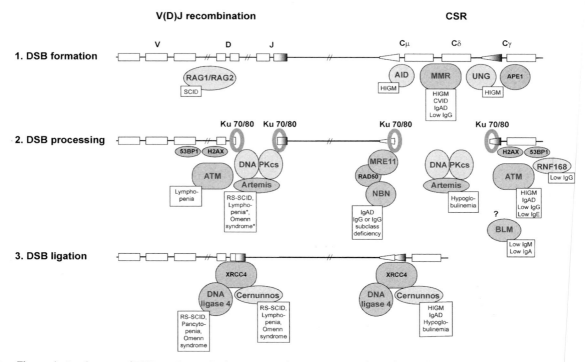

Figure 1. Involvement of DNA repair proteins in processes of antigen receptor diversification by V(D)J recombination and class switch recombination (CSR). Depending on their role on either V(D)J recombination or CSR, their deficiency relates to different PID phenotypes (text boxes). Proteins denoted in green were not previously associated with cancer whereas deficiency of DNA repair proteins denoted in red confer a risk or were associated to cancer onset. *, Artemis hypomorphic mutations; CVID, combined variable immunodeficiency; HIGM, Hyper-IgM; IgAD, IgA-deficiency; SCID, severe combined immunodeficiency; RS-SCID, severe combined immunodeficiency with sensitivity to ionizing radiation.

RS-SCID, is found in patients with null mutations in *DCLRE1C* (gene encoding Artemis), another important V(D)J factor.[30] Some patients with hypomorphic mutations in *DCLRE1C* can still mount V(D)J recombination but at much lower levels, resulting in a low number of B and T lymphocytes and reduced Ig production (Table 1).[42] RS-SCID, with a residual presence of T cells, has also been described in a few patients with hypomorphic mutations in *LIG4* (the gene encoding DNA ligase 4), although other patients have shown milder immunodeficiencies (Table 1).[45–47,51] The only DNA-PKcs–deficient patient described to date developed RS-SCID.[65] Finally, patients lacking Cernunnos present with radiosensitivity and immunodeficiency, ranging from B and T cell lymphopenia to SCID.[66–69]

Hyper-IgM disorders (HIGM) are characterized by normal or high levels of IgM, and low or absent levels of the remaining Ig classes, indicating that IgM positive cells were not able to switch to other isotypes—a hallmark of impaired CSR.[70,72] HIGM is seen in patients lacking AID,[72] as well as in patients missing other CSR proteins acting downstream of AID, such as UNG,[73] ATM,[31–33] and NBN (Table 1).[36,37] Immunodeficiencies in MMR patients are usually not very pronounced; only a few patients with homozygous or biallelic mutations in *MSH6*,[60,63] *PMS2*,[59] and *MSH2*[61] genes have been described, with decreased levels of IgA and/or IgG (Table 1). This could possibly be due to the existence of two pathways, BER and MMR, to process AID-induced mismatches.[13] Heterozygous mutations in *MSH5*, *MSH2*, and *MLH1* have been reported in patients with common variable immunodeficiency (CVID) and IgA-deficiency (IgAD), where production of one or two Ig classes is affected.[62,74] Less striking CSR defects were found in the only two RNF168-deficient patients described to date.[75–77]

Table 1. PID and cancer types occurring in different DNA repair deficiencies and associated syndromes

Gene	Syndrome	Role in V(D)J, CSR, SHM	PID phenotype	Associated cancers	Gene Cancer translocations in *Ig/TCR* loci
ATM	Ataxia-telangiectasia	V(D)J, CSR	HIGM, IgAD, reduced level of IgG or IgG subclasses,[31,] lymphopenia.[46,47]	Lymphomas and leukemias (T cell 5:1 B cell), other solid tumors.[34,35]	Yes[35]
NBN	Nijmegen breakage syndrome	V(D)J, CSR, SHM	HIGM, IgAD and IgG or IgG subclass deficiency, low B and T cell counts.[36–38]	Lymphomas (mainly B cell).[39,40]	Yes[36]
DCLRE1C (ARTEMIS)	–	V(D)J, CSR	Null mutants: RS-SCID.[30,41] Hypomorphic mutants: Hypoglobulinemia, lymphopenia,[42,43] Omenn syndrome.[44]	EBV-positive B cell lymphomas.[42]	Yes[42]
LIG4	Ligase IV syndrome	V(D)J, CSR	RS-SCID,[45,46] pancytopenia,[47] Omenn syndrome.[48]	EBV-positive lymphomas,[49,50] leukemias.[51,52]	?
LIG1	–	CSR?	IgAD, low IgG, and lymphopenia.[53]	Lymphoma.[53]	?
BLM	Bloom's syndrome	CSR?	Low IgM and IgA.[54–56]	Lymphomas, leukemias, carcinomas.[57]	?
FANC group	Fanconi Anemia	–	Pancytopenia.[58]	Acute myeloid leukemias, squamous cell carcinomas.[58]	No
MMR genes	CMMR-D	CSR, SHM	HIGM,[59] IgAD,[60–62] IgG deficiency,[63] CVID.[62]	Lymphomas, leukemias, brain tumors, colorectal cancer.[64]	?

CMMR-D, constitutional mismatch-repair deficiency syndrome; CSR, class-switch recombination; CVID, common variable immunodeficiency; EBV, Epstein-Barr virus; HIGM, hyper-IgM syndrome; IgAD, IgA-deficiency; SCID, severe combined immunodeficiency; SHM, somatic hypermutation.

RNF168 is an ubiquitin ligase involved in the recruitment of 53BP1 to DSB sites.[76] It is thought that 53BP1 plays an important role in the resolution of CSR-associated DSBs, which is concordant with the phenotype observed for the RNF168-deficient patients. Finally, a few patients lacking MRE11 presented with low levels of certain IgG-subclasses.[78]

To date, only one patient has been described with mutations in the *LIG1* gene, encoding DNA ligase 1. This patient presented with a typical immunodeficient phenotype characterized by IgAD, low IgG levels, and progressive lymphopenia.[53]

Two other DNA repair disorders that are sometimes associated with immunodeficiency are Bloom

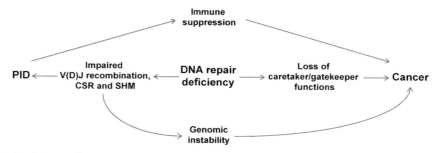

Figure 2. Relational diagram between DNA repair deficiencies, PID, and cancer. The generation of genomic instability, derived from defective antibody-diversification mechanisms and other DNA repair processes not specific to lymphocyte development, in addition to a lower state of alertness of the immune system, contributes toward cancer development.

syndrome (BS) and Fanconi Anemia (FA). BS is caused by inactivation of the *BLM* gene.[79] Ig deficiencies have been described for some BS patients, suggesting a potential role for BLM in CSR.[54–56] BLM is not involved in V(D)J recombination as such, but its inactivation may affect survival and development of lymphocytes.[80] FA is caused by germline inactivation of members of the FA pathway. The latter is most active during replicative stress and DNA repair that occurs through homologous recombination.[81] FA proteins are not believed to be involved in lymphocyte-specific genetic rearrangements. The immunodeficient phenotype of FA patients can be attributed to bone marrow failure, a hallmark of the FA syndrome.[58,82]

Some DNA repair proteins can affect lymphocyte development indirectly. Both V(D)J and CSR require cell proliferation and are dependent on faithful replication of genetic material and functional cell cycle checkpoints.[83–85] Furthermore, lymphocytes go through extensive cell proliferation, both during maturation and expansion, which brings about a greater demand for telomere maintenance, a process in which NBN, MRE11, and ATM participate.[86] Reactive metabolites produced during inflammation further increase the risk for DNA lesions.[6]

Cancer risk in DNA repair-associated PID patients

A considerable proportion of PID patients present with an increased predisposition for developing cancer,[87,88] where lymphoid cancers constitute the majority of malignancies diagnosed.[89] This is partly a consequence of the DNA lesions generated by impaired V(D)J recombination, CSR, and SHM processes, and/or activation of alt-EJ pathways in patients carrying DNA repair deficiencies.[8,21,90,91] As the function of PID-associated DNA repair proteins is not restricted to antigen receptor diversification, some PID patients also display an increased risk for developing non-lymphoid tumors. Affected tissues include brain, skin, breast, and the gastrointestinal tract that contain rapidly dividing cells and/or an increased metabolic activity.[87,88] Additionally, the predisposition of PID patients to cancer could be due to immunodeficiency itself, as tumor immune surveillance becomes impaired and infections by potentially oncogenic viruses are less likely to be dealt with effectively.[92] Some Artemis- and DNA ligase 4-deficient patients appear to be particularly prone to develop EBV-associated lymphomas.[42,49,50] CVID and IgAD patients also have a higher risk to develop gastric cancer than the general population, which may be related to their incapacity to clear *Heliobacter pylori* infections.[93] Similar mechanisms of disease probably underlie the predisposition of certain PIDs (not associated with DNA repair deficiencies) to develop cancer, as observed in X-linked agammaglobulinaemia, X-linked lymphoproliferative disease, or Wiskott–Aldrich syndrome patients.[88] As several steps are required for cancer development, a combination of all of the above might occur (Fig. 2). The type of tumors that develop in DNA repair-deficient PID patients, and the genetic characteristics of those tumors, may suggest which DNA recombination processes were involved in triggering tumorigenesis.[94]

Ataxia-telangiectasia

Ataxia-telangiectasia (AT) is caused by mutations in the *ATM* gene. At is characterized by cerebellar ataxia and other developmental defects, immunodeficiency, and radiosensitivity.[95] Approximately one-third of AT patients develop malignancies, with lymphomas and leukemias of T cell origin being predominant.[34] B cell neoplasias are less common and occur at an approximately 1:5 ratio to T cell cancers.[35] The *TCR* loci, at chromosomes 7p14, 7q34, and 14q11, are often found to be abnormally rearranged in a high proportion of T cells from AT individuals, even before the onset of malignancy.[96] The high incidence of T cell cancers and frequent involvement of the *TCR* loci in chromosomal rearrangements suggests that the tumorigenic trigger in AT is provided by impaired V(D)J recombination.[97,98] It is puzzling, though, why ATM deficiency primarily leads to malignant transformation of T cells instead of effects on T and B cells similarly. The development of B cell malignancies in AT patients might relate to defective CSR events, as IgA, IgG, and IgE deficiencies are common in those patients.[31,32,99] In addition to the role of ATM in antibody diversification, its involvement in the activation of cell cycle checkpoints and telomere maintenance must be considered.[86,100] ATM deficiency could function as a double-edge sword by promoting genomic instability on one hand and crippling tumor suppressor mechanisms on the other.

Nijmegen breakage syndrome

Nijmegen breakage syndrome (NBS) is caused by hypomorphic mutations in the *NBN* gene. NBS patient's phenotype greatly overlaps with that of AT patients, suggesting a functional relation between ATM and NBN.[101,102] Although lymphopenia (of B and T cells) is characteristic for both diseases, NBS patients have an extremely high risk ($>1,000\times$) for development of non-Hodgkin lymphomas, with the majority being of B cell origin and from diffuse large B cell type.[39,40] This suggests that, despite the functional overlap between ATM and NBN during B and T cell development, deficiency of the latter affects DNA repair processes specifically related to B cell transformation. Indeed this is supported by the pivotal role given to NBN in CSR[78,99,103,104] and by the frequent observation of IgA and IgG deficiencies associated with normal or high level of IgM in NBS patients.[36] Interestingly, Gregorek *et al.*[37] reported a group of NBS patients that presented with a sudden increase of IgM levels followed by the development of B cell lymphoma in a majority of cases, thus directly correlating antibody switching deficiencies with the onset of malignancy. NBN's role during V(D)J recombination processes might be less important, although some NBS patients do develop T cell tumors carrying translocated *TCR* loci.[40,105] NBN was also suggested to be a major player in the alt-EJ DNA repair pathway.[99,106] As the latter is mostly involved in CSR, and not in V(D)J recombination, it could contribute to the specific targeting of B cells by genomic instability.[26]

Artemis and DNA ligase 4 deficiencies

Artemis and DNA ligase 4 syndromes are less common than AT and NBS. Artemis and DNA ligase 4 proteins operate in subsequent steps of the NHEJ pathway, and the phenotypes of Artemis- and DNA ligase 4-deficient patients are somewhat related and characterized by profound immunodeficiencies.[30,45–47] EBV-positive B cell lymphomas have been diagnosed in two patients carrying hypomorphic *DCLRE1C* (encoding for Artemis) mutations. EBV transformation is supposedly facilitated by their strong immunodeficient background. Those tumors displayed clonal origin and pronounced genomic instability, suggesting a direct role for Artemis deficiency in tumorigenesis. EBV-associated B cell lymphomas were also described in two *LIG4* compound heterozygous patients.[49,50] Although those tumors were not described in detail, one can speculate that both EBV-mediated transformation and DNA ligase 4 deficiency could contribute toward tumorigenesis. A truncating mutation in the C-terminus of the *LIG4* gene was found in a PID patient who developed acute T cell leukemia.[52] Finally, a missense hypomorphic mutation in *LIG4* was described in an acute lymphoblastic leukemia patient who also presented with radiosensitivity.[51] Curiously, this patient did not reveal symptoms of immunodeficiency, and V(D)J recombination remained largely unaffected. In most cases, mice deficient for NHEJ factors need additional knockdown of *Trp53* in order to develop cancer.[107] Artemis/Trp53-deficient mice develop pro-B cell lymphomas presenting co-amplification of the *Igh* and *Mycn* loci but lacking translocations involving the *Igh* locus.[108] DNA ligase 4/Trp53-null mice succumb early to pro-B cell lymphomas but present characteristic translocations between chromosome 12, harboring the *Igh* locus, and chromosome 15, around the *Myc* oncogene.[109]

DNA ligase 1 deficiency

In addition to a typical immunodeficient phenotype, the only patient described with DNA ligase 1 deficiency developed a lymphoma.[53] The role of DNA ligase 1 in antibody diversification is not well established, but the onset at an early age of IgAD and low levels of IgG suggests its involvement in CSR. Mice carrying the same mutation encountered in the DNA ligase 1-deficient patient were also prone to develop lymphomas, thus supporting the role of DNA ligase 1 on lymphocyte development and lymphomagenesis.[110]

Other DNA repair defects associated with immunodeficiency

Although not generally classified as PIDs, there are other DNA repair-associated syndromes that simultaneously predispose for cancer development and immunodeficient phenotypes. BS and FA are two chromosomal instability syndromes caused by defects in proteins involved in maintenance of the cell's genomic stability. MMR deficiency also affects important cell caretaker systems essential for the fidelity of DNA replication.

BS

BS patients present with premature aging and a strong predisposition for cancer development as a consequence of widespread genomic instability.[111,112] *BLM* is a member of the RecQ helicase gene family involved in the unwinding and separation of DNA complementary strands and secondary structures, making the strands accessible for DNA replication and repair processes.[113] Hematological malignancies are common in BS patients, particularly non-Hodgkin lymphomas, which may support a role for BLM in lymphocyte development and lymphomagenesis.[57] To our knowledge, no data are available on the involvement of the *IgH* or *TCR* loci in BS-related malignancies.

FA

FA is a genetically heterogeneous disorder that produces a range of phenotypes that are highly variable between FA patients, including developmental defects and malformations, infertility, pancytopenia, and high prevalence of hematological malignancies

and solid tumors.[58] The most common hematological malignancies in FA are acute myeloid leukemias presenting with widespread clonal chromosomal aberrations. Notwithstanding, as observed for the spectrum of acute myeloid leukemia, chromosomal translocations involving the *TCR* or *IgH* loci are uncommon in FA; thus, a role for antibody diversification mechanisms in FA-associated acute myeloid leukemia onset is unlikely.[58]

Constitutional mismatch-repair deficiency syndrome

Biallelic germline mutations in *MLH1*, *MSH2*, *MSH6*, or *PMS2* cause what is referred to as constitutional mismatch-repair deficiency syndrome (CMMR-D).[64] CMMR-D patients present a high risk for developing childhood malignancies. Although hematological malignancies are common, the spectrum of tumors affecting CMMR-D patients is broad, with brain tumors and colorectal cancers being frequent.[64] This diversity of malignancies is probably related to the universal role of MMR as a cell caretaker system essential for dealing with the accumulation of point mutations during DNA replication.[114] Additionally, the fact that immunodeficiencies are not common in CMMR-D patients supports the notion that other pathways, such as the BER, might compensate for MMR loss during CSR.[13]

DNA repair-associated PIDs not yet associated to cancer predisposition

While mutations in *NHEJ1*, *DNA-PKcs*, *MRE11*, and *RNF168* have been described in PID patients, they apparently do not predispose to malignancies.[65,66,75,76,78] In mice, ATM was shown to compensate for Cernunnos deficiencies and could prevent lymphomagenesis.[115] Nevertheless, Cernunnos/Trp53-deficient mice succumb to thymic lymphomas at an early age and often develop medulloblastomas.[116] DNA-PKcs abrogation completely stalls B and T cell development and therefore does not provide patients with cellular precursors for malignant transformation.[65] In mice, on the other hand, DNA-PKcs deficiency alone predisposes to the development of T cell lymphomas.[117] MRE11-deficient patients possess a similar phenotype to that of AT and NBS patients, including developmental defects and radiosensitivity.[118] Although two siblings carrying *MRE11* mutations developed lung carcinomas, MRE11 deficiency does not appear to lead to increased risk for lymphoid cancer development.[119] MRE11 deficiency produces widespread genomic instability in mice but no increased risk for malignancy, independently of the *Trp53* mutation background.[120] Finally, the most recently described DNA repair gene associated with PIDs is *RNF168*. RNF168 is involved in the recruitment of DNA repair molecules upon the generation of DSBs. The only two patients described to date with RNF168 defects presented with low serum levels of IgG or IgA, which suggests an underlying CSR defect.[75–77] Interestingly, the father of one of the patients, a heterozygous RNF168 mutation carrier, developed B cell chronic lymphocytic leukemia.[76] Rnf168/Trp53-deficient mice develop thymomas and B cell lymphomas with reciprocal translocations between chromosomes 12 and 15 (*Igh* and *Myc* loci).[121] The recent discovery of these syndromes, in addition to the low number of cases described, might explain why any malignancy was not yet reported.

Cancer risk in heterozygous carriers

The role of DNA repair deficiencies in the onset of cancer in PID patients is partly related to faulty DNA recombination mechanisms during B and T cell development. Additionally, the involvement of DNA repair proteins in other DNA repair or damage response processes, not related to the generation of antibody diversity, might also contribute to the malignant transformation of cells. If such proteins possess a gatekeeper function, their targeting might implicate a loss of tumor suppressor functions, thereby allowing the propagation of genetic instability in cells. The observation of an increased risk for cancer development in heterozygous DNA repair mutation carriers provides insight into their tumorigenic potential. Furthermore, the somatic targeting of DNA repair genes during cancer development strengthens the assumption that they have an important role as cancer genes (Table 2).

Germline *ATM* heterozygous mutations might confer increased risk for breast cancer, although some reports contradicting this observation have been published.[117,118] Interestingly, the *ATM* locus is frequently targeted by loss of heterozygosity (LOH) at chromosome 11q in tumors, including breast and lymphoid malignancies.[119–121] Additionally, somatic *ATM* mutations in blood and lymphoid cancers have been described, thus supporting the role of *ATM* as a cancer gene.[122]

Similar to ATM, conflicting reports are available regarding the association of heterozygous germline *NBN* mutations with increased cancer risk.[123] The majority of studies have focused on the most

Table 2. Involvement of PID-related DNA repair genes in cancer

Gene	Cancer risk heterozygotes[a]	Somatic alterations in cancer
ATM	Breast cancer[122]	LOH in breast, ovarian, and lymphoid malignancies.[125–127] Mutations in lymphoid malignancies.[125]
NBN	Non-Hodgkin lymphomas, leukemias, melanomas, medulloblastomas, breast, prostate[123,124]	LOH in breast cancer, melanoma, and prostate cancer.[128–130]
DCLRE1C (Artemis)	ND	ND
LIG4	ND	ND
LIG1	ND	ND
BLM	Colorectal cancer[131]	Mutated in gastric cancer.[132]
FANC group	Breast, ovarian, and pancreatic cancer [133–135]	LOH and mutations of *BRCA2* in breast and ovarian cancer.[136–138]
MMR	Lynch syndrome: increased risk for colorectal, endometrial, and ovarian cancers.[139]	Hypermethylation of the *MLH1* gene.[140]

AT, ataxia-telangiectasia; LOH, loss of heterozygosity; ND, not determined.
[a]Association studies on genetic polymorphisms were not included.

common *NBN* founder mutation (*NBN 657del5*) and several of them described associations to a variety of cancers, including non-Hodgkin lymphomas and leukemias.[123,124] Associations are likely to be population-dependent. The potential role of NBN as a tumor suppressor was further assessed by investigating the occurrence of LOH at the *NBN* locus in tumors from *657del5* mutation carriers. The majority of tumors presented a physical loss of the wild-type allele, thereby silencing *NBN* expression.[128–150] Additional mutations, including missense amino acid substitutions were also associated with an increased risk for several cancers.[123]

The risk of heterozygous mutants for *DCLRE1C* and *LIG4* has not been assessed, probably due to the low number of carriers. Polymorphisms located within the *LIG4* associate with the risk for several cancers.[143–145]

Carriers of *BLM* heterozygous mutations might be at higher risk for developing colorectal cancer, as demonstrated in the Ashkenazi Jewish population, although conflicting reports have been published.[131,146] Frameshift somatic mutations have also been described in a polyadenine repeat present in the coding region of *BLM* in gastric carcinomas presenting microsatellite instability.[132]

The most prominent gene in the FA pathway is *BRCA2*. Monoallelic mutations in *BRCA2* are well-known to cause increased susceptibility to breast and other cancer types.[133] As for the remaining members of the FA complex, data on the risk of heterozygous carriers developing cancer are mainly provided from the study of FA families, but these were not found to be at higher risk to develop cancer.[147,148] Mutations in *PALB2* and *BRIP1*, associated with FA complementation groups N and J, respectively, were suggested to predispose for breast cancer.[134,135] *BRCA2* is targeted by LOH and found mutated in breast and ovarian carcinomas.[136–138]

Heterozygous, germline mutations in *MLH1*, *MSH2*, *MSH6*, and *PMS2* cause Lynch syndrome. Lynch syndrome is an autosomal dominant disease that confers an increased risk for colorectal cancer, as well as other tumor types.[139]

Clinical management of PID cancer patients carrying DNA repair defects

Cancer contributes greatly to the poor overall survival observed in PID patients carrying DNA repair defects. Additionally, DNA repair-deficient PID cancer patients display increased morbidity and mortality compared to the majority of cancer patients.[149–151] This is mostly due to the fact that PID DNA repair-deficient patients display increased toxicity to radiation and chemotherapeutic agents, the most common anticancer treatments.[11] Accordingly, the enrolling of PID cancer patients in standard therapy regimes is associated with a high risk for the development of new malignancies and intolerance to therapeutic agents.[152] Additionally, strategies based on the notion of synthetic lethality of DNA repair mechanisms will not provide specific targeting to cancer cells.[153] The fragility of many PID patients implies careful employment of therapeutic regimens. The utilization of ionizing radiation should be avoided and, when necessary, doses should be adapted appropriately. Hematopoietic stem cell transplantation performed under reduced-intensity conditioning regimes has proven successful in cancer treatment for a number of NBS patients.[154] Moreover, it is paramount that PID patients are diagnosed at an early age to provide better management of the disease and associated malignancies.

Future perspectives in the field

It is likely that some DNA repair defects underlying the development of PID are yet to be identified. Vajdic *et al.*[87] described that antibody deficiency alone was associated with an increased risk for cancer development, particularly non-Hodgkin lymphomas. CVID patients also displayed an increased risk for overall cancer development. If the described antibody deficiencies relate to faulty CSR events occurring in those patients, a background of genetic instability in the B cells from those patients may promote lymphomagenesis. Conversely, genes associated with CVID onset are generally involved in immune regulatory functions rather than in genetic mechanisms of lymphocyte maturation.[155] Their predisposition to a broader range of cancer types could relate to the decreased fitness of the host to deal with infections or cellular transformation.

The current state of technological development in the field of genetics is anticipated to lead to the discovery of novel disease-susceptibility genes in the coming years. The identification, by next-generation sequencing for example, of DNA repair deficiencies associated with PID development would give further insight into the genetics of immunogenesis, and into lymphocyte development in particular. From a clinical point of view, the discovery of such syndromes would facilitate the early diagnosis and adequate management of PID patients, crucial for a favorable prognosis. Additionally, when PIDs are accompanied by a predisposition to cancer, mechanisms of generation of genomic instability (e.g., required for in malignant transformation) might be elucidated and applied to cancer research in general. However, there is the likelihood that many PIDs do not follow a single-gene disease model. Genome-wide association studies (GWAS) on various PIDs of unknown genetic etiologies have reported several disease-associated loci.[156,157] Nevertheless, except for few loci, they often present with low effect sizes or have been located within gene deserts. Multifactorial genetic diseases will likely always constitute a challenge, despite the technological advances made. For a number of cases, next-generation sequencing techniques will likely give clues rather than definitive answers to the genetics behind PIDs. Yet, characterizing more cancer genomes by next-generation sequencing might provide further evidence for the involvement of PID-associated DNA repair genes in tumorigenesis.

Acknowledgments

This work was supported by the Swedish Cancer Society (Cancerfonden), the Swedish Research Council, the European Research Council (242551-ImmunoSwitch), and funds from the Karolinska Institutet.

Conflicts of interest

The authors have no conflicts of interests.

References

1. Zimmer, C. 2009. Origins. On the origin of sexual reproduction. *Science* 324: 1254–1256.
2. Caporale, L.H. 2000. Mutation is modulated: implications for evolution. *Bioessays* 22: 388–395.
3. Radman, M., I. Matic & F. Taddei. 1999. Evolution of evolvability. *Ann. N. Y. Acad. Sci.* 870: 146–155.
4. Howard, J.C. 1991. Immunology. Disease and evolution. *Nature* 352: 565–567.
5. Bonilla, F.A. & H.C. Oettgen. 2010. Adaptive immunity. *J. Allergy Clin. Immunol.* 125: S33–S40.
6. Revy, P., D. Buck, D.F. Le & J.P. de Villartay. 2005. The repair of DNA damages/modifications during the maturation of the immune system: lessons from human primary immunodeficiency disorders and animal models.' *Adv. Immunol.* 87: 237–295.

7. Moses, R.E. 2001. DNA damage processing defects and disease. *Annu. Rev. Genomics Hum. Genet.* 2: 41–68.
8. Puebla-Osorio, N. & C. Zhu. 2008. DNA damage and repair during lymphoid development: antigen receptor diversity, genomic integrity and lymphomagenesis. *Immunol. Res.* 41: 103–122.
9. Slatter, M.A. & A.R. Gennery. 2010. Primary immunodeficiency syndromes. *Adv. Exp. Med. Biol.* 685: 146–165.
10. Chistiakov, D.A., N.V. Voronova & P.A. Chistiakov. 2008. Genetic variations in DNA repair genes, radiosensitivity to cancer and susceptibility to acute tissue reactions in radiotherapy-treated cancer patients. *Acta Oncol.* 47: 809–824.
11. Nahas, S.A. & R.A. Gatti. 2009. DNA double strand break repair defects, primary immunodeficiency disorders, and 'radiosensitivity'. *Curr. Opin. Allergy Clin. Immunol.* 9: 510–516.
12. Lieber, M.R., C.P. Chang, M. Gallo, *et al.* 1994. The mechanism of V(D)J recombination: site-specificity, reaction fidelity and immunologic diversity. *Semin. Immunol.* 6: 143–153.
13. Stavnezer, J., J.E. Guikema & C.E. Schrader. 2008. Mechanism and regulation of class switch recombination. *Annu. Rev. Immunol.* 26: 261–292.
14. Peled, J.U., F.L. Kuang, M.D. Iglesias-Ussel, *et al.* 2008. The biochemistry of somatic hypermutation. *Annu. Rev. Immunol.* 26: 481–511.
15. Oettinger, M.A., D.G. Schatz, C. Gorka & D. Baltimore. 1990. RAG-1 and RAG-2, adjacent genes that synergistically activate V(D)J recombination. *Science* 248: 1517–1523.
16. Schatz, D.G., M.A. Oettinger & D. Baltimore. 1989. The V(D)J recombination activating gene, RAG-1. *Cell* 59: 1035–1048.
17. Lieber, M.R. 2010. The mechanism of double-strand DNA break repair by the nonhomologous DNA end-joining pathway. *Annu. Rev. Biochem.* 79: 181–211.
18. Muramatsu, M., K. Kinoshita, S. Fagarasan, *et al.* 2000. Class switch recombination and hypermutation require activation-induced cytidine deaminase (AID), a potential RNA editing enzyme. *Cell* 102: 553–563.
19. Stavnezer, J., A. Bjorkman, L. Du, *et al.* 2010. Mapping of switch recombination junctions, a tool for studying DNA repair pathways during immunoglobulin class switching. *Adv. Immunol.* 108: 45–109.
20. Kotnis, A., L. Du, C. Liu, *et al.* 2009. Non-homologous end joining in class switch recombination: the beginning of the end. *Philos. Trans. R. Soc. Lond B Biol. Sci.* 364: 653–665.
21. Zhang, Y., M. Gostissa, D.G. Hildebrand, *et al.* 2010. The role of mechanistic factors in promoting chromosomal translocations found in lymphoid and other cancers. *Adv. Immunol.* 106: 93–133.
22. Boboila, C., C. Yan, D.R. Wesemann, *et al.* 2010. Alternative end-joining catalyzes class switch recombination in the absence of both Ku70 and DNA ligase 4. *J. Exp. Med.* 207: 417–427.
23. Du, L., M. van der Burg, S.W. Popov, *et al.* 2008. Involvement of Artemis in nonhomologous end-joining during immunoglobulin class switch recombination. *J. Exp. Med.* 205: 3031–3040.

24. Pan-Hammarstrom, Q., A.M. Jones, A. Lahdesmaki, *et al.* 2005. Impact of DNA ligase IV on nonhomologous end joining pathways during class switch recombination in human cells. *J. Exp. Med.* **201:** 189–194.

25. Yan, C.T., C. Boboila, E.K. Souza, *et al.* 2007. IgH class switching and translocations use a robust non-classical end-joining pathway. *Nature* **449:** 478–482.

26. Corneo, B., R.L. Wendland, L. Deriano, *et al.* 2007. Rag mutations reveal robust alternative end joining. *Nature* **449:** 483–486.

27. Du, L., D.K. Dunn-Walters, K.H. Chrzanowska, *et al.* 2008. A regulatory role for NBS1 in strand-specific mutagenesis during somatic hypermutation. *PLoS One* **3:** e2482.

28. Niehues, T., R. Perez-Becker & C. Schuetz. 2010. More than just SCID–the phenotypic range of combined immunodeficiencies associated with mutations in the recombinase activating genes (RAG) 1 and 2. *Clin. Immunol.* **135:** 183–192.

29. Schwarz, K., G.H. Gauss, L. Ludwig, *et al.* 1996. RAG mutations in human B cell-negative SCID. *Science* **274:** 97–99.

30. Moshous, D., I. Callebaut, C.R. De, *et al.* 2001. Artemis, a novel DNA double-strand break repair/V(D)J recombination protein, is mutated in human severe combined immune deficiency. *Cell* **105:** 177–186.

31. Noordzij, J.G., N.M. Wulffraat, A. Haraldsson, *et al.* 2009. Ataxia-telangiectasia patients presenting with hyper-IgM syndrome. *Arch. Dis. Child.* **94:** 448–449.

32. Nowak-Wegrzyn, A., T.O. Crawford, J.A. Winkelstein, *et al.* 2004. Immunodeficiency and infections in ataxia-telangiectasia. *J. Pediatr.* **144:** 505–511.

33. Staples, E.R., E.M. McDermott, A. Reiman, *et al.* 2008. Immunodeficiency in ataxia telangiectasia is correlated strongly with the presence of two null mutations in the ataxia telangiectasia mutated gene. *Clin. Exp. Immunol.* **153:** 214–220.

34. Peterson, R.D., J.D. Funkhouser, C.M. Tuck-Muller & R.A. Gatti. 1992. Cancer susceptibility in ataxia-telangiectasia. *Leukemia* **6** (Suppl. 1): 8–13.

35. Taylor, A.M., J.A. Metcalfe, J. Thick & Y.F. Mak. 1996. Leukemia and lymphoma in ataxia telangiectasia. *Blood* **87:** 423–438.

36. van Engelen, B.G., J.A. Hiel, F.J. Gabreels, *et al.* 2001. Decreased immunoglobulin class switching in Nijmegen Breakage syndrome due to the DNA repair defect. *Hum. Immunol.* **62:** 1324–1327.

37. Gregorek, H., K.H. Chrzanowska, J. Michalkiewicz, *et al.* 2002. Heterogeneity of humoral immune abnormalities in children with Nijmegen breakage syndrome: an 8-year follow-up study in a single centre. *Clin. Exp. Immunol.* **130:** 319–324.

38. Demuth, I. & M. Digweed. 2007. The clinical manifestation of a defective response to DNA double-strand breaks as exemplified by Nijmegen breakage syndrome. *Oncogene* **26:** 7792–7798.

39. The International Nijmegen Breakage Syndrome Study Group. 2000. Nijmegen breakage syndrome. *Arch. Dis. Child.* **82:** 400–406.

40. Gladkowska-Dura, M., K. Dzierzanowska-Fangrat, W.T. Dura, *et al.* 2008. Unique morphological spectrum of lymphomas in Nijmegen breakage syndrome (NBS) patients with high frequency of consecutive lymphoma formation. *J. Pathol.* **216:** 337–344.

41. Noordzij, J.G., N.S. Verkaik, M. van der Burg, *et al.* 2003. Radiosensitive SCID patients with Artemis gene mutations show a complete B-cell differentiation arrest at the pre-B-cell receptor checkpoint in bone marrow. *Blood* **101:** 1446–1452.

42. Moshous, D., C. Pannetier, R.R. Chasseval, *et al.* 2003. Partial T and B lymphocyte immunodeficiency and predisposition to lymphoma in patients with hypomorphic mutations in Artemis. *J. Clin. Invest.* **111:** 381–387.

43. Ijspeert, H., A.C. Lankester, J.M. van den Berg, *et al.* 2011. Artemis splice defects cause atypical SCID and can be restored in vitro by an antisense oligonucleotide. *Genes Immun.* **12:** 434–444.

44. Ege, M., Y. Ma, B. Manfras, *et al.* 2005. Omenn syndrome due to ARTEMIS mutations. *Blood* **105:** 4179–4186.

45. Buck, D., D. Moshous, C.R. De, *et al.* 2006. Severe combined immunodeficiency and microcephaly in siblings with hypomorphic mutations in DNA ligase IV. *Eur. J. Immunol.* **36:** 224–235.

46. van der Burg, M., L.R. van Veelen, N.S. Verkaik, *et al.* 2006. A new type of radiosensitive T-B-NK+ severe combined immunodeficiency caused by a LIG4 mutation. *J. Clin. Invest.* **116:** 137–145.

47. O'Driscoll, M., K.M. Cerosaletti, P.M. Girard, *et al.* 2001. DNA ligase IV mutations identified in patients exhibiting developmental delay and immunodeficiency. *Mol. Cell* **8:** 1175–1185.

48. Grunebaum, E., A. Bates & C.M. Roifman. 2008. Omenn syndrome is associated with mutations in DNA ligase IV. *J. Allergy Clin. Immunol.* **122:** 1219–1220.

49. Enders, A., P. Fisch, K. Schwarz, *et al.* 2006. A severe form of human combined immunodeficiency due to mutations in DNA ligase IV. *J. Immunol.* **176:** 5060–5068.

50. Toita, N., N. Hatano, S. Ono, *et al.* 2007. Epstein-Barr virus-associated B-cell lymphoma in a patient with DNA ligase IV (LIG4) syndrome. *Am. J. Med. Genet. A.* **143:** 742–745.

51. Riballo, E., S.E. Critchlow, S.H. Teo, *et al.* 1999. Identification of a defect in DNA ligase IV in a radiosensitive leukaemia patient. *Curr. Biol.* **9:** 699–702.

52. Ben-Omran, T.I., K. Cerosaletti, P. Concannon, *et al.* 2005. A patient with mutations in DNA Ligase IV: clinical features and overlap with Nijmegen breakage syndrome. *Am. J. Med. Genet. A.* **137A:** 283–287.

53. Webster, A.D., D.E. Barnes, C.F. Arlett, *et al.* 1992. Growth retardation and immunodeficiency in a patient with mutations in the DNA ligase I gene. *Lancet* **339:** 1508–1509.

54. Kondo, N., F. Motoyoshi, S. Mori, *et al.* 1992. Long-term study of the immunodeficiency of Bloom's syndrome. *Acta Paediatr.* **81:** 86–90.

55. Van Kerckhove, C.W., J.L. Ceuppens, M. Vanderschueren-Lodeweyckx, *et al.* 1988. Bloom's syndrome. Clinical features and immunologic abnormalities of four patients. *Am. J. Dis. Child.* **142:** 1089–1093.

56. Etzioni, A., N. Lahat, A. Benderly, *et al.* 1989. Humoral and cellular immune dysfunction in a patient with Bloom's syndrome and recurrent infections. *J. Clin. Lab Immunol.* **28:** 151–154.

57. German, J. 1997. Bloom's syndrome. XX. The first 100 cancers. *Cancer Genet. Cytogenet.* **93:** 100–106.

58. Auerbach, A.D. 2009. Fanconi anemia and its diagnosis. *Mutat. Res.* **668:** 4–10.

59. Peron, S., A. Metin, P. Gardes, *et al.* 2008. Human PMS2 deficiency is associated with impaired immunoglobulin class switch recombination. *J. Exp. Med.* **205:** 2465–2472.

60. Ostergaard, J.R., L. Sunde & H. Okkels. 2005. Neurofibromatosis von Recklinghausen type I phenotype and early onset of cancers in siblings compound heterozygous for mutations in MSH6. *Am. J. Med. Genet. A.* **139A:** 96–105.

61. Whiteside, D., R. McLeod, G. Graham, *et al.* 2002. A homozygous germ-line mutation in the human MSH2 gene predisposes to hematological malignancy and multiple cafe-au-lait spots. *Cancer Res.* **62:** 359–362.

62. Offer, S.M., Q. Pan-Hammarstrom, L. Hammarstrom & R.S. Harris. 2010. Unique DNA repair gene variations and potential associations with the primary antibody deficiency syndromes IgAD and CVID. *PLoS One* **5:** e12260.

63. Scott, R.H., S. Mansour, K. Pritchard-Jones, *et al.* 2007. Medulloblastoma, acute myelocytic leukemia and colonic carcinomas in a child with biallelic MSH6 mutations. *Nat. Clin. Pract. Oncol.* **4:** 130–134.

64. Wimmer, K. & J. Etzler. 2008. Constitutional mismatch repair-deficiency syndrome: have we so far seen only the tip of an iceberg? *Hum. Genet.* **124:** 105–122.

65. van der Burg, M., H. Ijspeert, N.S. Verkaik, *et al.* 2009. A DNA-PKcs mutation in a radiosensitive T-B- SCID patient inhibits Artemis activation and nonhomologous end-joining. *J. Clin. Invest.* **119:** 91–98.

66. Buck, D., L. Malivert, C.R. De, *et al.* 2006. Cernunnos, a novel nonhomologous end-joining factor, is mutated in human immunodeficiency with microcephaly. *Cell* **124:** 287–299.

67. Cagdas, D., T.T. Ozgur, G.T. Asal, *et al.* 2011. Two SCID cases with Cernunnos-XLF deficiency successfully treated by hematopoietic stem cell transplantation. *Pediatr. Transplant.* 2011 Apr 27. doi: 10.1111/j.1399-3046.2011.01491.x. [Epub ahead of print].

68. Faraci, M., E. Lanino, C. Micalizzi, *et al.* 2009. Unrelated hematopoietic stem cell transplantation for Cernunnos-XLF deficiency. *Pediatr. Transplant.* **13:** 785–789.

69. Turul, T., I. Tezcan & O. Sanal. 2011. Cernunnos deficiency: a case report. *J. Investig. Allergol. Clin. Immunol.* **21:** 313–316.

70. Pan-Hammarstrom, Q. & L. Hammarstrom. 2008. Antibody deficiency diseases. *Eur. J. Immunol.* **38:** 327–333.

71. Durandy, A., N. Taubenheim, S. Peron & A. Fischer. 2007. Pathophysiology of B-cell intrinsic immunoglobulin class switch recombination deficiencies. *Adv. Immunol.* **94:** 275–306.

72. Revy, P., T. Muto, Y. Levy, *et al.* 2000. Activation-induced cytidine deaminase (AID) deficiency causes the autosomal recessive form of the Hyper-IgM syndrome (HIGM2). *Cell* **102:** 565–575.

73. Imai, K., G. Slupphaug, W.I. Lee, *et al.* 2003. Human uracil-DNA glycosylase deficiency associated with profoundly impaired immunoglobulin class-switch recombination. *Nat. Immunol.* **4:** 1023–1028.

74. Sekine, H., R.C. Ferreira, Q. Pan-Hammarstrom, *et al.* 2007. Role for Msh5 in the regulation of Ig class switch recombination. *Proc. Natl. Acad. Sci. USA* **104:** 7193–7198.

75. Stewart, G.S., T. Stankovic, P.J. Byrd, *et al.* 2007. RIDDLE immunodeficiency syndrome is linked to defects in 53BP1-mediated DNA damage signaling. *Proc. Natl. Acad. Sci. USA* **104:** 16910–16915.

76. Stewart, G.S., S. Panier, K. Townsend, *et al.* 2009. The RIDDLE syndrome protein mediates a ubiquitin-dependent signaling cascade at sites of DNA damage. *Cell* **136:** 420–434.

77. Devgan, S.S., O. Sanal, C. Doil, *et al.* 2011. Homozygous deficiency of ubiquitin-ligase ring-finger protein RNF168 mimics the radiosensitivity syndrome of ataxia-telangiectasia. *Cell Death Differ.* **18:** 1500–1506.

78. Lahdesmaki, A., A.M. Taylor, K.H. Chrzanowska & Q. Pan-Hammarstrom. 2004. Delineation of the role of the Mre11 complex in class switch recombination. *J. Biol. Chem.* **279:** 16479–16487.

79. Ellis, N.A., J. Groden, T.Z. Ye, *et al.* 1995. The Bloom's syndrome gene product is homologous to RecQ helicases. *Cell* **83:** 655–666.

80. Babbe, H., J. McMenamin, E. Hobeika, *et al.* 2009. Genomic instability resulting from Blm deficiency compromises development, maintenance, and function of the B cell lineage. *J. Immunol.* **182:** 347–360.

81. Kitao, H. & M. Takata. 2011. Fanconi anemia: a disorder defective in the DNA damage response. *Int. J. Hematol.* **93:** 417–424.

82. Krijger, P.H., N. Wit, P.C. van den Berk & H. Jacobs. 2010. The Fanconi anemia core complex is dispensable during somatic hypermutation and class switch recombination. *PLoS One* **5:** e15236.

83. Li, Z., D.I. Dordai, J. Lee & S. Desiderio. 1996. A conserved degradation signal regulates RAG-2 accumulation during cell division and links V(D)J recombination to the cell cycle. *Immunity* **5:** 575–589.

84. Lin, W.C. & S. Desiderio. 1994. Cell cycle regulation of V(D)J recombination-activating protein RAG-2. *Proc. Natl. Acad. Sci. USA* **91:** 2733–2737.

85. Rush, J.S., M. Liu, V.H. Odegard, *et al.* 2005. Expression of activation-induced cytidine deaminase is regulated by cell division, providing a mechanistic basis for division-linked class switch recombination. *Proc. Natl. Acad. Sci. USA* **102:** 13242–13247.

86. Andrews, N.P., H. Fujii, J.J. Goronzy & C.M. Weyand. 2010. Telomeres and immunological diseases of aging. *Gerontology* **56:** 390–403.

87. Vajdic, C.M., L. Mao, M.T. van Leeuwen, *et al.* 2010. Are antibody deficiency disorders associated with a narrower range of cancers than other forms of immunodeficiency? *Blood* **116:** 1228–1234.

88. Salavoura, K., A. Kolialexi, G. Tsangaris & A. Mavrou. 2008. Development of cancer in patients with primary immunodeficiencies. *Anticancer Res.* **28:** 1263–1269.

89. Filipovich, A.H., A. Mathur, D. Kamat & R.S. Shapiro. 1992. Primary immunodeficiencies: genetic risk factors for lymphoma. *Cancer Res.* **52:** 5465s–5467s.

90. Jankovic, M., A. Nussenzweig & M.C. Nussenzweig. 2007. Antigen receptor diversification and chromosome translocations. *Nat. Immunol.* **8:** 801–808.

91. Edry, E. & D. Melamed. 2007. Class switch recombination: a friend and a foe. *Clin. Immunol.* **123:** 244–251.

92. Rezaei, N., M. Hedayat, A. Aghamohammadi & K.E. Nichols. 2011. Primary immunodeficiency diseases associated with increased susceptibility to viral infections and malignancies. *J. Allergy Clin. Immunol.* **127:** 1329–1341.

93. Mellemkjaer, L., L. Hammarstrom, V. Andersen, *et al.* 2002. Cancer risk among patients with IgA deficiency or common variable immunodeficiency and their relatives: a combined Danish and Swedish study. *Clin. Exp. Immunol.* **130:** 495–500.

94. Arana, M.E. & T.A. Kunkel. 2010. Mutator phenotypes due to DNA replication infidelity. *Semin. Cancer Biol.* **20:** 304–311.

95. Chun, H.H. & R.A. Gatti. 2004. Ataxia-telangiectasia, an evolving phenotype. *DNA Repair (Amst).* **3:** 1187–1196.

96. Aurias, A., B. Dutrillaux, D. Buriot & J. Lejeune. 1980. High frequencies of inversions and translocations of chromosomes 7 and 14 in ataxia telangiectasia. *Mutat. Res.* **69:** 369–374.

97. Vacchio, M.S., A. Olaru, F. Livak & R.J. Hodes. 2007. ATM deficiency impairs thymocyte maturation because of defective resolution of T cell receptor alpha locus coding end breaks. *Proc. Natl. Acad. Sci. USA* **104:** 6323–6328.

98. Bredemeyer, A.L., G.G. Sharma, C.Y. Huang, *et al.* 2006. ATM stabilizes DNA double-strand-break complexes during V(D)J recombination. *Nature* **442:** 466–470.

99. Pan, Q., C. Petit-Frere, A. Lahdesmaki, *et al.* 2002. Alternative end joining during switch recombination in patients with ataxia-telangiectasia. *Eur. J. Immunol.* **32:** 1300–1308.

100. Khanna, K.K. 2000. Cancer risk and the ATM gene: a continuing debate. *J. Natl. Cancer Inst.* **92:** 795–802.

101. Shiloh, Y. 1997. Ataxia-telangiectasia and the Nijmegen breakage syndrome: related disorders but genes apart. *Annu. Rev. Genet.* **31:** 635–662.

102. Difilippantonio, S., A. Celeste, O. Fernandez-Capetillo, *et al.* 2005. Role of Nbs1 in the activation of the Atm kinase revealed in humanized mouse models. *Nat. Cell Biol.* **7:** 675–685.

103. Kracker, S., Y. Bergmann, I. Demuth, *et al.* 2005. Nibrin functions in Ig class-switch recombination. *Proc. Natl. Acad. Sci. USA* **102:** 1584–1589.

104. Reina-San-Martin, B., M.C. Nussenzweig, A. Nussenzweig & S. Difilippantonio. 2005. Genomic instability, endoreduplication, and diminished Ig class-switch recombination in B cells lacking Nbs1. *Proc. Natl. Acad. Sci. USA* **102:** 1590–1595.

105. Harfst, E., S. Cooper, S. Neubauer, *et al.* 2000. Normal V(D)J recombination in cells from patients with Nijmegen breakage syndrome. *Mol. Immunol.* **37:** 915–929.

106. Dinkelmann, M., E. Spehalski, T. Stoneham, *et al.* 2009. Multiple functions of MRN in end-joining pathways during isotype class switching. *Nat. Struct. Mol. Biol.* **16:** 808–813.

107. Ferguson, D.O. & F.W. Alt. 2001. DNA double strand break repair and chromosomal translocation: lessons from animal models. *Oncogene* **20:** 5572–5579.

108. Rooney, S., J. Sekiguchi, S. Whitlow, *et al.* 2004. Artemis and p53 cooperate to suppress oncogenic N-myc amplification in progenitor B cells. *Proc. Natl. Acad. Sci. USA* **101:** 2410–2415.

109. Frank, K.M., N.E. Sharpless, Y. Gao, *et al.* 2000. DNA ligase IV deficiency in mice leads to defective neurogenesis and embryonic lethality via the p53 pathway. *Mol. Cell* **5:** 993–1002.

110. Harrison, C., A.M. Ketchen, N.J. Redhead, *et al.* 2002. Replication failure, genome instability, and increased cancer susceptibility in mice with a point mutation in the DNA ligase I gene. *Cancer Res.* **62:** 4065–4074.

111. Furuichi, Y. 2001. Premature aging and predisposition to cancers caused by mutations in RecQ family helicases. *Ann. N. Y. Acad. Sci.* **928:** 121–131.

112. Vijayalaxmi, H., J. Evans, J.H. Ray & J. German. 1983. Bloom's syndrome: evidence for an increased mutation frequency in vivo. *Science* **221:** 851–853.

113. Hickson, I.D. 2003. RecQ helicases: caretakers of the genome. *Nat. Rev. Cancer* **3:** 169–178.

114. Kunkel, T.A. & D.A. Erie. 2005. DNA mismatch repair. *Annu. Rev. Biochem.* **74:** 681–710.

115. Zha, S., C. Guo, C. Boboila, *et al.* 2011. ATM damage response and XLF repair factor are functionally redundant in joining DNA breaks. *Nature* **469:** 250–254.

116. Li, G., F.W. Alt, H.L. Cheng, *et al.* 2008. Lymphocyte-specific compensation for XLF/cernunnos end-joining functions in V(D)J recombination. *Mol. Cell* **31:** 631–640.

117. Jhappan, C., H.C. Morse, III, R.D. Fleischmann, *et al.* 1997. DNA-PKcs: a T-cell tumour suppressor encoded at the mouse scid locus. *Nat. Genet.* **17:** 483–486.

118. Stracker, T.H. & J.H. Petrini. 2011. The MRE11 complex: starting from the ends. *Nat. Rev. Mol. Cell Biol.* **12:** 90–103.

119. Uchisaka, N., N. Takahashi, M. Sato, *et al.* 2009. Two brothers with ataxia-telangiectasia-like disorder with lung adenocarcinoma. *J. Pediatr.* **155:** 435–438.

120. Theunissen, J.W., M.I. Kaplan, P.A. Hunt, *et al.* 2003. Checkpoint failure and chromosomal instability without lymphomagenesis in Mre11(ATLD1/ATLD1) mice. *Mol. Cell* **12:** 1511–1523.

121. Bohgaki, T., M. Bohgaki, R. Cardoso, *et al.* 2011. Genomic instability, defective spermatogenesis, immunodeficiency, and cancer in a mouse model of the RIDDLE syndrome. *PLoS Genet.* **7:** e1001381.

122. Ahmed, M. & N. Rahman. 2006. ATM and breast cancer susceptibility. *Oncogene* **25:** 5906–5911.

123. Dzikiewicz-Krawczyk, A. 2008. The importance of making ends meet: mutations in genes and altered expression of proteins of the MRN complex and cancer. *Mutat. Res.* **659:** 262–273.

124. Ciara, E., D. Piekutowska-Abramczuk, E. Popowska, *et al.* 2010. Heterozygous germ-line mutations in the NBN gene predispose to medulloblastoma in pediatric patients. *Acta Neuropathol.* **119:** 325–334.

125. Gumy-Pause, F., P. Wacker & A.P. Sappino. 2004. ATM gene and lymphoid malignancies. *Leukemia* **18:** 238–242.

126. Kerangueven, F., F. Eisinger, T. Noguchi, *et al.* 1997. Loss of heterozygosity in human breast carcinomas in the ataxia

telangiectasia, Cowden disease and BRCA1 gene regions. *Oncogene* **14**: 339–347.

127. Koike, M., S. Takeuchi, S. Park, *et al.* 1999. Ovarian cancer: loss of heterozygosity frequently occurs in the ATM gene, but structural alterations do not occur in this gene. *Oncology* **56**: 160–163.

128. Cybulski, C., B. Gorski, T. Debniak, *et al.* 2004. NBS1 is a prostate cancer susceptibility gene. *Cancer Res.* **64**: 1215–1219.

129. Gorski, B., T. Debniak, B. Masojc, *et al.* 2003. Germline 657del5 mutation in the NBS1 gene in breast cancer patients. *Int. J. Cancer* **106**: 379–381.

130. Plisiecka-Halasa, J., A. Dansonka-Mieszkowska, A. Rembiszewska, *et al.* 2002. Nijmegen breakage syndrome gene (NBS1) alterations and its protein (nibrin) expression in human ovarian tumours. *Ann. Hum. Genet.* **66**: 353–359.

131. Gruber, S.B., N.A. Ellis, K.K. Scott, *et al.* 2002. BLM heterozygosity and the risk of colorectal cancer. *Science* **297**: 2013.

132. Calin, G., G.N. Ranzani, D. Amadori, *et al.* 2001. Somatic frameshift mutations in the Bloom syndrome BLM gene are frequent in sporadic gastric carcinomas with microsatellite mutator phenotype. *BMC Genet.* **2**: 14.

133. D'Andrea, A.D. 2010. Susceptibility pathways in Fanconi's anemia and breast cancer. *N. Engl. J. Med.* **362**: 1909–1919.

134. Seal, S., D. Thompson, A. Renwick, *et al.* 2006. Truncating mutations in the Fanconi anemia J gene BRIP1 are low-penetrance breast cancer susceptibility alleles. *Nat. Genet.* **38**: 1239–1241.

135. Hellebrand, H., C. Sutter, E. Honisch, *et al.* 2011. Germline mutations in the PALB2 gene are population specific and occur with low frequencies in familial breast cancer. *Hum. Mutat.* **32**: E2176–E2188.

136. Cleton-Jansen, A.-M., N. Collins, S.R. Lakhani, *et al.* 1995. Loss of heterozygosity in sporadic breast tumours at the BRCA2 locus on chromosome 13q12-q13. *Br. J. Cancer* **72**: 1241–1244.

137. Hilton, J.L., J.P. Geisler, J.A. Rathe, *et al.* 2002. Inactivation of BRCA1 and BRCA2 in ovarian cancer. *J. Natl. Cancer Inst.* **94**: 1396–1406.

138. Lancaster, J.M., R. Wooster, J. Mangion, *et al.* 1996. BRCA2 mutations in primary breast and ovarian cancers. *Nat. Genet.* **13**: 238–240.

139. Lynch, H.T., P.M. Lynch, S.J. Lanspa, *et al.* 2009. Review of the Lynch syndrome: history, molecular genetics, screening, differential diagnosis, and medicolegal ramifications. *Clin. Genet.* **76**: 1–18.

140. Cunningham, J.M., E.R. Christensen, D.J. Tester, *et al.* 1998. Hypermethylation of the hMLH1 promoter in colon cancer with microsatellite instability. *Cancer Res.* **58**: 3455–3460.

141. Dombernowsky, S.L., M. Weischer, K.H. Allin, *et al.* 2008. Risk of cancer by ATM missense mutations in the general population. *J. Clin. Oncol.* **26**: 3057–3062.

142. Boultwood, J. 2001. Ataxia telangiectasia gene mutations in leukaemia and lymphoma. *J. Clin. Pathol.* **54**: 512–516.

143. Andreae, J., R. Varon, K. Sperling & K. Seeger. 2007. Polymorphisms in the DNA ligase IV gene might influence the risk of acute lymphoblastic leukemia in children. *Leukemia* **21**: 2226–2227.

144. Pearce, C.L., A.M. Near, D.J. Van Den Berg, *et al.* 2009. Validating genetic risk associations for ovarian cancer through the international Ovarian Cancer Association Consortium. *Br. J. Cancer* **100**: 412–420.

145. Tseng, R.C., F.J. Hsieh, C.M. Shih, *et al.* 2009. Lung cancer susceptibility and prognosis associated with polymorphisms in the nonhomologous end-joining pathway genes: a multiple genotype-phenotype study. *Cancer* **115**: 2939–2948.

146. Cleary, S.P., W. Zhang, N.N. Di, *et al.* 2003. Heterozygosity for the BLM(Ash) mutation and cancer risk. *Cancer Res.* **63**: 1769–1771.

147. Berwick, M., J.M. Satagopan, L. Ben-Porat, *et al.* 2007. Genetic heterogeneity among Fanconi anemia heterozygotes and risk of cancer. *Cancer Res.* **67**: 9591–9596.

148. Mathew, C.G. 2006. Fanconi anaemia genes and susceptibility to cancer. *Oncogene* **25**: 5875–5884.

149. Dembowska-Baginska, B., D. Perek, A. Brozyna, *et al.* 2009. Non-Hodgkin lymphoma (NHL) in children with Nijmegen Breakage syndrome (NBS). *Pediatr. Blood Cancer* **52**: 186–190.

150. Kutler, D.I., A.D. Auerbach, J. Satagopan, *et al.* 2003. High incidence of head and neck squamous cell carcinoma in patients with Fanconi anemia. *Arch. Otolaryngol. Head Neck Surg.* **129**: 106–112.

151. Micol, R., S.L. Ben, F. Suarez, *et al.* 2011. Morbidity and mortality from ataxia-telangiectasia are associated with ATM genotype. *J. Allergy Clin. Immunol.* **128**: 382–389.

152. Pollard, J.M. & R.A. Gatti. 2009. Clinical radiation sensitivity with DNA repair disorders: an overview. *Int. J. Radiat. Oncol. Biol. Phys.* **74**: 1323–1331.

153. Shaheen, M., C. Allen, J.A. Nickoloff & R. Hromas. 2011. Synthetic lethality: exploiting the addiction of cancer to DNA repair. *Blood* **117**: 6074–6082.

154. Albert, M.H., A.R. Gennery, J. Greil, *et al.* 2010. Successful SCT for Nijmegen breakage syndrome. *Bone Marrow Transplant.* **45**: 622–626.

155. Eibel, H., U. Salzer & K. Warnatz. 2010. Common variable immunodeficiency at the end of a prospering decade: towards novel gene defects and beyond. *Curr. Opin. Allergy Clin. Immunol.* **10**: 526–533.

156. Ferreira, R.C., Q. Pan-Hammarstrom, R.R. Graham, *et al.* 2010. Association of IFIH1 and other autoimmunity risk alleles with selective IgA deficiency. *Nat. Genet.* **42**: 777–780.

157. Orange, J.S., J.T. Glessner, E. Resnick, *et al.* 2011. Genome-wide association identifies diverse causes of common variable immunodeficiency. *J. Allergy Clin. Immunol.* **127**: 1360–1367.

Ann. N.Y. Acad. Sci. ISSN 0077-8923

ANNALS OF THE NEW YORK ACADEMY OF SCIENCES
Issue: *The Year in Human and Medical Genetics: Inborn Errors of Immunity*

Inherited defects causing hemophagocytic lymphohistiocytic syndrome

Geneviève de Saint Basile,[1,2,3] Gaël Ménasché,[1,2] and Sylvain Latour[1,2]

[1]Institut National de la Santé et de la Recherche Médicale INSERM, U768, Paris, France. [2]Université Paris Descartes, Sorbone Paris Cité, Faculté de Médecine, Necker Hospital, 75015 Paris, France. [3]Centre d'Etudes des Déficits Immunitaires, Assistance Publique-Hôpitaux de Paris (AP-HP) Hôpital Necker, 75015 Paris, France

Address for correspondence: Geneviève de Saint Basile, INSERM U768-Hôpital Necker-Enfants Malades-Bâtiment Pasteur – Porte P2, 149 rue de Sèvres, F-75015 Paris, France. genevieve.de-saint-basile@inserm.fr

Hemophagocytic lymphohistiocytosis (HLH) manifests as the uncontrolled activation of T lymphocytes and macrophages infiltrating multiple organs. Molecular studies of individuals with HLH have demonstrated in most of these conditions a critical role of granule-dependent cytotoxic activity in the regulation of lymphocyte homeostasis, and have allowed the characterization of key effectors regulating cytotoxic granule release. The cytolytic process may now be considered a multistep process, including cell activation; the polarization of cytotoxic granules toward the conjugated target cell; the tethering, priming, and fusion of the cytotoxic granules with the plasma membrane; and the release of their contents (perforin and granzymes) into the intercellular cleft, leading to target cell death. Cytolytic cells have a second effector function involving the production of cytokines, principally γ-interferon, which is secreted independently of the exocytosis cytotoxic granule pathway. An analysis of the mechanisms underlying HLH has identified γ-interferon as a key cytokine inducing uncontrolled macrophage activation, and thus represents a potential therapeutic target.

Keywords: hemophagocytic; syndrome; cytotoxicity; apoptosis; γ-interferon; immune regulation

The signs of HLH

Hemophagocytic lymphohistiocytic syndrome (HLH) is characterized by a high, nonremitting fever associated with hepatosplenomegaly and neurological signs ranging from confusion and seizures to coma.[1] These clinical signs are associated with pancytopenia, including anemia and thrombocytopenia in particular, hepatitis with high levels of liver enzymes, hypertriglyceridemia, hypofibrinogenemia, hyponatremia, and high ferritin levels.[2] HLH results from an abnormal, uncontrolled immune response involving the continual expansion and activation of the polyclonal CD8$^+$ T cell, histiocyte, and macrophage populations responsible for the phagocytosis of blood cells (hemophagocytosis) in various organs (Fig. 1). The strong activation of histiocytes and macrophages results mostly from the release of IFN-γ from activated T cells. Activated CD8$^+$ T lymphocytes and macrophages infiltrate multiple organs, including the bone marrow, the lymph nodes, the spleen, the liver, and the brain.[3–5] Activated cells produce large amounts of a number of inflammatory cytokines including IFN-γ, interleukin 6 (IL-6), IL-18, and tumor necrosis factor alpha (TNF-α).[2,6] This "hypercytokinemia" probably contributes to the set of clinical and biological signs typical of HLH. In infiltrated tissues, these molecules induce cell necrosis and organ failure. HLH in humans can be triggered by infection, especially with viruses of the herpes group, such as Epstein–Barr virus (EBV) in particular. The signs of HLH result largely from the production of large amounts of cytokines by macrophages in response to the sustained activation of T lymphocytes. In humans, several inborn errors, most affecting the cytotoxic activity of lymphocytes, have been

doi: 10.1111/j.1749-6632.2011.06307.x

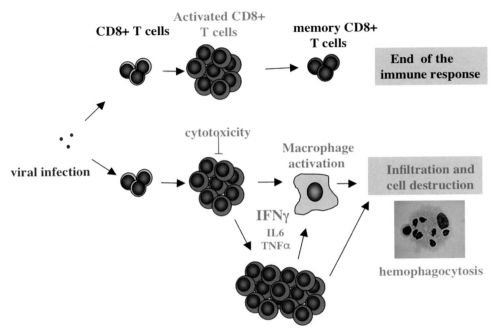

Figure 1. HLH pathophysiology. In a normal subject, viral infection leads to the stimulation of antigen-specific CD8[+] T cells, which transiently undergo clonal expansion, produce IFN-γ, and carry out cell-mediated cytolysis to eliminate the infected cells. Following pathogen clearance, most of the effector cells die, leaving a small number of memory CD8[+] T cells. Patients with HLH display uncontrolled strong expansion of antigen-specific effector T cells, which secrete high levels of IFN-γ, further activating macrophages. High levels of secretion are observed for inflammatory cytokines, including TNF, interleukin-6 (IL-6), and IL-18, leading to an uncontrolled systemic inflammatory response. Activated macrophages take up bystander hematopoietic cells by phagocytosis (a process known as hemophagocytosis). Activated lymphocytes and macrophages infiltrate various organs, resulting in massive tissue necrosis and organ failure. One of the principal mechanisms underlying HLH is a defect in the granule-dependent cytotoxic activity of lymphocytes, which fail to deplete antigen-presenting cells and infected cells, resulting in a sustained immune response.

shown to lead to the development of signs of HLH.

HLH may result from defects in lymphocyte cytotoxic activity

The granule-dependent cytotoxic activity of lymphocytes

Cytotoxic T lymphocytes (CTLs) and NK cells employ similar target cell killing methods, involving the polarized release of perforin and granzymes from lytic granules toward the target cell. CTLs recognizing a target cell form a transient CTL-target cell conjugate. A sequence of coordinated events then culminates in the killing of the target cell within 20–30 min (Fig. 2). These steps include the formation of an immunological synapse (IS) at the site of cell–cell contact, the movement of cytotoxic granules toward the microtubule organizing center

(MTOC), and the reorientation of the MTOC toward the target cell. Polarized lytic granules then dock at the plasma membrane, in a secretory domain adjacent to the area in which the T cell receptor and signaling molecules are found. The lytic granules are then released into an intercellular cleft that forms transiently between the two cells. The pore-forming activity of perforin allows proapoptotic granzymes to reach the cytoplasm of the target cell, where they cleave key substrates to initiate apoptotic cell death.[7]

Inherited defects of lymphocyte cytotoxic activity

Familial hemophagocytic lymphohistiocytosis (FHL) is inherited as an autosomal recessive disease[5] with an estimated incidence of 1/50,000 live births.[8] Overwhelming HLH is the distinguishing and only feature of this condition, no other

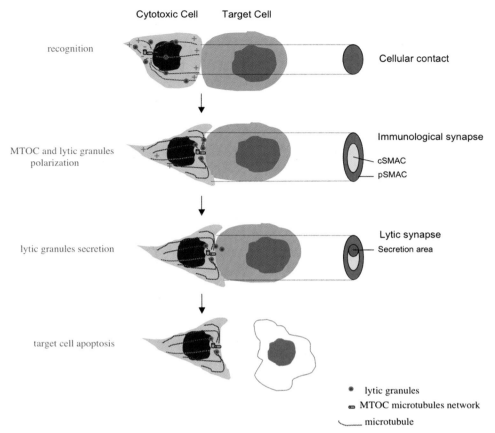

Figure 2. The granule-dependent cytotoxic activity of lymphocytes. Following cognate target cell recognition, the CTL forms a transient conjugate with the target cell. The CTL rapidly polarizes its MTOC and the microtubule network toward the contact site, where an IS is formed. This synapse is organized into a central supramolecular activation complex (cSMAC) (yellow) containing signaling molecules and the TCR, surrounded by a peripheral integrin-rich ring, the pSMAC (red). Cytotoxic granules move along microtubules toward the IS, where they dock and fuse with the plasma membrane to release their contents (perforin and granzymes) into a small secretory area (shown in gray). The release of perforin triggers granzyme entry into the target cell and the apoptosis of that cell.

associated signs being observed, by contrast to other inherited conditions causing HLH (Table 1). The symptoms of HLH usually become evident within the first six months of life and may, in rare cases, even develop *in utero*[9] or at birth.[10] However, familial forms with a later onset, at any time up to adulthood, have also been reported.[11,12] One of the characteristics of FHL is defective NK cell cytotoxicity.[13] Defects in T cell cytotoxicity induced by anti-CD3 are also observed in most cases.

FHL2 due to perforin deficiency

A deficiency of the cytolytic effector perforin (PRF1), which is present in cytotoxic granules, was

the first genetic defect causing FHL[14] to be identified (Table 1 and Fig. 1). Perforin deficiency accounts for about 30–35% of FHL cases. This molecule plays a crucial role in regulating the access of granzymes to the cytosol of the target cell, where they cleave key substrates to initiate apoptotic cell death. More than 70 different recessive mutations have been found in the perforin genes of FHL2 patients. Most of these mutations result in perforin protein being barely detectable or present in only small amounts in cytotoxic granules,[7,14,15] impairing cytotoxic activity. In addition, several unusual missense mutations of the perforin gene have been identified that specifically affect the processing or calcium-binding function of the protein.[16,17] In these cases, the mutated

Table 1. Genetic disorders associated with occurrence of HLH and their murine counterparts

	Gene locus	Hemophagocytic syndrome	Cytotoxic activity	Hypopigmentation	Mouse model
Familial hemophagocytic lymphohistiocytosis (FHL): gene					
FHL type 2: perforin	10q21-22	+	−	−	*Pko*
FHL type 3: Munc13-4	17q25	+	−	−	*Jinx*
FHL type 4: syntaxin 11	6q24	+	+/	−	
FHL type 5: Munc18-2	19q13	+	+/	−	
Griscelli syndrome type 2					
Rab27a	15q21	+	−	+	*Ashen*
Chediak–Higashi syndrome					
LYST	1q42-43	+	−	+[b]	*Beige*
X-linked lymphoproliferative syndrome					
XLP 1: SH2D1A (SAP)	Xq25	±	±[a]	−	*Sap*
XLP 2: XIAP	Xq25	+	+	−	*Xiap*

[a]Defect in SLAM-mediated toxicity.
[b]Abnormal granule size.

protein can be synthesized, packaged, and released in normal amounts, but this protein is not cytotoxic to the target cell. Missense mutations causing the partial impairment of perforin production and function have also been reported. They are frequently associated with atypical (mostly late-onset) HLH disease. One of these mutations, the Ala91Val substitution, is found at high frequency in healthy individuals (about 4–8%) and was initially considered to be a neutral polymorphism.[18] Nevertheless, additional studies demonstrated that the Ala91Val variant was associated with a partial loss (50%) of PRF1-dependent cytotoxicity, strongly suggesting that the Ala91Val allele conferred a predisposition to late-onset disease, the homozygous state being associated with susceptibility to lymphoma and the heterozygous state (with a second "null" perforin allele present) being associated with HLH.[19–21] Recent reports have also provided convincing evidence that temperature-sensitive mutations of the PFR1 gene may be associated with a late onset of FHL and predisposition to hematological malignancies (discussed below).[11] It has thus become clear that there is a genotype/phenotype correlation in perforin deficiency, with a correlation between age at onset and the residual functional activity of the protein. Phenotypes range from very early-onset HLH to predisposition to blood cancers.[11] However, expression levels may be further modified by the en-

vironment (i.e., infection with virus) or potential modifier genes.

Given the limited function of perforin in cytotoxic cells, the identification of perforin deficiency as a cause of HLH provided direct evidence of the importance of the cytotoxic function of T and NK cells in the control of lymphocyte homeostasis during immune responses. It also led to the identification of additional causes of genetically determined HLH, all of which were found to involve impairment of the granule-dependent cytotoxic function of lymphocytes.

FHL3 due to Munc13-4 deficiency

Munc13-4 deficiency was the second cause of FHL (FHL3) to be identified. It results from mutations in *UNC13D* (Table 1).[22] Munc13-4 deficiency accounts for 30–35% of FHL cases. The exocytosis of cytotoxic granules from Munc13-4–deficient T and NK lymphocytes is impaired, whereas other secretory pathways, including the polarized secretion of IFN-γ, function normally.[22–24] Munc13-4–deficient lymphocytes form normal stable conjugates with target cells and polarize the lytic machinery. However, Munc13-4 is required for the priming of lytic granules docked at the plasma membrane, probably through regulation of the interaction between the vesicle (v)- and target (t)-SNARE required for fusion of the granule with the plasma membrane.[22,25]

Indeed, the role of Munc13-4 in this step is probably similar to that of Munc13-1 as a priming factor for synaptic vesicle secretion at the neurological synapse.[26,27]

Munc13-4 production is detected in many tissues, but the phenotype of FHL3 patients is similar to that of patients with perforin deficiency. We cannot entirely exclude the possibility that subtle defects in these tissues induce mild clinical signs that have been missed to date, or that the functional characteristics of the Munc13-4–dependent exocytosis pathway may be strictly limited to the regulated secretory function of CTLs and NK cells.

FHL4 due to syntaxin 11 deficiency

Patients with FHL4 carry mutations in the syntaxin 11 gene (STX11),[28] encoding a member of the soluble *N*-ethylmaleimide-sensitive factor attachment protein receptor (t-SNARE) family involved in membrane fusion events (Table 1). Syntaxin 11 is phylogenetically related to the target membrane SNARE proteins (t-SNARE) syntaxins 1–4.[25,29] The selective pairing of t-SNARE, v-SNARE, and synaptosome-associated proteins (SNAP) from opposing membranes results in the formation of a very stable bundle of four parallel helices regulating membrane fusion during intracellular trafficking.[30] Syntaxin 11 is produced in large amounts in blood cells, including CTLs, NK cells, and myeloid cells in particular.[28,31,32] All the deleterious mutations in STX11 reported in FHL4 patients to date have been null mutations. Most were identified in Turkish and Kurdish populations, in which they account for about 20% of FHL cases.[31] The identification of syntaxin 11 deficiency as a cause of FHL led to investigations of the role of this member of the SNARE family in cytotoxic granule exocytosis. Defects were found in the cytotoxic activity of NK cells from patients with FHL4, but it was more difficult to demonstrate any impairment of the cytotoxic activity of syntaxin 11-deficient CTLs, at least by standard techniques. Stimulation with IL-2 partly restores cytotoxic activity stimulation.[32,33] Syntaxin 11 is present not only in lymphocytes, but also in monocytes and macrophages, in which it is produced in large amounts. This led to the suggestion that syntaxin 11 is also involved in downregulating the phagocytic activity of macrophages.[34] Further studies are required to assess the significance of this observation and to clarify the potential contribution of syntaxin 11-deficient monocytes to the develop-

ment of immune deregulation in FHL4 patients. However, the FHL4 phenotype is not significantly different from those of FHL2 or FHL3.

Thus, syntaxin 11 is thought to be another key effector of the cytotoxic machinery required for the release of the contents of cytotoxic granules, probably through involvement in the regulation of membrane fusion events.[35] The precise step of the cytotoxic pathway regulated by syntaxin 11 remains to be determined, although a role in the fusion of cytotoxic granules to the plasma membrane at the immunological synapse is thought to be the most likely.

FHL5 due to Munc18-2 deficiency

The most recently identified cause of FHL, FHL5, is a deficiency of the syntaxin-binding–protein-2 (*STXBP2*) gene, which encodes Munc18-2.[33,36] STXBP2/Munc18-2 belongs to the SM family of fusion accessory proteins. These proteins are partners of SNARE protein, playing a complementary role in membrane fusion.[37,38] Like syntaxin 11, STXBP2/Munc18-2 is widely expressed. The various mutations identified in this gene affect protein stability.[33,36] These mutations seems to be correlated with phenotype, in terms of age at onset and disease severity.[33] Syntaxin 11 levels are very low in STXBP2/Munc18-2–deficient lymphoblasts and these two proteins can be coimmunoprecipitated. Thus, syntaxin 11 is probably the main partner of Munc18-2 in lymphocytes, requiring Munc18-2 for stable expression. Consistent with the pathophysiological features of FHL, Munc18-2–deficient NK cells have impaired cytotoxic activity that is partially restored by IL2 stimulation, as previously reported for syntaxin 11-deficient NK cells.[33,36] A role for Munc18-2 in late stages of the exocytosis pathway is supported by the observation that the perforin-containing granules of Munc18-2–deficient NK cells are normally polarized toward cognate target cells, despite the impairment of exocytosis preventing them from releasing their contents.[33] Thus, the same defective cytotoxic phenotype characterizes both syntaxin 11 and STXBP2 deficiencies, providing support for the existence of a functional interaction between these two proteins in the degranulation process.

The role of Munc18 protein in vesicle exocytosis has been deduced principally through studies of STXBP1/Munc18-1 in neurons, in which the elimination of this protein leads to a complete loss of neurotransmitter secretion in mice.[39,40] The identification of Munc18-2 deficiency as the cause of FHL5 strongly suggests that the STXBP2–syntaxin 11 complex at the IS of a cytotoxic cell conjugated with its target may play a role similar to that of the STXBP1-syntaxin 1 complex at the neurological synapse, by regulating granule docking and the initiation of SNARE complex formation upstream from the priming step.

HLH associated with pigmentary dilution

The same signs of HLH observed in FHL are also associated with pigmentary dilution in two inherited conditions: type 2 Griscelli syndrome (GS2) and Chediak-Higashi syndrome (CHS) (Table 1).

GS2 results from biallelic mutations in the gene encoding Rab27a, a ubiquitous small GTP-binding GTPase protein[41] (Table 1). Nonsense, frameshift, and missense mutations in Rab27a have been characterized in more than 100 independent patients. Rab27a-deficient NK cells and CTLs display impairment of the mediated exocytosis of cytotoxic granules, although polarization is preserved. Electron microscopy has shown that, in the absence of Rab27a, cytotoxic granules cannot reach the IS to dock with the plasma membrane.[42] Munc13-4 interacts with Rab27a in cytotoxic cells.[43] This molecular interaction is probably involved in co-ordination of the final step of exocytosis, between the docking and priming of lytic granules. Pigmentary dilution in GS2 can be accounted for by defects in the release of the content of melanosomes from melanocyte dendrites. In melanocytes, Rab27a associates with melanophilin, which in turn interacts with the molecular motor protein myosin-Va. This tripartite complex (Rab27a-melanophilin-myosin-Va) links the melanosomes to the actin network, facilitating their targeting to the tips of melanocyte dendrites, from whence they can be transferred to adjacent keratinocytes.[44] A deficiency of any of these three proteins has been shown to impair melanosome transport and to result in the same hypopigmentation phenotype.[45] Such deficiencies cause the following diseases: GS1 (myosin-Va defect), GS2 (Rab27a defect), and GS3 (melanophilin defect). However, only Rab27a plays a crucial role in the cytotoxic machinery; deficiencies in this protein thus result in an HLH immune phenotype.

CHS (Table 1) was the first condition characterized by pigmentation dilution, defective T and NK lymphocyte cytotoxic activity, and the occurrence of HLH of relatively late-onset (2–10 years of age).[45,46] One particularly striking phenotypic feature of this autosomal recessive condition is the presence of giant intracytoplasmic lysosomal structures in all granulated cells, including hematopoietic cells and melanocytes. The cytotoxic granules of cytotoxic cells are also enlarged, and they do not release their content at the IS, despite normal polarization upon activation. Progressive primary neurological disease is another hallmark of CHS.[47] Mutations in *CHS1/LYST*, encoding LYST, a huge (425 kDa) ubiquitous cytosolic protein, account for this disease (Table 1).[48,49] However, the precise function of LYST remains unknown, although this protein is thought to act as a vesicle trafficking regulatory protein, through interactions in which it binds to other protein partners.[50,51]

HLH and normal cytotoxic activity

Several forms of HLH are characterized by normal granule exocytosis and normal cytolytic granule activity. These forms (unlike FHL, GS2, and CHS) are characterized by normal NK cell cytotoxicity against K562 target cells and the induction of normal T cell cytotoxicity by anti-CD3 antibody. Disease onset may occur from the age of one year into adulthood, and is frequently triggered by EBV infection. The best characterized form is X-linked lymphoproliferative syndrome (XLP).

XLP syndrome

XLP is a very rare immunodeficiency with an estimated incidence of 1/1,000,000 live births. This condition is characterized principally by extreme vulnerability to EBV infection, which triggers HLH (also known as virus-associated hemophagocytic syndrome or fulminant mononucleosis) and/or malignant lymphoproliferation.[52] Two genetic causes of XLP have been identified. XLP type 1 (XLP-1) is caused by hemizygous mutations in the *SH2D1A* gene encoding the signaling lymphocyte activation molecule (SLAM)–associated protein (SAP),[53–55] whereas hemizygous mutations in the gene encoding the X-linked inhibitor of apoptosis (XIAP) (also known as *BIRC4*) are responsible for XLP type 2.[56] The *SH2D1A* and *XIAP* genes are located in close proximity at the same gene locus (in Xq25); they are separated by only 0.4 Mb.

HLH is the most frequent and severe clinical outcome observed in XLP-1 and XLP-2 patients, and EBV infection is a common trigger.[57–60] However, some differences in the clinical presentation of HLH have been reported between XLP-1 and XLP-2.[59] HLH is more severe—often with a lethal outcome—in XLP-1, whereas recurrent splenomegaly associated with cytopenia and fever is found in XLP-2 patients (even in the absence of EBV infection), potentially corresponding to a minimal form of HLH. Full-blown HLH can develop in the absence of EBV infection, and this occurs more frequently in XLP-2.[61] In addition to HLH, patients with XLP display other clinical phenotypes, which can be used to distinguish between XLP-1 and XLP-2.[59] Hypogammaglobulinemia is observed in both XLP-1 (65%) and XLP-2 (30%). Predisposition to lymphoma is associated only with XLP-1 (30%), and chronic hemorrhagic colitis is found only in patients with XLP-2 (20%).

XLP-1 due to SAP deficiency

The product of the *SH2D1A* gene, SAP, is a small adaptor protein produced exclusively in T, NK, and NKT cells. More than 80 mutations in the *SH2D1A* gene causing XLP-1 have been identified, including missense, nonsense, and splice-site mutations, and micro- and macrodeletions. Most of the missense mutations markedly decrease the stability of the SAP protein and impair its adaptor function. No correlation has been found between *SH2D1A* gene mutations and XLP-1 clinical phenotypes.

SAP consists of a unique SH2 domain fused to a short *C*-terminal tail. SAP uses its SH2 domain to bind with high affinity and specificity to immunoreceptor tyrosine-based switch motifs (ITSM) present in the cytoplasmic domains of SLAM receptors (SLAM-R).[62,63] The SLAM-R family includes SLAM, 2B4, NTB-A, CD84, Ly-9, and CRACC, all of which have a similar structural organization, consisting of an extracellular domain with two or four immunoglobulin (Ig)–like domains, a single transmembrane portion, and an intracytoplasmic tail with ITSMs. SLAM-R are involved in the regulation of immunity in the context of homotypic cell–cell interactions, with the exception of 2B4, which binds to CD48. SAP couples SLAM-family receptors to downstream signaling pathways through the recruitment and activation of the tyrosine kinase Fyn, enabling SLAM receptors to transmit various activating or regulatory signals[63,64] (Fig. 3). It has also been suggested that SAP functions as a competitor or regulator of SH2-containing molecules, binding to SLAM receptors.[63] Multiple cellular defects have been documented in SAP-deficient humans and mice, including altered CD8[+] T cell and NK cell cytotoxic responses, CD4[+] T helper cell cytokine production and function, a blockade of CD1d-restricted NKT cell development, defective antibody production associated with small numbers of switched memory B cells, and defects in germinal center formation.[62,65] These studies support the notion that the immune dysfunctions seen in patients with SAP deficiency result mostly from changes to signal transduction via SLAM-family receptors.

Immune defects leading to HLH and lymphomas in XLP-1 patients are thought to result principally from SLAM-R dysfunction, leading to defects in cytotoxicity (Fig. 3). In NK cells and CD8[+] T cells, SLAM-R are activating or costimulating receptors for cytotoxic function. Studies of human NK and CD8[+] T cells from XLP-1 patients have shown that, in the absence of SAP, the activating function of SLAM-R, 2B4, and NTB-A shifts toward the inhibition of cell-mediated cytotoxicity to EBV-infected B cells.[66–69] This inhibition is dependent on SLAM ligand expression by the target cells, and the recognition and killing of these cells is restored by blocking interactions with SLAM receptors.[70] Similar observations have been reported for SAP-deficient mice,[71] which develop clinical signs of HLH when infected with LCMV and MHV-68.[72] A recent study showed that cytotoxicity is further reduced in mice lacking the three SAP family adaptors: SAP, EAT-2, and ERT.[65] In the absence of these three adaptors, 2B4, NTB-A, Ly-9, CD84, and CRACC become inhibitory receptors in NK cells, repressing activating receptors such as NKG2D and CD16. The biochemical mechanism underlying this inhibition remains unclear, but it seems to involve inositol–phosphatase SHIP-1, which associates with SLAM-R.[65]

A proapoptotic role for SAP in T cells has also recently been suggested.[73] The induction of cell death via T cell receptor (TCR) activation is defective in the T cells of XLP-1 patients, although this defect can be overcome by increasing the strength of TCR activation. This pathway involves the SLAM receptor NTB-A. The contribution of this defect to the immune deregulation observed in response to EBV infection in XLP-1 patients remains unclear.

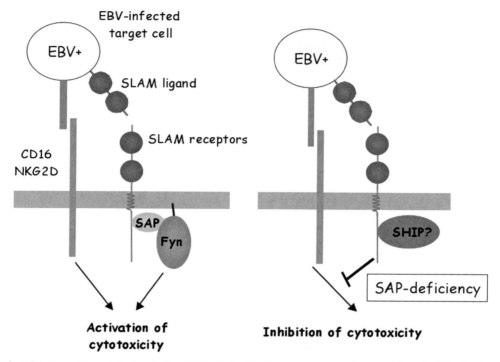

Figure 3. Inhibition of the cytotoxic activity of NK cells by SLAM receptors in the absence of SAP. In NK cells, the adaptor molecule SAP mediates activating signals from SLAM family receptors by recruiting and activating the protein tyrosine kinase Fyn. These signals mediate the cytotoxic activity of NK cells, by acting in synergy with signals emanating from activating NK cell receptors, such as NKG2D and CD16. SLAM receptors are triggered by SLAM ligands, which are expressed on EBV-infected B cells. The expression of the ligands of NKG2D on infected cells is induced by the viral infection. CD16 binds to the Fc portion of IgG antibodies raised against infected cells. In the absence of SAP, SLAM receptors deliver signals that inhibit activating NK cell receptors, such as NKG2D and CD16. The mechanism of inhibition remains poorly understood, but may involve the inhibitory molecule SHIP, which is known to associate with SLAM receptors.

Another feature of XLP-1 is the almost complete absence of CD1d-restricted invariant NKT lymphocytes.[74,75] Studies in mice have shown that, in the absence of SAP, the development of NKT cells is blocked early, at the positive selection step in the thymus.[74] NKT cells have been implicated in the initiation and regulation of various immune responses. It is therefore also possible that their absence contributes to the susceptibility to EBV of XLP-1 patients.[76,77]

XLP-2 due to XIAP deficiency

XIAP mutations were originally identified in a cohort of patients with clinical XLP without identified mutations in *SH2D1A* and with normal SAP levels.[56] More than 20 mutations in *XIAP* have been described, including missense, nonsense, and frameshift mutations and deletions.[56,59–61] XIAP belongs to the inhibitors of apoptosis proteins (IAP)

family and is known to be a potent physiological inhibitor of caspases 3, 7, and 9.[78] *XIAP* is ubiquitously expressed. In proliferating human T cells, XIAP binds to and inhibits caspases 3 and 7.[79] In addition to its antiapoptotic function, XIAP is also involved in multiple signaling pathways, including that for copper metabolism, activation of the NF-κB and MAP kinase pathways and signal transduction via the TGF-β receptor, the BMP receptor, and the intracellular pattern recognition receptor NOD2.[80,81] Consistent with the antiapoptotic role of XIAP, human XIAP–deficient lymphocytes display enhanced activation-induced cell death (AICD).[56,61] XLP-2 patients do not display lymphopenia, but XIAP probably contributes to their survival, as a nonrandom X-chromosome inactivation is observed in the leukocytes of female carriers of *XIAP* mutations, with cells preferentially expressing the wild-type *XIAP* allele.[56,61] XIAP-deficient mice were initially reported to have no major phenotypic abnormalities, and there is currently no evidence to suggest that they could constitute a valid model for XLP-2.[82,83]

The physiopathology of HLH in XLP-2 is not understood and does not currently seem to be consistent with the paradigm of HLH resulting from defects in the cytotoxic pathway. Indeed, NK cells from XIAP-deficient patients display normal 2B4-mediated cytotoxicity with anti-2B4 antibodies, and their overall cytotoxic function is normal when assessed with K562 target cells.[56,61] Cytotoxicity and the degranulation of CD8$^+$ T cells in response to anti-CD3 antibodies are also normal in the absence of XIAP (S. Latour, unpublished observations). Further studies are required to determine the precise mechanisms underlying HLH in patients with XIAP deficiency.

Studies of murine models of HLH

Studies of animal models of HLH have contributed to our understanding of the link between the genetic defects of the cytotoxic machinery and the aberrant immune response observed in patients with HLH (Table 1 and Fig. 1). LCMV (lymphocytic choriomeningitis virus)–infected perforin-deficient, Unc13-deficient (the mouse ortholog of human Munc13-4), SAP-deficient, and Rab27a-deficient mice develop the body temperature changes, splenomegaly, pancytopenia, hypercytokinemia, and histological features characteristic of HLH.[84–87] These LCMV-infected, cytotoxicity-deficient mice may therefore be considered to be reliable models of human HLH. Studies in perforin-deficient mice have shown that CD8$^+$ T cells and γ-interferon production play a key role in HLH pathogenesis, because HLH was prevented in these studies only by the administration of anti-CD8 or the neutralization of γ-interferon, whereas antibodies against CD4 and the neutralization of other inflammatory cytokines, including TNF-α, had no effect.[85] These findings are consistent with the larger numbers of activated CD8$^+$ T effector cells in the blood and tissues of HLH patients and the much higher serum concentrations of γ-interferon in patients with inherited and acquired HLH during active disease[2,88] (and our own unpublished observations). Thus, the pathogenesis of HLH in patients with impaired cytotoxicity is probably based on the inability of CD8$^+$ T cytotoxic effector cells

to eliminate the infecting pathogen (Fig. 1). The infected cells are recognized, leading to cytotoxic cell activation and clonal expansion, but the resulting cytotoxic cell population fails to kill the infected, antigen-presenting cells and to remove the source of stimulation. The ever-expanding population of cytotoxic lymphocytes produces large quantities of cytokines, such as γ-interferon, which sustain macrophage activation. There is a striking resemblance between the biological changes induced by inflammatory cytokines, such as TNF-α in particular, and the clinical and laboratory findings typical of HLH.[2]

Future directions

Defective cytotoxic function and immune surveillance

Evidence for a link between functional defects in granule-dependent cytotoxicity and cancer susceptibility has been provided by analyses of the mouse model of perforin deficiency, which is particularly susceptible to the development of spontaneous B cell lymphomas.[89,90] In humans, the role of perforin, and of granule-dependent lymphocyte cytotoxicity in general, in controlling susceptibility to cancer remains difficult to assess. In recent years, several correlative studies have attempted to demonstrate such a link.[20,91–93] However, given the small size of the cohorts of patients screened in these studies, these results should be interpreted with caution. The most compelling evidence currently available for a link between perforin and immune surveillance in humans is the recent observation that temperature-sensitive perforin missense mutations are frequently inherited in patients with late-onset FHL and a high level of susceptibility to hematological malignancies. Thus, by contrast to what is observed with true null mutations, residual levels of protein activity at permissive temperature are closely correlated with age at onset of HLH and the occurrence of lymphoma or leukemia.[11] Low levels of perforin activity probably enable patients to survive long enough without developing HLH to unmask their predisposition to cancer.

By extrapolation, we can suggest that hypomorphic mutations may also be associated with a higher susceptibility to lymphomagenesis in other genetically determined defects of the cytotoxic activity of lymphocytes.

Another important issue is the minimal level of cytotoxic activity required to maintain immune homeostasis and prevent predisposition to cancer. Clearly, a single normal perforin allele expressed in the parents of children with inherited HLH is sufficient to maintain good health. None of these obligate carriers has ever been reported to have a higher predisposition to cancers, although no exhaustive studies have yet been carried out on this population.

Alternative treatment based on pathophysiology

A γ-interferon blockade not only prevents HLH, but also has a therapeutic effect in experimental HLH.[94] The therapeutic administration of an anti-γ-interferon antibody has been shown to induce recovery from HLH in two different murine models of human HLH (perforin-deficient and Rab27a-deficient mice, both infected with LCMV). Recovery was demonstrated by the higher levels of survival in perforin-deficient mice and a moderation of body temperature changes, the correction of blood cytopenia, lower cytokinemia, the restoration of splenic architecture, and lower levels of hemophagocytosis in the liver in both murine models. The neutralization of γ-interferon or of the γ-interferon receptor signaling pathway could therefore be considered in the future as a potential alternative treatment for alleviating the clinical signs of HLH in humans. This treatment may be particularly beneficial in patients with inherited HLH, as the drugs currently used to treat HLH, such as etoposide[95] and antithymoglobulin agents[96] are potentially toxic and have a much stronger immunosuppressive effect than a transient γ-interferon blockade. Another potential advantage of a γ-interferon blockade for managing inherited HLH would be the possibility of increasing engraftment following hematopoietic stem cell transplantation, because γ-interferon has a myelosuppressive effect. The neutralization of γ-interferon might also be an efficient and safe way to treat patients with acquired HLH, provided that the T cell activation trigger is also amenable to therapy.

Acknowledgments

This work was supported by the French National Institute for Health (INSERM), the French National Research Agency (ANR/Genopath), the European Research Council (ERC), and the Imagine Foundation.

Conflicts of interest

The authors declare no conflicts of interest.

References

1. Henter, J.I., G. Elinder & A. Ost. 1991. Diagnostic guidelines for hemophagocytic lymphohistiocytosis. The FHL Study Group of the Histiocyte Society. *Semin. Oncol.* **18:** 29–33.
2. Henter, J.I., G. Elinder, O. Soder, *et al.* 1991. Hypercytokinemia in familial hemophagocytic lymphohistiocytosis. *Blood* **78:** 2918–2922.
3. Billiau, A.D., T. Roskams, R. Van Damme-Lombaerts, *et al.* 2005. Macrophage activation syndrome: characteristic findings on liver biopsy illustrating the key role of activated, IFN-gamma-producing lymphocytes and IL-6- and TNF-alpha-producing macrophages. *Blood* **105:** 1648–1651.
4. Henter, J.I., M. Arico, G. Elinder, *et al.* 1998. Familial hemophagocytic lymphohistiocytosis: primary hemophagocytic lymphohistiocytosis. *Hematol. Oncol. Clin. N. Am.* **12:** 417–433.
5. Farquhar, J. & A. Claireaux. 1952. Familial haemophagocytic reticulosis. *Arch. Dis. Child* **27:** 519–525.
6. Osugi, Y., J. Hara, S. Tagawa, *et al.* 1997. Cytokine production regulating Th1 and Th2 cytokines in hemophagocytic lymphohistiocytosis. *Blood* **89:** 4100–4103.
7. Voskoboinik, I., M.J. Smyth & J.A. Trapani. 2006. Perforin-mediated target-cell death and immune homeostasis. *Nat. Rev. Immunol.* **6:** 940–952.
8. Henter, J.I., G. Elinder, O. Soder & A. Ost. 1991. Incidence in Sweden and clinical features of familial hemophagocytic lymphohistiocytosis diagnostic guidelines for hemophagocytic lymphohistiocytosis. The FHL Study Group of the Histiocyte Society. *Acta. Paediatr. Scand.* **80:** 428–435.
9. Bechara, E., F. Dijoud, G. de Saint Basile, *et al.* 2011. Hemophagocytic lymphohistiocytosis with Munc13-4 mutation: a cause of recurrent fatal hydrops fetalis. *Pediatrics* **128:** e251–e254.
10. Lipton, J.M., S. Westra, C.E. Haverty, *et al.* 2004. Case records of the Massachusetts General Hospital. Weekly clinicopathological exercises: case 28-2004. Newborn twins with thrombocytopenia, coagulation defects, and hepatosplenomegaly. *N. Engl. J. Med.* **351:** 1120–1130.
11. Chia, J., K.P. Yeo, J.C. Whisstock, *et al.* 2009. Temperature sensitivity of human perforin mutants unmasks subtotal loss of cytotoxicity, delayed FHL, and a predisposition to cancer. *Proc. Natl. Acad. Sci. USA* **106:** 9809–9814.
12. Rohr, J., K. Beutel, A. Maul-Pavicic, *et al.* 2010. Atypical familial hemophagocytic lymphohistiocytosis due to mutations in UNC13D and STXBP2 overlaps with primary immunodeficiency diseases. *Haematologica* **95:** 2080–2087.
13. Schneider, E.M., I. Lorenz, M. Muller-Rosenberger, *et al.* 2002. Hemophagocytic lymphohistiocytosis is associated with deficiencies of cellular cytolysis but normal expression of transcripts relevant to killer-cell-induced apoptosis. *Blood* **100:** 2891–2898.

14. Stepp, S., R. Dufourcq-Lagelouse, F. Le Deist, *et al.* 1999. Perforin gene defects in familial hemophagocytic lymphohistiocytosis. *Science* **286:** 1957–1959.

15. Feldmann, J., F. Le Deist, M. Ouachee-Chardin, *et al.* 2002. Functional consequences of perforin gene mutations in 22 patients with familial haemophagocytic lymphohistiocytosis. *Br. J. Haematol.* **117:** 965–972.

16. Voskoboinik, I., M.C. Thia, A. De Bono, *et al.* 2004. The functional basis for hemophagocytic lymphohistiocytosis in a patient with co-inherited missense mutations in the perforin (PFN1) gene. *J. Exp. Med.* **200:** 811–816.

17. Feldmann, J., G. Menasche, I. Callebaut, *et al.* 2005. Severe and progressive encephalitis as a presenting manifestation of a novel missense perforin mutation and impaired cytolytic activity. *Blood* **105:** 2658–2663.

18. Zur Stadt, U., K. Beutel, B. Weber, *et al.* 2004. A91V is a polymorphism in the perforin gene not causative of an FHLH phenotype. *Blood* **104:** 1909; author reply 1910.

19. Trambas, C., F. Gallo, D. Pende, *et al.* 2005. A single amino acid change, A91V, leads to conformational changes that can impair processing to the active form of perforin. *Blood* **106:** 932–937.

20. Santoro, A., S. Cannella, A. Trizzino, *et al.* 2005. A single amino acid change A91V in perforin: a novel, frequent predisposing factor to childhood acute lymphoblastic leukemia? *Haematologica* **90:** 697–698.

21. Voskoboinik, I., V.R. Sutton, A. Ciccone, *et al.* 2007. Perforin activity and immune homeostasis: the common A91V polymorphism in perforin results in both presynaptic and postsynaptic defects in function. *Blood* **110:** 1184–1190.

22. Feldmann, J., I. Callebaut, G. Raposo, *et al.* 2003. Munc13-4 is essential for cytolytic granules fusion and is mutated in a form of familial hemophagocytic lymphohistiocytosis (FHL3). *Cell* **115:** 461–473.

23. Ueda, I., E. Ishii, A. Morimoto, *et al.* 2006. Correlation between phenotypic heterogeneity and gene mutational characteristics in familial hemophagocytic lymphohistiocytosis (FHL). *Pediatr. Blood Can.* **46:** 482–488.

24. Marcenaro, S., F. Gallo, S. Martini, *et al.* 2006. Analysis of natural killer-cell function in familial hemophagocytic lymphohistiocytosis (FHL): defective CD107a surface expression heralds Munc13-4 defect and discriminates between genetic subtypes of the disease. *Blood* **108:** 2316–2323.

25. Hong, W. 2005. Cytotoxic T lymphocyte exocytosis: bring on the SNAREs! *Trends Cell Biol.* **15:** 644–650.

26. Brose, N., K. Hofmann, Y. Hata & T.C. Sudhof. 1995. Mammalian homologues of *Caenorhabditis elegans unc-13* gene define novel family of C2-domain proteins. *J. Biol. Chem.* **270:** 25273–25280.

27. Brose, N., C. Rosenmund & J. Rettig. 2000. Regulation of transmitter release by Unc-13 and its homologues. *Curr. Opin. Neurobiol.* **10:** 303–311.

28. zur Stadt, U., S. Schmidt, B. Kasper, *et al.* 2005. Linkage of familial hemophagocytic lymphohistiocytosis (FHL) type-4 to chromosome 6q24 and identification of mutations in syntaxin 11. *Hum. Mol. Genet.* **14:** 827–834.

29. Prekeris, R., J. Klumperman & R.H. Scheller. 2000. Syntaxin 11 is an atypical SNARE abundant in the immune system. *Eur. J. Cell. Biol.* **79:** 771–780.

30. Jahn, R. & R.H. Scheller. 2006. SNAREs—engines for membrane fusion. *Nat. Rev. Mol. Cell. Biol.* **7:** 631–643.

31. Zur Stadt, U., K. Beutel, S. Kolberg, *et al.* 2006. Mutation spectrum in children with primary hemophagocytic lymphohistiocytosis: molecular and functional analyses of PRF1, UNC13D, STX11, and RAB27A. *Hum. Mutat.* **27:** 62–68.

32. Bryceson, Y.T., E. Rudd, C. Zheng, *et al.* 2007. Defective cytotoxic lymphocyte degranulation in syntaxin-11 deficient familial hemophagocytic lymphohistiocytosis 4 (FHL4) patients. *Blood* **110:** 1906–1915.

33. Cote, M., M.M. Menager, A. Burgess, *et al.* 2009. Munc18-2 deficiency causes familial hemophagocytic lymphohistiocytosis type 5 and impairs cytotoxic granule exocytosis in patient NK cells. *J. Clin. Invest.* **119:** 3765–3773.

34. Zhang, S., D. Ma, X. Wang, *et al.* 2008. Syntaxin-11 is expressed in primary human monocytes/macrophages and acts as a negative regulator of macrophage engulfment of apoptotic cells and IgG-opsonized target cells. *Br. J. Haematol.* **142:** 469–479.

35. Arneson, L.N., A. Brickshawana, C.M. Segovis, *et al.* 2007. Cutting edge: syntaxin 11 regulates lymphocyte-mediated secretion and cytotoxicity. *J. Immunol.* **179:** 3397–3401.

36. zur Stadt, U., J. Rohr, W. Seifert, *et al.* 2009. Familial hemophagocytic lymphohistiocytosis type 5 (FHL-5) is caused by mutations in Munc18-2 and impaired binding to syntaxin 11. *Am. J. Hum. Genet.* **85:** 482–492.

37. Toonen, R.F. & M. Verhage. 2003. Vesicle trafficking: pleasure and pain from SM genes. *Trends Cell. Biol.* **13:** 177–186.

38. Sudhof, T.C. & J.E. Rothman. 2009. Membrane fusion: grappling with SNARE and SM proteins. *Science* **323:** 474–477.

39. Verhage, M., A.S. Maia, J.J. Plomp, *et al.* 2000. Synaptic assembly of the brain in the absence of neurotransmitter secretion. *Science* **287:** 864–869.

40. Toonen, R.F. & M. Verhage. 2007. Munc18-1 in secretion: lonely Munc joins SNARE team and takes control. *Trends Neurosci.* **30:** 564–572.

41. Ménasché, G., E. Pastural, J. Feldmann, *et al.* 2000. Mutations in RAB27A cause Griscelli syndrome associated with hemophagocytic syndrome. *Nat. Genet.* **25:** 173–176.

42. Stinchcombe, J.C., D.C. Barral, E.H. Mules, *et al.* 2001. Rab27a is required for regulated secretion in cytotoxic t lymphocytes. *J. Cell. Biol.* **152:** 825–834.

43. Menager, M.M., G. Menasche, M. Romao, *et al.* 2007. Secretory cytotoxic granule maturation and exocytosis require the effector protein hMunc13-4. *Nat. Immunol.* **8:** 257–267.

44. Wu, X.S., K. Rao, H. Zhang, *et al.* 2002. Identification of an organelle receptor for myosin-Va. *Nat. Cell. Biol.* **4:** 271–278.

45. Menasche, G., J. Feldmann, A. Fischer & G. de Saint Basile. 2005. Primary hemophagocytic syndromes point to a direct link between lymphocyte cytotoxicity and homeostasis. *Immunol. Rev.* **203:** 165–179.

46. Stinchcombe, J., G. Bossi & G.M. Griffiths. 2004. Linking albinism and immunity: the secrets of secretory lysosomes. *Science* **305:** 55–59.

47. Tardieu, M., C. Lacroix, B. Neven, *et al.* 2005. Progressive neurologic dysfunctions 20 years after allogeneic bone marrow transplantation for Chediak-Higashi syndrome. *Blood* **106:** 40–42.

48. Nagle, D.L., A.M. Karim, E.A. Woolf, *et al.* 1996. Identification and mutation analysis of the complete gene for Chediak–Higashi syndrome. *Nat. Genet.* **14:** 307–311.

49. Barbosa, M.D.F.S., Q.A. Nguyen, V.T. Tchernev, *et al.* 1996. Identification of the homologous beige and Chediak–Higashi syndrome genes. *Nature* **382:** 262–265.

50. Gebauer, D., J. Li, G. Jogl, *et al.* 2004. Crystal structure of the PH-BEACH domains of human LRBA/BGL. *Biochemistry* **43:** 14873–14880.

51. Jogl, G., Y. Shen, D. Gebauer, *et al.* 2002. Crystal structure of the BEACH domain reveals an unusual fold and extensive association with a novel PH domain. *EMBO J.* **21:** 4785–4795.

52. Purtilo, D.T., C.K. Cassel, J.P. Yang & R. Harper. 1975. X-linked recessive progressive combined variable immunodeficiency (Duncan's disease). *Lancet* **1:** 935–940.

53. Coffey, A.J., R.A. Brooksbank, O. Brandau, *et al.* 1998. Host response to EBV infection in X-linked lymphoproliferative disease results from mutations in an SH2-domain encoding gene [see comments]. *Nat. Genet.* **20:** 129–135.

54. Nichols, K.E., D.P. Harkin, S. Levitz, *et al.* 1998. Inactivating mutations in an SH2 domain-encoding gene in X-linked lymphoproliferative syndrome. *Proc. Natl. Acad. Sci. USA* **95:** 13765–13770.

55. Sayos, J., C. Wu, M. Morra, *et al.* 1998. The X-linked lymphoproliferative-disease gene product SAP regulates signals induced through the co-receptor SLAM. *Nature* **395:** 462–469.

56. Rigaud, S., M.C. Fondaneche, N. Lambert, *et al.* 2006. XIAP deficiency in humans causes an X-linked lymphoproliferative syndrome. *Nature* **444:** 110–114.

57. Seemayer, T.A., T.G. Gross, R.M. Egeler, *et al.* 1995. X-linked lymphoproliferative disease: twenty-five years after the discovery. *Pediatr. Res.* **38:** 471–478.

58. Gaspar, H.B., R. Sharifi, K.C. Gilmour & A.J. Thrasher. 2002. X-linked lymphoproliferative disease: clinical, diagnostic and molecular perspective. *Br. J. Haematol.* **119:** 585–595.

59. Pachlopnik Schmid, J., D. Canioni, D. Moshous, *et al.* 2011. Clinical similarities and differences of patients with X-linked lymphoproliferative syndrome type 1 (XLP-1/SAP deficiency) versus type 2 (XLP-2/XIAP deficiency). *Blood* **117:** 1522–1529.

60. Horn, P.C., B.H. Belohradsky, C. Urban, *et al.* 2011. Two new families with X-linked inhibitor of apoptosis deficiency and a review of all 26 published cases. *J. Allergy. Clin. Immunol.* **127:** 544–546.

61. Marsh, R.A., L. Madden, B.J. Kitchen, *et al.* 2010. XIAP deficiency: a unique primary immunodeficiency best classified as X-linked familial hemophagocytic lymphohistiocytosis and not as X-linked lymphoproliferative disease. *Blood* **7:** 1079–1082.

62. Schwartzberg, P.L., K.L. Mueller, H. Qi & J.L. Cannons. 2009. SLAM receptors and SAP influence lymphocyte interactions, development and function. *Nat. Rev. Immunol.* **9:** 39–46.

63. Veillette, A., Z. Dong, L.A. Perez-Quintero, *et al.* 2009. Importance and mechanism of 'switch' function of SAP family adapters. *Immunol. Rev.* **232:** 229–239.

64. Latour, S., G. Gish, C.D. Helgason, *et al.* 2001. Regulation of SLAM-mediated signal transduction by SAP, the X-linked lymphoproliferative gene product. *Nat. Immunol.* **2:** 681–690.

65. Dong, Z., M.E. Cruz-Munoz, M.C. Zhong, *et al.* 2009. Essential function for SAP family adaptors in the surveillance of hematopoietic cells by natural killer cells. *Nat. Immunol.* **10:** 973–980.

66. Bottino, C., M. Falco, S. Parolini, *et al.* 2001. NTB-A [correction of GNTB-A], a novel SH2D1A-associated surface molecule contributing to the inability of natural killer cells to kill Epstein-Barr virus-infected B cells in X-linked lymphoproliferative disease. *J. Exp. Med.* **194:** 235–246.

67. Parolini, S., C. Bottino, M. Falco, *et al.* 2000. X-linked lymphoproliferative disease. 2B4 molecules displaying inhibitory rather than activating function are responsible for the inability of natural killer cells to kill Epstein–Barr virus-infected cells. *J. Exp. Med.* **192:** 337–346.

68. Dupre, L., G. Andolfi, S.G. Tangye, *et al.* 2005. SAP controls the cytolytic activity of CD8+ T cells against EBV-infected cells. *Blood* **105:** 4383–4389.

69. Sharifi, R., J.C. Sinclair, K.C. Gilmour, *et al.* 2004. SAP mediates specific cytotoxic T-cell functions in X-linked lymphoproliferative disease. *Blood* **103:** 3821–3827.

70. Hislop, A.D., U. Palendira, A.M. Leese, *et al.* 2010. Impaired Epstein-Barr virus-specific CD8+ T cell function in X-linked lymphoproliferative disease is restricted to SLAM family-positive B cell targets. *Blood* **116:** 3249–3257.

71. Bloch-Queyrat, C., M.C. Fondaneche, R. Chen, *et al.* 2005. Regulation of natural cytotoxicity by the adaptor SAP and the Src-related kinase Fyn. *J. Exp. Med.* **202:** 181–192.

72. Yin, L., U. Al-Alem, J. Liang, *et al.* 2003. Mice deficient in the X-linked lymphoproliferative disease gene *sap* exhibit increased susceptibility to murine gammaherpesvirus-68 and hypo-gammaglobulinemia. *J. Med. Virol.* **71:** 446–455.

73. Snow, A.L., R.A. Marsh, S.M. Krummey, *et al.* 2009. Restimulation-induced apoptosis of T cells is impaired in patients with X-linked lymphoproliferative disease caused by SAP deficiency. *J. Clin. Invest.* **119:** 2976–2989.

74. Pasquier, B., L. Yin, M.C. Fondaneche, *et al.* 2005. Defective NKT cell development in mice and humans lacking the adapter SAP, the X-linked lymphoproliferative syndrome gene product. *J. Exp. Med.* **201:** 695–701.

75. Nichols, K.E., J. Hom, S.Y. Gong, *et al.* 2005. Regulation of NKT cell development by SAP, the protein defective in XLP. *Nat. Med.* **11:** 340–345.

76. Latour, S. 2007. Natural killer T cells and X-linked lymphoproliferative syndrome. *Curr. Opin. Allergy Clin. Immunol.* **7:** 510–514.

77. Bendelac, A., P.B. Savage & L. Teyton. 2007. The biology of NKT cells. *Annu. Rev. Immunol.* **25:** 297–336.

78. Eckelman, B.P., G.S. Salvesen & F.L. Scott. 2006. Human inhibitor of apoptosis proteins: why XIAP is the black sheep of the family. *EMBO Rep.* **7:** 988–994.

79. Paulsen, M., S. Ussat, M. Jakob, *et al.* 2008. Interaction with XIAP prevents full caspase-3/-7 activation in proliferating human T lymphocytes. *Eur. J. Immunol.* **38:** 1979–1987.

80. Dubrez-Daloz, L., A. Dupoux, & J. Cartier. 2008. IAPs: more than just inhibitors of apoptosis proteins. *Cell Cycle* **7:** 1036–1046.

81. Krieg, A., R.G. Correa, J.B. Garrison, *et al.* 2009. XIAP mediates NOD signaling via interaction with RIP2. *Proc. Natl. Acad. Sci. USA* **106:** 14524–14529.

82. Harlin, H., S.B. Reffey, C.S. Duckett, *et al.* 2001. Characterization of XIAP-deficient mice. *Mol. Cell. Biol.* **21:** 3604–3608.

83. Olayioye, M.A., H. Kaufmann, M. Pakusch, *et al.* 2005. XIAP-deficiency leads to delayed lobuloalveolar development in the mammary gland. *Cell Death Differ.* **12:** 87–90.

84. Badovinac, V.P., S.E. Hamilton & J.T. Harty. 2003. Viral infection results in massive CD8+ T cell expansion and mortality in vaccinated perforin-deficient mice. *Immunity* **18:** 463–474.

85. Jordan, M.B., D. Hildeman, J. Kappler & P. Marrack. 2004. An animal model of hemophagocytic lymphohistiocytosis (HLH): CD8+ T cells and interferon gamma are essential for the disorder. *Blood* **104:** 735–743.

86. Crozat, K., K. Hoebe, S. Ugolini, *et al.* 2007. Jinx, an MCMV susceptibility phenotype caused by disruption of Unc13d: a mouse model of type 3 familial hemophagocytic lymphohistiocytosis. *J. Exp. Med.* **204:** 853–863.

87. Pachlopnik Schmid, J., C.H. Ho, J. Diana, *et al.* 2008. A Griscelli syndrome type 2 murine model of hemophagocytic lymphohistiocytosis (HLH). *Eur. J. Immunol.* **38:** 3219–3225.

88. Mazodier, K., V. Marin, D. Novick, *et al.* 2005. Severe imbalance of IL-18/IL-18BP in patients with secondary hemophagocytic syndrome. *Blood* **106:** 3483–3489.

89. Smyth, M.J., K.Y. Thia, S.E. Street, *et al.* 2000. Perforin-mediated cytotoxicity is critical for surveillance of spontaneous lymphoma. *J. Exp. Med.* **192:** 755–760.

90. Bolitho, P., S.E. Street, J.A. Westwood, *et al.* 2009. Perforin-mediated suppression of B-cell lymphoma. *Proc. Natl. Acad. Sci. USA* **106:** 2723–2728.

91. Cannella, S., A. Santoro, G. Bruno, *et al.* 2007. Germline mutations of the perforin gene are a frequent occurrence in childhood anaplastic large cell lymphoma. *Cancer* **109:** 2566–2571.

92. Mehta, P.A., S.M. Davies, A. Kumar, *et al.* 2006. Perforin polymorphism A91V and susceptibility to B-precursor childhood acute lymphoblastic leukemia: a report from the Children's Oncology Group. *Leukemia* **20:** 1539–1541.

93. Clementi, R., F. Locatelli, L. Dupre, *et al.* 2005. A proportion of patients with lymphoma may harbor mutations of the perforin gene. *Blood* **105:** 4424–4428.

94. Pachlopnik Schmid, J., C.H. Ho, F. Chrétien, *et al.* 2009. Neutralization of IFNγ defeats hemophagocytosis in LCMV-infected perforin- and Rab27a-deficient mice. *EMBO Mol. Med.* **1:** 112–124.

95. Henter, J.I., A. Horne, M. Arico, *et al.* 2007. HLH-2004: diagnostic and therapeutic guidelines for hemophagocytic lymphohistiocytosis. *Pediatr. Blood Can.* **48:** 124–131.

96. Mahlaoui, N., M. Ouachee-Chardin, G. de Saint Basile, *et al.* 2007. Immunotherapy of familial hemophagocytic lymphohistiocytosis with antithymocyte globulins: a single-center retrospective report of 38 patients. *Pediatrics* **120:** e622–e628.

· Ann. N.Y. Acad. Sci. ISSN 0077-8923

ANNALS OF THE NEW YORK ACADEMY OF SCIENCES

Issue: *The Year in Human and Medical Genetics: Inborn Errors of Immunity*

Autoimmune polyendocrinopathy candidiasis ectodermal dystrophy: known and novel aspects of the syndrome

Kai Kisand and Pärt Peterson

Institute of General and Molecular Pathology, University of Tartu, Tartu, Estonia

Address for correspondence: Kai Kisand, Institute of General and Molecular Pathology, University of Tartu, 19 Ravila Str., Tartu
EE 50411, Estonia. kai.kisand@ut.ee

Autoimmune polyendocrinopathy candidiasis ectodermal dystrophy (APECED) is a monogenic autosomal recessive disease caused by mutations in the autoimmune regulator (AIRE) gene and, as a syndrome, is characterized by chronic mucocutaneous candidiasis and the presentation of various autoimmune diseases. During the last decade, research on APECED and AIRE has provided immunologists with several invaluable lessons regarding tolerance and autoimmunity. This review describes the clinical and immunological features of APECED and discusses emerging alternative models to explain the pathogenesis of the disease.

Keywords: APECED; AIRE; chronic mucocutaneous candidiasis; IL-17; IL-22

History

Autoimmune polyendocrinopathy candidiasis ectodermal dystrophy (APECED) is classified as a type IV primary immunodeficiency: a disease of immune dysregulation.[1] The first description of the syndrome dates back to 1929, when the association between hypoparathyroidism and chronic candidiasis was published by Thorpe and Handley.[2] In 1946, a clinical triad of chronic mucocutaneous candidiasis (CMC), hypoparathyroidism, and adrenal insufficiency was reported,[3] which was recognized in 1956 as the Whitaker syndrome.[4] In 1980, Neufeld *et al.* classified three types of autoimmune polyendocrine syndromes (APS) with different combinations of endocrinopathies and other manifestations. Of these, APS1 was used to describe the syndrome that is the topic of this review.[5] To describe the disease more precisely, the acronym APECED was introduced by the Finnish pediatrician Professor Jaakko Perheentupa, who significantly contributed to the clinical characterization of the syndrome by leading studies investigating a large cohort of Finnish patients.[6,7]

Diagnosis

APECED is more prevalent in some historically isolated populations, such as Iranian Jews (1:9,000),[8] Sardinians (1:14,000),[9] and Finns (1:25,000).[10] Lower prevalence has been also determined for Slovenia (1:43,000),[11] Norway (1:80,000),[12] and Poland (1:129,000),[13] which may hamper a clinician's ability to recognize it. The first sign of the syndrome is usually a chronic *Candida* infection during early childhood, followed by autoimmune hypoparathyroidism and adrenocortical failure (Addison's disease).[10,14,15] Classical diagnosis requires the presence of at least two of these three major components or only one component if a sibling has already been diagnosed.[6,14] However, following the identification of causal genetic mutations in the autoimmune regulator (AIRE),[16,17] molecular methods can facilitate diagnosis of cases with atypical clinical presentations.[18–20] More recently, the discovery that autoantibodies specific for type I interferons (especially IFN-ω and IFN-α) correlate with AIRE deficiency has allowed their surrogate use as a specific and sensitive diagnostic tool for

doi: 10.1111/j.1749-6632.2011.06308.x
Ann. N.Y. Acad. Sci. 1246 (2011) 77–91 © 2011 New York Academy of Sciences.

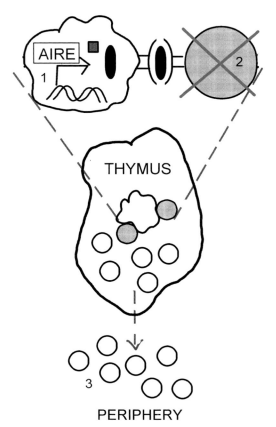

Figure 1. (1) In medullary thymic epithelial cells, AIRE drives the expression of peripheral tissue-specific antigens (black oval, dark rectangle) that are presented to developing thymocytes. (2) Self-reactive thymocytes (gray circles) are deleted and (3) only non-self-reactive thymocytes (white circles) are exported to the periphery.

APECED,[21–26] especially in cases where mutational analysis is complicated (for example, large deletions, duplications, or mutations in regulatory or intronic regions).

AIRE: function and mutations

The AIRE gene is mainly expressed by thymic medullary epithelial cells (mTECs) that play an important role in the presentation of the self-antigens to developing thymocytes and in establishing self-tolerance.[27] In addition, AIRE expression has been reported in lymph nodes and tonsils.[28,29] In mTECs, the AIRE protein has the unique property of directing the expression of hundreds or thousands of tissue-specific proteins, a process known as promiscuous or ectopic gene expression (Fig. 1).[30]

AIRE is subcellularly located in the nucleus forming nuclear bodies that resemble, but are distinct from, the nuclear dots containing the promyelocytic leukemia (PML) protein.[31] These nuclear bodies are known to associate with transcriptionally active, or chromatin-associated, proteins.[32] In agreement with its role in transcription, AIRE contains a combination of functional domains: the N-terminal CARD (caspase-recruitment) domain; the SAND (SP100, AIRE, Nuc p41/75, DEAF) domain, located in the middle; and two PHD (plant homeodomain) fingers at the C-terminal region of the protein, which indicates that AIRE plays a role in transcription (Fig. 2). The structure of AIRE is highly conserved among mammalian species and shares close similarity with the SP140 and SP110 proteins.[33]

Over 60 APECED-associated mutations have been reported in the AIRE gene, and two disease-causing mutations are found in over 95% of patients.[14] Most of these mutations, distributed throughout the coding region, are either nonsense or frameshift mutations that result in truncated polypeptides or in single amino acid–changing missense mutations.[15] These include single nucleotide substitutions, small insertions, deletions, and mutations affecting splice consensus sequences. Moreover, large genomic deletions that can escape conventional mutation analysis have been described in the AIRE gene.[34,35] The R257X mutation in exon 6 and a 13 base-pair deletion (967-979del13bp) in exon 8 are the most prevalent mutations.[16,17] R257X accounts for 83% of Finnish disease alleles and is frequently found in other patients of European descent;[31,36,37] 967-979del13bp is common among North American, British, and Norwegian APECED patients;[24,38] Y85C is common in Iranian Jews; and R139X is common in Sardinian APECED patients.[8,9,31] Several mutations have been described to affect either AIRE transcriptional activity or its localization to nuclear bodies. For example, the 6-helix CARD domain is involved in homodimerization, and missense mutations in this region often affect AIRE multimerization or localization to nuclear bodies.[39] Similarly, the dominant negative mutation G228W, located within the SAND domain, prevents AIRE localization to nuclear bodies and severely affects the intracellular localization and transcriptional activity of the wild-type AIRE protein.[18,40] Patients with a heterozygous G228W

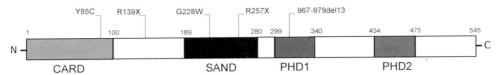

Figure 2. Schematic representation of the human AIRE protein. The localization of selected APECED-causing mutations is indicated. CARD, caspase-recruitment domain; SAND, SP100, AIRE1, NucP41/P75, and DEAF1 domain; PHD, plant homeodomain.

mutation present with APECED associated with hypothyroid autoimmune thyroiditis, and multiorgan autoimmune diseases are also present in the corresponding mouse model.[18,41] The SAND domain is a putative DNA binding region whose binding to DNA has been suggested in SP100 protein;[42] however, whether the G228W mutation affects DNA binding remains undetermined at this time. In the *C*-terminus, AIRE has two PHD fingers that interact with proteins involved in transcriptional control at the chromatin level. The first PHD domain may function as a histone code reader because it interacts with the unmethylated histone H3 lysine residue 4.[43,44] The interaction is also necessary for the regulation of tissue-specific genes; however, additional factors may be required for transcriptional activation at the chromatin level. Most of the missense mutations in PHD domains destroy the structure of the zinc-finger fold and thus severely decrease AIRE's transcriptional activation capacity.[44,45]

Significant variation in clinical presentations of APECED has been described for patients carrying a homozygous R257X mutation, and intrafamilial differences have been reported between siblings of the identical AIRE genotype.[46] Therefore, despite considerable variations in the APECED phenotype, correlations with respective genotypes are far from clear. A correlation seems to exist, however, with *Candida* infections. In our analysis of 160 APECED patients, mostly homozygous for one of the three recurring AIRE truncations (R139X, R257X, or 967-979del13bp), candidiasis was significantly less prevalent in patients homozygous for 967-979del13bp than in patients carrying the R257X or R139X mutations.[47,48] This suggests that AIRE proteins truncated before the SAND domain might render individuals more susceptible to this type of infection. Interestingly, candidiasis has also been reported to be rare among Iranian Jewish patients carrying the Y85C mutation.[31]

Clinical features

The APECED clinical picture varies in severity and in the number of disease components—with up to 10 abnormalities per patient.[10] However, the order in which these symptoms and/or diseases present is strikingly consistent.[6,10,14] CMC is the first sign of APECED in 75–93% of cases,[6,10,49] followed by hypoparathyroidism, with peak incidence between four and five years of age, and then by Addison's disease (also in childhood).[6,14] The complete triad develops in up to two-thirds of patients.[6,49] Other early manifestations that can present prior to the symptoms and/or diseases described above include hepatitis, keratoconjunctivitis, periodic rashes with fever, chronic diarrhea, severe obstipation, alopecia, or vitiligo.[10] Additional clinical manifestations develop up to the fifth decade of life of these patients.[6]

Endocrine manifestations

Apart from hypoparathyroidism and Addison's disease, the spectrum of endocrinopathies associated with APECED includes hypergonadotropic hypogonadism, type 1 diabetes, autoimmune thyroid diseases, and pituitary defects,[10,14] disorders regarded to be of autoimmune origin. The appearance of these manifestations is often associated with a specific set of organ-specific autoantibodies (Table 1). However, it should be noted that the correlation of autoantibodies is purely statistical, meaning that the prevalence of the antibodies is higher in the group of patients presenting with the certain manifestation compared to patients without this manifestation. In certain cases, the antibodies can be predictive of future disease manifestations. For example autoantibodies specific for steroidogenic enzymes (P450c21, P450c17, and P450scc; see Table 1 for abbreviations) correlate well with the adrenocortical and hypogonadal dysfunction;[49,53–56,67,68] in contrast, autoantibodies specific for GAD65, which can be considered relatively good markers for isolated type 1

Table 1. APECED manifestations and associated autoantibodies

Manifestation and autoantibody targets	Prevalence (%)	References
Hypoparathyroidism[a]	85	
• NACHT leucine-rich repeat protein 5 (NALP5)	32–49	50, 51
• Calcium-sensing receptor (CaSR)	86[b]	52
Addison's disease	78	
• Steroid 17-α–hydroxylase (P450c17)	44	53, 54
• Steroid 21-hydroxylase (P450c21)	60–66	50, 51, 53
• Side-chain cleavage enzyme (P450scc)	38–52	50, 53, 56
Ovarian failure	60	
• P450scc and P450c17		53
Diabetes mellitus	13	
• Islet antigen-2 (IA-2)	7	53, 57
• Glutamic acid decarboxylase-65 (GAD65)[c]	27–36	50, 53, 57
Hypothyroidism	14	
• Thyroglobulin (TG)	15–18	57, 58
• Thyroid peroxidase (TPO)	21–36	57, 58
Testicular failure	8	
• Testis-specific gene 10 protein (TSGA10)[c]	8	59
Hypopituitarism	5	
• Tudor domain-containing protein 6 (TDRD6)	49	60
Gastritis/pernicious anemia	20	
• Intrinsic factor (IF)	15–30	49, 57
Autoimmune hepatitis	18	
• Aromatic L-amino acid decarboxylase (AADC)	39–51	53, 61
• Cytochrome P450 1A2 (P450 1A2)	8	53, 62
Intestinal dysfunction	22	
• Tryptophan hydroxylase (TPH)	48	53, 63
• Histidine decarboxylase (HDC)	37	64
Alopecia	39	
• Tyrosine hydroxylase (TH)	44	53, 65
Vitiligo	27	
SOX9/SOX10	15–22	66
Rash with fever	14	
Lung manifestations	Rare	
• Potassium channel-regulating protein (KCNRG)	6	67
Tubulointerstitial nephritis	9	
Asplenia	20	
Keratoconjunctivitis	22	
Dental enamel dysplasia	77	
Nail dystropy	50	

[a]Prevalence of APECED manifestations is presented according to data from the biggest cohort available (Finnish patients) at 30 years of age of Ref. 10

[b]Prevalence in patients with hypoparathyroidism.

[c]Autoantibodies, although their target is expressed in respective tissue, are not associated with the manifestation.

diabetes, are not associated with diabetes in APECED patients.[53,70] Furthermore, the high prevalence of some APECED-related autoantibodies, like those specific for TDRD6[60] or AADC,[61] contrasts with the rarity of the related manifestations (for example, hypopituitarism and chronic active hepatitis respectively) (Table 1). Pathogenic roles can be attributed to antibodies binding to cell surface molecules, such as the calcium-sensing receptor (CaSR) that is the autoantigen associated with hypoparathyroidism.[52] Interestingly, CaSR antibodies from two anti-CaSR–positive APECED patients were able to stimulate the CaSR.[71] CaSR stimulation, then, might inhibit parathyroid hormone secretion and lower calcium levels, which provides an alternative explanation for hypoparathyroidism other than mere destruction of the glands.[71,72]

Many autoantibodies associated with APECED are specific for intracellular enzymes involved in hormone or neurotransmitter biosynthesis.[26] Although these antibodies can often neutralize their target enzymes *in vitro*,[56,73] they possess little direct pathogenic potential *in vivo* since their targets are sequestered within the cell. It is conceivable that the presence of autoantibodies specific for intracellular enzymes is indicative of ongoing T cell reactivity. Therefore, autoantibodies serve as a valuable disease marker since autoimmune endocrine diseases are believed to be mostly mediated by T cells. For example, circulating autoantigen-specific T cells that react to P450c21, or its epitopes, have been detected in patients presenting with Addison's disease.[74–76] Due to the rarity of APECED, however, tissue samples of affected organs are not typically available for study. Furthermore, the number of blood samples available for T cell studies is also very limited. These facts help explain the paucity of data describing antigen-specific T cell responses in APECED patients in spite of the critical role of the thymus and T cells in mediating disease pathogenesis.

Gastrointestinal manifestations

While an autoimmune etiology of the endocrinopathies seems likely, the origin of other APECED-associated abnormalities is less well defined; for example, the rather prevalent gastrointestinal manifestations in APECED patients can be of variable etiology.[10,14] Chronic atrophic gastritis and pernicious anemia are often associated with autoantibodies specific for parietal cells and intrinsic

factor.[10] Chronic active hepatitis is also regarded to be autoimmune in origin and is accompanied by autoantibodies specific for liver-expressed antigens P450 1A2 and AADC.[62,73] In some cases, chronic diarrhea is the result of hypocalcemia in patients with hypoparathyroidism,[14] and in others, diarrhea alternates with obstipation.[10] Malabsorption and steatorrhea can be the result of exocrine pancreatic failure.[10] Interestingly, the intestinal endocrine cells are also the targets of autoimmune attack, and it has been suggested that intestinal dysfunction can also be considered to be an endocrinopathy.[77] Autoantibodies to TPH and HDC have been associated with gastrointestinal dysfunction in APECED and with the destruction of serotonin-producing enterocromaffin and endocromaffin-like cells, respectively.[64,65] Cholecystokinin-producing cells were absent in one patient with malabsorption.[78] Alternatively, intestinal candidiasis can induce severe diarrhea, even in the absence of overt oral infection. Candida enteritis can be diagnosed if the symptoms subside subsequent to antifungal treatment.[10]

Ectodermal manifestations

Ectodermal manifestations associated with APECED include autoimmune skin diseases, such as vitiligo and alopecia, keratoconjunctivitis, dental enamel hypoplasia, pitted nail dystrophy, and tympanic membrane calcification.[6,10] Nail dystrophy is reported frequently in APECED patients;[10] however, others have found differentiating onychomycosis from nail dystrophy to be difficult.[24,79] Collins *et al.* suggested that nail dystrophy in Irish APECED patients is a consequence of ungular candidiasis.[79] Dental enamel hypoplasia affects about three quarters of APECED patients,[10] and while originally thought to involve only permanent teeth, recent studies have revealed that hypoplastic changes also affect decidual teeth.[80] The proposed hypothesis of hypoparathyroidism causing enamel hypoplasia in APECED seems unlikely, since these two phenomena do not always present together.[6,80,81] Moreover, dentin appears normal in APECED patient teeth samples, thereby ruling out a mineralization defect as the predominant etiological factor associated with enamel hypoplasia.[80] However, dental defects may be secondary to recurrent oral infections and malnutrition.[79] Although the pathogenesis of ectodermal dystrophies is still open,[38] the primary failure of morphogenesis of ectodermal tissues is extremely unlikely in APECED since these aberrations are not present at birth but develop over time.[79] The autoimmune origin of these manifestations seems conceivable even though no autoantigens associated with ectodermal dystrophies have been reported to date.

Other manifestations

Asplenia, tubulointestinal nephritis, obstructive lung disease, vasculitis, Sjögren's syndrome, cutaneous vasculitis, hemolytic anemia, scleroderma, metaphyseal dysplasia, and celiac disease have also been reported to be associated with APECED.[49,82] Autoimmune bronchiolitis and tubulointestinal nephritis have successfully been treated with immunosuppressive regimens.[14,67] An autoantigen present in bronchial epithelial cells has been identified,[67] and the autoimmune nature of renal destruction has been confirmed by examining biopsy samples and by determining antiproximal tubular autoantibodies.[14,83,84] Asplenia, presenting in up to 20% of APECED patients,[10] results in impaired immune responses to encapsulated bacteria and is a serious risk factor for developing septicemia.[85] The pathogenesis of asplenia remains unknown.

CMC

Intriguingly, the most prevalent (and the earliest) disease manifestation associated with APECED is CMC, a selective immunodeficiency that is distinct from the multiple autoimmune manifestations characteristic for APECED patients.[6] CMC usually appears first as oral thrush, although some parents recall recurrent napkin dermatitis during the first two years of life.[6,14,79] The course and severity of candidiasis varies significantly. In some cases, it presents as a mild and remittent infection, compared to patients who develop chronic hypertrophic and/or atrophic lesions.[6,14] CMC can dominate the presentation profile associated with APECED for several years, together with some less common manifestations, before the endocrinopathies develop.[6] Oral Candida infection may spread to the esophagus and cause substernal pain, especially upon swallowing, and in rare cases may cause esophageal stricture.[14] Accordingly, oral and esophageal candidiasis must be strictly controlled to avoid development of squamous cell carcinoma.[86] Symptomatic intestinal candidiasis may also be present even in the absence of oral disease. The skin of the hands and sometimes

Table 2. The prevalences of autoantibodies specific for cytokines in APECED and thymoma patients

Autoantibodies to	Prevalence (%) in	
	APECED	Thymoma/MG
IFN-ω	100	60
IFN-α	95	70
IFN-β	22	Rare
IFN-λ	14	Rare
IL-22	91	5–10
IL-17F	75	5–10
IL-17A	41	5–10

MG, myasthenia gravis.

face may be also affected. The fingernails are more commonly affected than toenails, a presentation that can be explained by the spreading of the infection from the mouth to fingers during infancy.[79] Vaginal Candida infection can also be present.[14]

Cytokines as autoantigens and their role in CMC pathogenesis

The hallmark of APECED is the variety of different autoantibodies that develop in association with the disease.[15] Among these, the anticytokine autoantibodies stand out due to their high prevalence and early emergence (even before clinical manifestations develop), suggesting that these antibodies are intimately associated with disease pathogenesis.[48] Neutralizing autoantibodies specific for type I IFNs in APECED were discovered in 2006 by Meager et al.,[21] and their diagnostic value was rapidly appreciated.[22,24,25,87] Thymoma, with associated myasthenia gravis (MG), is the only other disease among many others screened that have shown reactivity against type I IFNs.[21,48,88,89] The prevalence of anticytokine autoantibodies in APECED and thymoma patients is described in Table 2. Although these autoantibodies influence interferon-stimulated gene expression in vivo and in vitro,[90] there is no clear evidence indicating that APECED patients have an increased susceptibility to viral diseases, as has been described for genetic causes for impaired type I and III IFN secretion.[90,91] This can be explained by the paracrine function of high concentrations of IFNs after their secretion and compensation by IFN-γ.[21,90] The notion that neutralization of type I

IFNs is not associated with an inability to clear *Candida* infections is supported by the fact that CMC does not manifest in patients with genetic causes of type I IFN dysfunction;[91] instead, increased levels of IFNs seem to downmodulate Th17 differentiation, the cell type believed to be responsible for protection against *Candida* infection.[92,93]

More recently, autoantibodies against the Th17-related cytokines (IL-22, IL-17F, and IL-17A) were identified in APECED patients.[47,94] These autoantibodies are very specific, highly prevalent, neutralizing, and develop very early in the disease course.[47,94–96] Importantly, *Candida* infections in APECED patients have been associated with autoantibodies against IL-22 and/or IL-17F.[47,96] Remarkably, rare thymoma patients presenting with CMC were also positive for neutralizing autoantibodies against Th17-related cytokines, which supports a pathogenic role for these autoantibodies.[47] The link between the Th17 pathway and anticandidal immunity has been substantiated by studies examining certain monogenic disorders associated with CMC and by using mice with disrupted Th17 pathways (reviewed in Refs. 97 and 98). IL-17A and IL-22 synergistically exert their function on epithelial cells by inducing the production of chemokines and antimicrobial peptides (S100A7, S100A8, S100A9, β-defensins, and histatins) that have direct antifungal activity.[99,100] IL-22 in addition promotes epithelial barrier integrity, especially in synergy with TNF-α if cosecreted by Th22 cells (a skin-homing cell type).[101,102] In contrast to several other syndromes associated with CMC,[93,103] the PBMCs of APECED patients produce normal or even increased amounts of IL-17A[95,104] but are deficient in IL-22 and IL-17F secretion.[47,95,104] As this defect is not *Candida*-specific, we suspect that an autoimmune response against IL-17F– and IL-22–producing cells is mounted.[48] Interestingly, IL-22 was recently shown to be surface-bound to Th cells that secrete IL-22 in response to *Mycobacterium tuberculosis* infections.[105] Since the amount of secreted IL-22 was found to be inversely correlated with autoantibody titers in APECED patients, we hypothesize that antibody-mediated cytotoxicity might be responsible for the depletion of IL-22–producing cells. Complement-mediated destruction seems unlikely, as the differentiation of IL-17A– and IL-22–secreting cells *in vitro* remained unaltered in the presence of sera collected from APECED patients.[47]

Collectively, these findings show that CMC in APECED is essentially autoimmune and therefore similar to most disease manifestations associated with APECED. This has led to the suggestion that gradual immunosuppressive treatments in conjunction with administration of antifungal agents might be (paradoxically) beneficial even in cases of apparent immunodeficiency.[48]

Other infections

The fact that protective immune responses are targeted in APECED prompted a reevaluation of the manifestations associated with this syndrome. Specifically, we asked if susceptibility to other infections had been overlooked in these patients. A review of the literature revealed several cases of unusual or severe infections. In a French study of 19 patients, eight presented with episodes of recurrent isolated fever, recurrent pneumonia, corneal abscess, recurrent otitis and sinusitis, recurrent pyodermitis, septicemia from intestinal origin, or encephalitis following a case of the mumps.[57] The septicemia case occurred during immunosuppressive treatment, but all of the other infections described were unrelated to either immunosuppression or asplenia. A Japanese patient presented with severe HSV-1 stomatitis with viral reactivation occurring 2–3 times per year.[106] A recent Italian survey of 24 patients reported encephalitis in two of them,[101] and a case of chronic otitis media was described by Podkrajsek.[34] Together, these clinical findings suggest that the neutralization of type I IFNs and Th17-related cytokines may have effects that together with other predisposing environmental factors may lead to severe or atypical infections. We thus propose that infectious complications in APECED patients need more attention and additional surveillance.

Although the following suggestion is hypothetical, other manifestations where impaired defensive mechanisms (e.g., neutralization of cytokines) may have contributed to the pathogenesis of APECED include keratoconjunctivitis, bronchiolitis, gastrointestinal dysfunction, and rash with fever. Some of these manifestations, such as bronchiolitis, malabsorption, and keratoconjunctivitis, have been reported to respond well to immunosuppressive treatments that have supported their autoimmune origin.[57,67,108,109] However, immunosuppression can also restrain autoimmunity to protective antimicrobial mechanisms that help to control the infections contributing to these manifestations.

Studies of immune cell subpopulations

Studies of immune cell subtypes of APECED patients have often provided contradicting results. Monocyte numbers have been reported to be increased in APECED patients[110–112] or to remain unaffected.[56] Wolff et al. described a decreased percentage of $CD16^+$ monocytes in APECED patients,[56] whereas the dendritic cell subpopulations remained unchanged.[56,111] Also, functional analyses of myeloid cells yielded conflicting results. Brännström et al. reported that monocytes from APECED patients displayed a decreased and delayed internalization of zymosan and decreased phoshotyrosine kinase activation following exposure to Candida antigen.[113] In contrast, monocyte and neutrophil phagocytosis of Candida was found to be unaltered by Perniola et al.[110] Subtle changes in dendritic cell functions have also been characterized; however, most of the changes in antigen presenting cell populations are moderate and found in a small number of adult patients.[114–116] It seems likely that these aberrations could be secondary to chronic inflammation and depend on the clinical status of the recruited patients.

Total $CD4^+$ T cell numbers and the proportion of $CD4^+$ T cells expressing memory or activation markers have been reported to be increased or to remain at normal levels in APECED patients.[56,57,117–119] Data derived from studies examining iNKT cells have also resulted in controversial findings, for example, iNKT cell numbers were found to be decreased in one study[120] and unchanged in another.[56] The most consistent data concern regulatory T cells. Their deficient number, impaired function, or diminished FOXP3 expression has been found in four different studies.[56,121–123] However, whether this defect in regulatory T cells is a result of thymic aberrations or peripheral events (e.g., increased homing to inflammatory tissues) remains unknown.[124]

While many of the described abnormalities are modest and possibly secondary to inflammation, more profound changes to naive $CD8^+$ T cells have recently been described in APECED patients.[125] In a group of 12 patients, a significant decrease in CD127 and CD5 surface expression and an almost complete lack of a conventional naive population ($CD45RA^+$

$CD62L^+$ $CCR7^+$ perforin$^-$) was reported.[125] Recent thymic emigrants (recognized by surface CD31 expression) were also abnormal.[125] In light of these data, it is tempting to speculate that AIRE-deficient thymic tissues resulted in the selection of aberrant $CD8^+$ T cells. However, the study was performed in adults (mean age of 40 years) who already had a severely reduced thymic T cell output. It is also conceivable that peripheral $CD8^+$ T cells are sensitive to cytokine or chemokine imbalances present in these patients. These results need to be confirmed in pediatric patients and further tested in patients with APS2 and chronic CMC to exclude effects of chronic inflammation.

Mechanisms of APECED pathogenesis

A question puzzling researchers for years is the target-organ specificity in APECED. Although AIRE controls expression of thousands of peripheral antigens in the thymus, the organs affected are limited and so is the number of autoantigens present in each.[124] Moreover, the first symptoms and development of autoantibodies in these patients are not related to organ-specific autoimmunity. Instead, the most prevalent and earliest targets of the immune response are cytokines (type I IFNs and Th17-related cytokines) that seemingly are not AIRE dependent and are most likely produced by non-mTEC sources in the thymus or elsewhere.[48] In theory, all secreted antigens (cytokines included) should be processed by thymic dendritic cells and presented during the process of negative selection to developing thymocytes to ensure central tolerance. These discrepancies have provoked a reevaluation of the current model of disease pathogenesis of APECED.[48,126]

The current AIRE function model is based on convincing experiments using T cell receptor (TCR) transgenic mouse models that showed impaired negative selection of autoreactive thymocytes in an AIRE-deficient thymus.[127,128] However, in this scenario self-reactive T cells escaping from an AIRE-deficient thymus are naive and in low numbers in the setting of nonmanipulated TCR repertoire (Fig. 3A). The tolerization of potential autoreactive T cells that have escaped thymic negative selection is more likely to occur by multiple peripheral tolerogenic back-up mechanisms than would be their immediate activation.[129,130] The activation of naive self-reactive T cells in the periphery should take time, and would depend on multiple

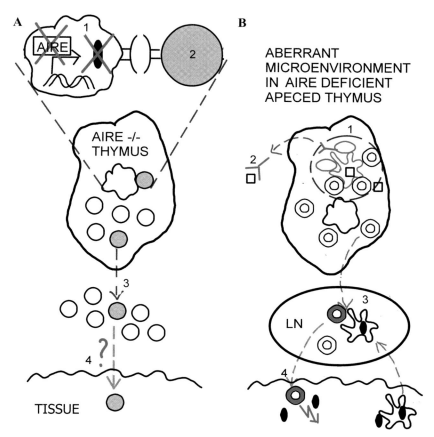

Figure 3. Current and alternative model of AIRE deficiency. (A) Current model: deficient negative selection (1) in medullary thymic epithelial cells AIRE deficiency leads to downregulation of the expression of tissue-specific autoantigens (dark oval) that are not presented to thymocytes; (2) self-reactive thymocytes (gray circles) are not negatively selected; (3) they are exported to the periphery together with non-self-reactive thymocytes (white circles); (4) how these rare, naive autoreactive T cells become activated to cause early tissue destruction remains unexplained by this model. (B) According to an alternative model, aberrant microenvironment in APECED thymus leads to the formation of (1) tertiary lymphoid tissue where cytokines (rectangles) are presented in immunogenic manner to T and B cells; (2) neutralizing autoantibodies against cytokines are released directly from the thymus; (3) CD8 single positive thymocytes are affected by the aberrant thymic microenvironment (e.g., due to cytokine dysbalance) and are exported to the periphery with lower activation threshold leading to their activation after tissue specific antigen (dark oval) release and presentation by dendritic cells followed by (4) immune attack toward tissues.

predisposing and triggering factors that are different between individuals.[48] This pathway is consistent with the varied APECED-related manifestations that develop during adulthood. However, to date there are no satisfactory explanations for the early autoimmune response raised against cytokines or to the early targeting of parathyroid and adrenal glands during disease progression in humans. Endocrine organs have a great functional reserve, for example, adrenal hormone deficiencies do not manifest clinically until at least 90% of the functioning cortical cells have been destroyed.[75,131] Therefore,

it should take several years before the symptoms appear following the initiation of immune attack—meaning that the rare, naive autoreactive cells likely became activated soon after birth if hypoparathyroidism or adrenocortical failure are to manifest at three or four years of age.

To explain these discrepancies we suggest that the thymic microenvironment is affected by an AIRE deficiency resulting in the export of preactivated or abnormal T cells and priming of autoantibody producing B cells (Fig. 3B). This hypothesis is based on (1) the identification of an irregular population of naive CD8$^+$ cells in APECED patients[125] (see section "Studies of immune cell subpopulations") and (2) the striking analogy between disease presentation in APECED and thymoma patients.[126] Aberrant CD8$^+$ thymic emigrants might be more resistant to tolerance induction in the periphery due to a lower activation threshold and thus they might become activated under conditions of excessive autoantigen releases, for example, during postnatal remodeling of fetal type of endocrine tissues.[132] The similarity between APECED and thymoma, two syndromes affecting the thymus, is provocative. One clear link is that the TEC in almost all thymomas fail to express AIRE.[133] Among the many diseases that have been screened for autoantibodies to type I IFNs only these two have been identified,[48,134] leading to the idea that the thymus itself may be the site for autoimmunization against cytokines, as these autoantibodies are clearly not the result of peripheral manifestations associated with APECED. Despite being a primary lymphoid organ, the thymus can develop tertiary lymphoid tissue and become a site where active immune responses can be initiated. In young MG patients, the thymus regularly develops germinal centers containing plasma cells that spontaneously produce anti-acetylcholine receptor autoantibodies.[135] Similarly, thymomas also contain perivascular infiltrates and even intraparenchymal germinal centers with plasma cells spontaneously producing auto-antibodies against IFN-α and IL-12 that show antigen-driven somatic mutations.[89,136] We predict that in the aberrant AIRE-deficient microenvironment, tertiary lymphoid tissue can develop in the thymus of APECED patients and generate preactivated autoreactive T cells and autoantibody producing plasma cells that target cytokines and cytokine-producing cells. Cell types and mechanisms responsible for this process remain undefined to date, although there is evidence that type I IFNs and IL-22 are expressed by cells residing in thymus.[48] Whether this mechanism of active autoimmunization can be extended to include endocrine and ectodermal antigens that might be also present in the thymus needs to be further evaluated.

The validity of the current and emerging models of disease pathogenesis in APECED should be further evaluated by any means available for human studies, as the results obtained using transgenic mouse models cannot be directly applied to human disease. One set of experiments that could substantiate the role of impaired negative selection in human AIRE deficiency would be to determine the precursor frequency of autoreactive T cells using MHC tertramer-based techniques. This approach should identify the presence of autoreactive T cells even if they have become anergic by peripheral tolerogenic mechanisms.

Conclusions

APECED has proven to be an extremely useful disease model for better understanding mechanisms of self-tolerance and the development of autoimmunity. Continuing research in the field will likely reveal additional observations that will improve our understanding of the processes associated with central and peripheral tolerance.

Acknowledgments

We would like to thank Nick Willcox and Tony Meager for fruitful discussions and bright ideas. The study was supported by the European Regional Development Fund and Archimedes Foundation, Estonian Science Foundation (Grants 8358, 8169), and the Estonian Ministry of Education and Research Targeted Funding Grant SF0180021s07.

Conflicts of interest

The authors declare no conflicts of interest.

References

1. Notarangelo, L., J.L. Casanova, M.E. Conley, et al. 2006. Primary immunodeficiency diseases: an update from the International Union of Immunological Societies Primary Immunodeficiency Diseases Classification Committee Meeting in Budapest, 2005. J. Allergy Clin. Immunol. 117: 883–896.
2. Thorpe, E.S. & H.E. Handley. 1929. Chronic tetany and chronic mycelial stomatitis in a child aged four and one-half years. Am. J. Dis. Child 38: 328–338.
3. Leonard, M.F. 1946. Chronic idiopathic hypoparathyroidism with superimposed Addison's disease in a child. J. Clin. Endocrinol. Metab. 6: 493–506.
4. Esselborn, V.M., B.H. Landing, J. Whitaker, et al. 1956. The syndrome of familial juvenile hypoadrenocorticism, hypoparathyroidism and superficial moniliasis. J. Clin. Endocrinol. Metab. 16: 1374–1387.
5. Neufeld, M., N. Maclaren & R. Blizzard. 1980. Autoimmune polyglandular syndromes. Pediatr. Ann. 9: 154–162.
6. Ahonen, P., S. Myllarniemi, I. Sipila, et al. 1990. Clinical variation of autoimmune polyendocrinopathy–candidiasis–ectodermal dystrophy (APECED) in a series of 68 patients. N. Engl. J. Med. 322: 1829–1836.

7. Perheentupa, J. 2002. APS-I/APECED: the clinical disease and therapy. *Endocrinol. Metab. Clin. North Am.* **31:** 295–320, vi.

8. Zlotogora, J. & M.S. Shapiro. 1992. Polyglandular autoimmune syndrome type I among Iranian Jews. *J. Med. Genet.* **29:** 824–886.

9. Rosatelli, M.C., A. Meloni, A. Meloni, *et al.* 1998. A common mutation in Sardinian autoimmune polyendocrinopathy–candidiasis–ectodermal dystrophy patients. *Hum. Genet.* **103:** 428–434.

10. Perheentupa, J. 2006. Autoimmune polyendocrinopathy–candidiasis–ectodermal dystrophy. *J. Clin. Endocrinol. Metab.* **91:** 2843–2850.

11. Podkrajsek, K.T., N. Bratanic, C. Krzisnik, *et al.* 2005. Autoimmune regulator-1 messenger ribonucleic acid analysis in a novel intronic mutation and two additional novel AIRE gene mutations in a cohort of autoimmune polyendocrinopathy–candidiasis–ectodermal dystrophy patients. *J. Clin. Endocrinol. Metab.* **90:** 4930–4935.

12. Myhre, A.G., M. Halonen, P. Eskelin, *et al.* 2001. Autoimmune polyendocrine syndrome type 1 (APS I) in Norway. *Clin. Endocrinol.* **54:** 211–217.

13. Stolarski, B., E. Pronicka, L. Korniszewski, *et al.* 2006. Molecular background of polyendocrinopathy–candidiasis–ectodermal dystrophy syndrome in a Polish population: novel AIRE mutations and an estimate of disease prevalence. *Clin. Genet.* **70:** 348–354.

14. Husebye, E.S., J. Perheentupa, R. Rautemaa, *et al.* 2009. Clinical manifestations and management of patients with autoimmune polyendocrine syndrome type I. *J. Intern. Med.* **265:** 514–529.

15. Peterson, P. & L. Peltonen. 2005. Autoimmune polyendocrinopathy syndrome type 1 (APS1) and AIRE gene: new views on molecular basis of autoimmunity. *J. Autoimmun.* **25**(Suppl): 49–55.

16. Nagamine, K., P. Peterson, H.S. Scott, *et al.* 1997. Positional cloning of the APECED gene. *Nat. Genet.* **17:** 393–398.

17. Consortium, F.-G.A. 1997. An autoimmune disease, APECED, caused by mutations in a novel gene featuring two PHD-type zinc-finger domains. *Nat. Genet.* **17:** 399–403.

18. Cetani, F., G. Barbesino, S. Borsari, *et al.* 2001. A novel mutation of the autoimmune regulator gene in an Italian kindred with autoimmune polyendocrinopathy–candidiasis–ectodermal dystrophy, acting in a dominant fashion and strongly cosegregating with hypothyroid autoimmune thyroiditis. *J. Clin. Endocrinol. Metab.* **86:** 4747–4752.

19. Boe, A.S., P.M. Knappskog, A.G. Myhre, *et al.* 2002. Mutational analysis of the autoimmune regulator (AIRE) gene in sporadic autoimmune Addison's disease can reveal patients with unidentified autoimmune polyendocrine syndrome type I. *Eur. J. Endocrinol.* **146:** 519–522.

20. Cervato, S., L. Morlin, M.P. Albergoni, *et al.* 2010. AIRE gene mutations and autoantibodies to interferon omega in patients with chronic hypoparathyroidism without APECED. *Clin. Endocrinol.* **73:** 630–636.

21. Meager, A., K. Visvalingam, P. Peterson, *et al.* 2006. Anti-interferon autoantibodies in autoimmune polyendocrinopathy syndrome type 1. *PLoS Med.* **3:** e289.

22. Meloni, A., M. Furcas, F. Cetani, *et al.* 2008. Autoantibodies against type I interferons as an additional diagnostic criterion for autoimmune polyendocrine syndrome type I. *J. Clin. Endocrinol. Metab.* **93:** 4389–4397.

23. Toth, B., A.S. Wolff, Z. Halasz, *et al.* 2010. Novel sequence variation of AIRE and detection of interferon-omega antibodies in early infancy. *Clin. Endocrinol.* **72:** 641–647.

24. Wolff, A.S., M.M. Erichsen, A. Meager, *et al.* 2007. Autoimmune polyendocrine syndrome type 1 in Norway: phenotypic variation, autoantibodies, and novel mutations in the autoimmune regulator gene. *J. Clin. Endocrinol. Metab.* **92:** 595–603.

25. Zhang, L., J.M. Barker, S. Babu, *et al.* 2007. A robust immunoassay for anti-interferon autoantibodies that is highly specific for patients with autoimmune polyglandular syndrome type 1. *Clin. Immunol.* **125:** 131–137.

26. Husebye, E.S. & M.S. Anderson. 2011. Autoimmune polyendocrine syndromes: clues to type 1 diabetes pathogenesis. *Immunity* **32:** 479–487.

27. Heino, M., P. Peterson, J. Kudoh, *et al.* 1999. Autoimmune regulator is expressed in the cells regulating immune tolerance in thymus medulla. *Biochem. Biophys. Res. Commun.* **257:** 821–825.

28. Gardner, J.M., J.J. Devoss, R.S. Friedman, *et al.* 2008. Deletional tolerance mediated by extrathymic Aire-expressing cells. *Science* **321:** 843–847.

29. Poliani, P.L., K. Kisand, V. Marrella, *et al.* 2010. Human peripheral lymphoid tissues contain autoimmune regulator-expressing dendritic cells. *Am. J. Pathol.* **176:** 1104–1112.

30. Kyewski, B. & J. Derbinski. 2004. Self-representation in the thymus: an extended view. *Nat. Rev. Immunol.* **4:** 688–698.

31. Bjorses, P., M. Halonen, J.J. Palvimo, *et al.* 2000. Mutations in the AIRE gene: effects on subcellular location and transactivation function of the autoimmune polyendocrinopathy-candidiasis-ectodermal dystrophy protein. *Am. J. Hum. Genet.* **66:** 378–392.

32. Bernardi, R. & P.P. Pandolfi. 2007. Structure, dynamics and functions of promyelocytic leukaemia nuclear bodies. *Nat. Rev. Mol. Cell. Biol.* **8:** 1006–1016.

33. Peterson, P., T. Org & A. Rebane. 2008. Transcriptional regulation by AIRE: molecular mechanisms of central tolerance. *Nat. Rev. Immunol.* **8:** 948–957.

34. Podkrajsek, K.T., T. Milenkovic, R.J. Odink, *et al.* 2008. Detection of a complete autoimmune regulator gene deletion and two additional novel mutations in a cohort of patients with atypical phenotypic variants of autoimmune polyglandular syndrome type 1. *Eur. J. Endocrinol.* **159:** 633–639.

35. Boe Wolff, A.S., B. Oftedal, S. Johansson, *et al.* 2008. AIRE variations in Addison's disease and autoimmune polyendocrine syndromes (APS): partial gene deletions contribute to APS I. *Genes Immun.* **9:** 130–136.

36. Cihakova, D., K. Trebusak, M. Heino, *et al.* 2001. Novel AIRE mutations and P450 cytochrome autoantibodies in Central and Eastern European patients with APECED. *Hum. Mutat.* **18:** 225–232.

37. Scott, H.S., M. Heino, P. Peterson, *et al.* 1998. Common mutations in autoimmune polyendocrinopathy–candidiasis–ectodermal dystrophy patients of different origins. *Mol. Endocrinol.* **12:** 1112–1119.

38. Peterson, P., J. Pitkanen, N. Sillanpaa, *et al.* 2004. Autoimmune polyendocrinopathy candidiasis ectodermal dystrophy (APECED): a model disease to study molecular aspects of endocrine autoimmunity. *Clin. Exp. Immunol.* **135:** 348–357.

39. Ferguson, B.J., C. Alexander, S.W. Rossi, *et al.* 2008. AIRE's CARD revealed, a new structure for central tolerance provokes transcriptional plasticity. *J. Biol. Chem.* **283:** 1723–1731.

40. Ilmarinen, T., P. Eskelin, M. Halonen, *et al.* 2005. Functional analysis of SAND mutations in AIRE supports dominant inheritance of the G228W mutation. *Hum. Mutat.* **26:** 322–331.

41. Su, M.A., K. Giang, K. Zumer, *et al.* 2008. Mechanisms of an autoimmunity syndrome in mice caused by a dominant mutation in AIRE. *J. Clin. Invest.* **118:** 1712–1726.

42. Bottomley, M.J., M.W. Collard, J.I. Huggenvik, *et al.* 2001. The SAND domain structure defines a novel DNA-binding fold in transcriptional regulation. *Nat. Struct. Biol.* **8:** 626–633.

43. Org, T., F. Chignola, C. Hetenyi, *et al.* 2008. The autoimmune regulator PHD finger binds to non-methylated histone H3K4 to activate gene expression. *EMBO Rep.* **9:** 370–376.

44. Koh, A.S., A.J. Kuo, S.Y. Park, *et al.* 2008. AIRE employs a histone-binding module to mediate immunological tolerance, linking chromatin regulation with organ-specific autoimmunity. *Proc. Natl. Acad. Sci. USA* **105:** 15878–15883.

45. Chignola, F., M. Gaetani, A. Rebane, *et al.* 2009. The solution structure of the first PHD finger of autoimmune regulator in complex with non-modified histone H3 tail reveals the antagonistic role of H3R2 methylation. *Nucleic. Acids Res.* **37:** 2951–2961.

46. Halonen, M., P. Eskelin, A.G. Myhre, *et al.* 2002. AIRE mutations and human leukocyte antigen genotypes as determinants of the autoimmune polyendocrinopathy–candidiasis–ectodermal dystrophy phenotype. *J. Clin. Endocrinol. Metab.* **87:** 2568–2574.

47. Kisand, K., A.S. Boe Wolff, K.T. Podkrajsek, *et al.* 2010. Chronic mucocutaneous candidiasis in APECED or thymoma patients correlates with autoimmunity to Th17-associated cytokines. *J. Exp. Med.* **207:** 299–308.

48. Kisand, K., D. Lilic, J.L. Casanova, *et al.* 2011. Mucocutaneous candidiasis and autoimmunity against cytokines in APECED and thymoma patients: clinical and pathogenetic implications. *Eur. J. Immunol.* **41:** 1517–1527.

49. Betterle, C., N.A. Greggio & M. Volpato. 1998. Clinical review 93: autoimmune polyglandular syndrome type 1. *J. Clin. Endocrinol. Metab.* **83:** 1049–1055.

50. Wolff, A.S., B.E. Oftedal, K. Kisand, *et al.* 2010. Flow cytometry study of blood cell subtypes reflects autoimmune and inflammatory processes in autoimmune polyendocrine syndrome type I. *Scand. J. Immunol.* **71:** 459–467.

51. Alimohammadi, M., P. Bjorklund, A. Hallgren, *et al.* 2008. Autoimmune polyendocrine syndrome type 1 and NALP5, a parathyroid autoantigen. *N. Engl. J. Med.* **358:** 1018–1028.

52. Gavalas, N.G., E.H. Kemp, K.J. Krohn, *et al.* 2007. The calcium-sensing receptor is a target of autoantibodies in patients with autoimmune polyendocrine syndrome type 1. *J. Clin. Endocrinol. Metab.* **92:** 2107–2114.

53. Soderbergh, A., A.G. Myhre, O. Ekwall, *et al.* 2004. Prevalence and clinical associations of 10 defined autoantibodies in autoimmune polyendocrine syndrome type I. *J. Clin. Endocrinol. Metab.* **89:** 557–562.

54. Krohn, K., R. Uibo, E. Aavik, *et al.* 1992. Identification by molecular cloning of an autoantigen associated with Addison's disease as steroid 17 alpha-hydroxylase. *Lancet* **339:** 770–773.

55. Winqvist, O., F.A. Karlsson & O. Kampe. 1992. 21-Hydroxylase, a major autoantigen in idiopathic Addison's disease. *Lancet* **339:** 1559–1562.

56. Winqvist, O., J. Gustafsson, F. Rorsman, *et al.* 1993. Two different cytochrome P450 enzymes are the adrenal antigens in autoimmune polyendocrine syndrome type I and Addison's disease. *J. Clin. Invest.* **92:** 2377–2385.

57. Proust-Lemoine, E., P. Saugier-Veber, D. Lefranc, *et al.* 2010. Autoimmune polyendocrine syndrome type 1 in north-western France: AIRE gene mutation specificities and severe forms needing immunosuppressive therapies. *Horm. Res. Paediatr.* **74:** 275–284.

58. Perniola, R., A. Falorni, M.G. Clemente, *et al.* 2000. Organ-specific and non-organ-specific autoantibodies in children and young adults with autoimmune polyendocrinopathy-candidiasis-ectodermal dystrophy (APECED). *Eur. J. Endocrinol.* **143:** 497–503.

59. Reimand, K., J. Perheentupa, M. Link, *et al.* 2008. Testis-expressed protein TSGA10 an auto-antigen in autoimmune polyendocrine syndrome type I. *Int. Immunol.* **20:** 39–44.

60. Bensing, S., S.O. Fetissov, J. Mulder, *et al.* 2007. Pituitary autoantibodies in autoimmune polyendocrine syndrome type 1. *Proc. Natl. Acad. Sci. USA* **104:** 949–954.

61. Husebye, E.S., G. Gebre-Medhin, T. Tuomi, *et al.* 1997. Autoantibodies against aromatic L-amino acid decarboxylase in autoimmune polyendocrine syndrome type I. *J. Clin. Endocrinol. Metab.* **82:** 147–150.

62. Clemente, M.G., P. Obermayer-Straub, A. Meloni, *et al.* 1997. Cytochrome P450 1A2 is a hepatic autoantigen in autoimmune polyglandular syndrome type 1. *J. Clin. Endocrinol. Metab.* **82:** 1353–1361.

63. Ekwall, O., H. Hedstrand, L. Grimelius, *et al.* 1998. Identification of tryptophan hydroxylase as an intestinal autoantigen. *Lancet* **352:** 279–283.

64. Skoldberg, F., G.M. Portela-Gomes, L. Grimelius, *et al.* 2003. Histidine decarboxylase, a pyridoxal phosphate-dependent enzyme, is an autoantigen of gastric enterochromaffin-like cells. *J. Clin. Endocrinol. Metab.* **88:** 1445–1452.

65. Hedstrand, H., O. Ekwall, J. Haavik, *et al.* 2000. Identification of tyrosine hydroxylase as an autoantigen in autoimmune polyendocrine syndrome type I. *Biochem. Biophys. Res. Commun.* **267:** 456–461.

66. Hedstrand, H., O. Ekwall, M.J. Olsson, *et al.* 2001. The transcription factors SOX9 and SOX10 are vitiligo autoantigens

in autoimmune polyendocrine syndrome type I. *J. Biol. Chem.* **276**: 35390–35395.

67. Alimohammadi, M., N. Dubois, F. Skoldberg, *et al.* 2009. Pulmonary autoimmunity as a feature of autoimmune polyendocrine syndrome type 1 and identification of KC-NRG as a bronchial autoantigen. *Proc. Natl. Acad. Sci. USA* **106**: 4396–4401.

68. Uibo, R., E. Aavik, P. Peterson, *et al.* 1994. Autoantibodies to cytochrome P450 enzymes P450scc, P450c17, and P450c21 in autoimmune polyglandular disease types I and II and in isolated Addison's disease. *J. Clin. Endocrinol. Metab.* **78**: 323–328.

69. Furmaniak, J., S. Kominami, T. Asawa, *et al.* 1994. Autoimmune Addison's disease—evidence for a role of steroid 21-hydroxylase autoantibodies in adrenal insufficiency. *J. Clin. Endocrinol. Metab.* **79**: 1517–1521.

70. Gylling, M., T. Tuomi, P. Bjorses, *et al.* 2000. ss-cell autoantibodies, human leukocyte antigen II alleles, and type 1 diabetes in autoimmune polyendocrinopathy-candidiasis-ectodermal dystrophy. *J. Clin. Endocrinol. Metab.* **85**: 4434–4440.

71. Kemp, E.H., N.G. Gavalas, K.J. Krohn, *et al.* 2009. Activating autoantibodies against the calcium-sensing receptor detected in two patients with autoimmune polyendocrine syndrome type 1. *J. Clin. Endocrinol. Metab.* **94**: 4749–4756.

72. Husebye, E.S. 2009. Functional autoantibodies cause hypoparathyroidism. *J. Clin. Endocrinol. Metab.* **94**: 4655–4657.

73. Gebre-Medhin, G., E.S. Husebye, J. Gustafsson, *et al.* 1997. Cytochrome P450IA2 and aromatic L-amino acid decarboxylase are hepatic autoantigens in autoimmune polyendocrine syndrome type I. *FEBS Lett.* **412**: 439–445.

74. Bratland, E., B. Skinningsrud, D.E. Undlien, *et al.* 2009. T cell responses to steroid cytochrome P450 21-hydroxylase in patients with autoimmune primary adrenal insufficiency. *J. Clin. Endocrinol. Metab.* **94**: 5117–5124.

75. Bratland, E. & E.S. Husebye. 2011. Cellular immunity and immunopathology in autoimmune Addison's disease. *Mol. Cell. Endocrinol.* **336**: 180–190.

76. Rottembourg, D., C. Deal, M. Lambert, *et al.* 2010. 21-Hydroxylase epitopes are targeted by CD8 T cells in autoimmune Addison's disease. *J. Autoimmun.* **35**: 309–315.

77. Gianani, R. & G.S. Eisenbarth. 2003. Autoimmunity to gastrointestinal endocrine cells in autoimmune polyendocrine syndrome type I. *J. Clin. Endocrinol. Metab.* **88**: 1442–1444.

78. Hogenauer, C., R.L. Meyer, G.J. Netto, *et al.* 2001. Malabsorption due to cholecystokinin deficiency in a patient with autoimmune polyglandular syndrome type I. *N. Engl. J. Med.* **344**: 270–274.

79. Collins, S.M., M. Dominguez, T. Ilmarinen, *et al.* 2006. Dermatological manifestations of autoimmune polyendocrinopathy–candidiasis–ectodermal dystrophy syndrome. *Br. J. Dermatol.* **154**: 1088–1093.

80. Pavlic, A. & J. Waltimo-Siren. 2009. Clinical and microstructural aberrations of enamel of deciduous and permanent teeth in patients with autoimmune polyendocrinopathy-candidiasis-ectodermal dystrophy. *Arch. Oral. Biol.* **54**: 658–665.

81. Perniola, R., G. Tamborrino, S. Marsigliante, *et al.* 1998. Assessment of enamel hypoplasia in autoimmune polyendocrinopathy–candidiasis–ectodermal dystrophy (APECED). *J. Oral. Pathol. Med.* **27**: 278–282.

82. Orlova, E.M., A.M. Bukina, E.S. Kuznetsova, *et al.* 2010. Autoimmune polyglandular syndrome 1 in Russian patients: clinical variants and autoimmune regulator mutations. *Horm. Res. Paediatr.* **73**: 449–457.

83. Al-Owain, M., N. Kaya, H. Al-Zaidan, *et al.* 2010. Renal failure associated with APECED and terminal 4q deletion: evidence of autoimmune nephropathy. *Clin. Dev. Immunol.* **2010**: 586342.

84. Ulinski, T., L. Perrin, M. Morris, *et al.* 2006. Autoimmune polyendocrinopathy-candidiasis-ectodermal dystrophy syndrome with renal failure: impact of posttransplant immunosuppression on disease activity. *J. Clin. Endocrinol. Metab.* **91**: 192–195.

85. Di Sabatino, A., R. Carsetti & G.R. Corazza. 2011. Postsplenectomy and hyposplenic states. *Lancet* **378**: 86–97.

86. Rautemaa, R., J. Hietanen, S. Niissalo, *et al.* 2007. Oral and oesophageal squamous cell carcinoma—a complication or component of autoimmune polyendocrinopathy–candidiasis–ectodermal dystrophy (APECED, APS-I). *Oral. Oncol.* **43**: 607–613.

87. Oftedal, B.E., A.S. Wolff, E. Bratland, *et al.* 2008. Radioimmunoassay for autoantibodies against interferon omega; its use in the diagnosis of autoimmune polyendocrine syndrome type I. *Clin. Immunol.* **129**: 163–169.

88. Meager, A., A. Vincent, J. Newsom-Davis, *et al.* 1997. Spontaneous neutralising antibodies to interferon-alpha and interleukin-12 in thymoma-associated autoimmune disease. *Lancet* **350**: 1596–1597.

89. Marx, A., N. Willcox, M.I. Leite, *et al.* 2010. Thymoma and paraneoplastic myasthenia gravis. *Autoimmunity* **43**: 413–427.

90. Kisand, K., M. Link, A.S. Wolff, *et al.* 2008. Interferon autoantibodies associated with AIRE deficiency decrease the expression of IFN-stimulated genes. *Blood* **112**: 2657–2666.

91. Zhang, S.Y., S. Boisson-Dupuis, A. Chapgier, *et al.* 2008. Inborn errors of interferon (IFN)-mediated immunity in humans: insights into the respective roles of IFN-alpha/beta, IFN-gamma, and IFN-lambda in host defense. *Immunol. Rev.* **226**: 29–40.

92. Moschen, A.R., S. Geiger, I. Krehan, *et al.* 2008. Interferon-alpha controls IL-17 expression in vitro and in vivo. *Immunobiology* **213**: 779–787.

93. Liu, L., S. Okada, X.F. Kong, *et al.* 2011. Gain-of-function human STAT1 mutations impair IL-17 immunity and underlie chronic mucocutaneous candidiasis. *J. Exp. Med.* **208**: 1635–1648.

94. Puel, A., R. Doffinger, A. Natividad, *et al.* 2010. Autoantibodies against IL-17A, IL-17F, and IL-22 in patients with chronic mucocutaneous candidiasis and autoimmune polyendocrine syndrome type I. *J. Exp. Med.* **207**: 291–297.

95. Ahlgren, K.M., S. Moretti, B.A. Lundgren, *et al.* 2011. Increased IL-17A secretion in response to Candida albicans in autoimmune polyendocrine syndrome type 1 and its animal model. *Eur. J. Immunol.* **41**: 235–245.

96. Oftedal, B.E., O. Kampe, A. Meager, *et al*. 2011. Measuring autoantibodies against IL-17F and IL-22 in autoimmune polyendocrine syndrome type I by radioligand binding assay using fusion proteins. *Scand. J. Immunol.* **74:** 327–333.

97. Gaffen, S.L., N. Hernandez-Santos & A.C. Peterson. 2011. IL-17 signaling in host defense against Candida albicans. *Immunol. Res.* **50:** 181–187.

98. Puel, A., S. Cypowyj, J. Bustamante, *et al*. 2011. Chronic mucocutaneous Candidiasis in humans with inborn errors of interleukin-17 immunity. *Science* **332:** 65–68.

99. Liang, S.C., X.Y. Tan, D.P. Luxenberg, *et al*. 2006. Interleukin (IL)-22 and IL-17 are coexpressed by Th17 cells and cooperatively enhance expression of antimicrobial peptides. *J. Exp. Med.* **203:** 2271–2279.

100. Conti, H.R., O. Baker, A.F. Freeman, *et al*. 2011. New mechanism of oral immunity to mucosal candidiasis in hyper-IgE syndrome. *Mucosal. Immunol.* **4:** 448–455.

101. Sonnenberg, G.F., L.A. Fouser & D. Artis. 2011. Border patrol: regulation of immunity, inflammation and tissue homeostasis at barrier surfaces by IL-22. *Nat. Immunol.* **12:** 383–390.

102. Eyerich, S., J. Wagener, V. Wenzel, *et al*. 2011. IL-22 and TNF-alpha represent a key cytokine combination for epidermal integrity during infection with Candida albicans. *Eur. J. Immunol.* **41:** 1894–1901.

103. Eyerich, K., S. Foerster, S. Rombold, *et al*. 2008. Patients with chronic mucocutaneous candidiasis exhibit reduced production of Th17-associated cytokines IL-17 and IL-22. *J. Invest. Dermatol.* **128:** 2640–2645.

104. Ng, W.F., A. von Delwig, A.J. Carmichael, *et al*. 2010. Impaired T(H)17 responses in patients with chronic mucocutaneous candidiasis with and without autoimmune polyendocrinopathy–candidiasis–ectodermal dystrophy. *J. Allergy Clin. Immunol.* **126:** 1006–1015 e4.

105. Zeng, G., C.Y. Chen, D. Huang, *et al*. 2011. Membrane-bound IL-22 after de novo production in tuberculosis and anti-Mycobacterium tuberculosis effector function of IL-22+ CD4+ T cells. *J. Immunol.* **187:** 190–199.

106. Nagafuchi, S., K. Umene, F. Yamanaka, *et al*. 2007. Recurrent herpes simplex virus infection in a patient with autoimmune polyendocrinopathy–candidiasis–ectodermal dystrophy associated with L29P and IVS9-1G>C compound heterozygous autoimmune regulator gene mutations. *J. Intern. Med.* **261:** 605–610.

107. Mazza, C., F. Buzi, F. Ortolani, *et al*. 2011. Clinical heterogeneity and diagnostic delay of autoimmune polyendocrinopathy–candidiasis–ectodermal dystrophy syndrome. *Clin. Immunol.* **139:** 6–11.

108. Ward, L., J. Paquette, E. Seidman, *et al*. 1999. Severe autoimmune polyendocrinopathy–candidiasis–ectodermal dystrophy in an adolescent girl with a novel AIRE mutation: response to immunosuppressive therapy. *J. Clin. Endocrinol. Metab.* **84:** 844–852.

109. Padeh, S., R. Theodor, A. Jonas, *et al*. 1997. Severe malabsorption in autoimmune polyendocrinopathy–candidosis–ectodermal dystrophy syndrome successfully treated with immunosuppression. *Arch. Dis. Child* **76:** 532–534.

110. Perniola, R., M. Congedo, A. Rizzo, *et al*. 2008. Innate and adaptive immunity in patients with autoimmune polyendocrinopathy–candidiasis–ectodermal dystrophy. *Mycoses* **51:** 228–235.

111. Hong, M., K.R. Ryan, P.D. Arkwright, *et al*. 2009. Pattern recognition receptor expression is not impaired in patients with chronic mucocutanous candidiasis with or without autoimmune polyendocrinopathy candidiasis ectodermal dystrophy. *Clin. Exp. Immunol.* **156:** 40–51.

112. Ramsey, C., S. Hassler, P. Marits, *et al*. 2006. Increased antigen presenting cell-mediated T cell activation in mice and patients without the autoimmune regulator. *Eur. J. Immunol.* **36:** 305–317.

113. Brannstrom, J., S. Hassler, L. Peltonen, *et al*. 2006. Defect internalization and tyrosine kinase activation in AIRE deficient antigen presenting cells exposed to Candida albicans antigens. *Clin. Immunol.* **121:** 265–273.

114. Pontynen, N., M. Strengell, N. Sillanpaa, *et al*. 2008. Critical immunological pathways are downregulated in APECED patient dendritic cells. *J. Mol. Med.* **86:** 1139–1152.

115. Ryan, K.R., M. Hong, P.D. Arkwright, *et al*. 2008. Impaired dendritic cell maturation and cytokine production in patients with chronic mucocutaneous candidiasis with or without APECED. *Clin. Exp. Immunol.* **154:** 406–414.

116. Lindh, E., S.M. Lind, E. Lindmark, *et al*. 2008. AIRE regulates T-cell-independent B-cell responses through BAFF. *Proc. Natl. Acad. Sci. USA* **105:** 18466–18471.

117. Perniola, R., G. Lobreglio, M.C. Rosatelli, *et al*. 2005. Immunophenotypic characterisation of peripheral blood lymphocytes in autoimmune polyglandular syndrome type 1: clinical study and review of the literature. *J. Pediatr. Endocrinol. Metab.* **18:** 155–164.

118. Tuovinen, H., N. Pontynen, M. Gylling, *et al*. 2009. Gammadelta T cells develop independently of AIRE. *Cell Immunol.* **257:** 5–12.

119. Sediva, A., D. Cihakova & J. Lebl. 2002. Immunological findings in patients with autoimmune polyendocrinopathy–candidiasis–ectodermal dystrophy (APECED) and their family members: are heterozygotes subclinically affected? *J. Pediatr. Endocrinol. Metab.* **15:** 1491–1496.

120. Lindh, E., E. Rosmaraki, L. Berg, *et al*. 2010. AIRE deficiency leads to impaired iNKT cell development. *J. Autoimmun.* **34:** 66–72.

121. Kekalainen, E., H. Tuovinen, J. Joensuu, *et al*. 2007. A defect of regulatory T cells in patients with autoimmune polyendocrinopathy–candidiasis–ectodermal dystrophy. *J. Immunol.* **178:** 1208–1215.

122. Laakso, S.M., T.T. Laurinolli, L.H. Rossi, *et al*. 2010. Regulatory T cell defect in APECED patients is associated with loss of naive FOXP3(+) precursors and impaired activated population. *J. Autoimmun.* **35:** 351–357.

123. Ryan, K.R., C.A. Lawson, A.R. Lorenzi, *et al*. 2005. CD4+CD25+ T-regulatory cells are decreased in patients with autoimmune polyendocrinopathy candidiasis ectodermal dystrophy. *J. Allergy Clin. Immunol.* **116:** 1158–1159.

124. Mathis, D. & C. Benoist. 2009. AIRE. *Annu. Rev. Immunol.* **27:** 287–312.

125. Laakso, S.M., E. Kekalainen, L.H. Rossi, *et al*. 2011. IL-7 dysregulation and loss of CD8+ T cell homeostasis

in the monogenic human disease autoimmune polyendocrinopathy–candidiasis–ectodermal dystrophy. *J. Immunol.* **187:** 2023–2030.

126. Meager, A., P. Peterson & N. Willcox. 2008. Hypothetical review: thymic aberrations and type-I interferons; attempts to deduce autoimmunizing mechanisms from unexpected clues in monogenic and paraneoplastic syndromes. *Clin. Exp. Immunol.* **154:** 141–151.

127. Anderson, M.S. & M.A. Su. 2010. AIRE and T cell development. *Curr. Opin. Immunol.* **23:** 198–206.

128. Liston, A., S. Lesage, J. Wilson, *et al.* 2003. AIRE regulates negative selection of organ-specific T cells. *Nat. Immunol.* **4:** 350–354.

129. Goodnow, C.C., J. Sprent, B. Fazekas de St Groth, *et al.* 2005. Cellular and genetic mechanisms of self-tolerance and autoimmunity. *Nature* **435:** 590–597.

130. Teh, C.E., S.R. Daley, A. Enders, *et al.* 2010. T-cell regulation by casitas B-lineage lymphoma (Cblb) is a critical failsafe against autoimmune disease due to autoimmune regulator (Aire) deficiency. *Proc. Natl. Acad. Sci. USA* **107:** 14709–14714.

131. Rosenthal, F.D., M.K. Davies & A.C. Burden. 1978. Malig-nant disease presenting as Addison's disease. *Br. Med. J.* **1:** 1591–1592.

132. Spencer, S.J., S. Mesiano, J.Y. Lee, *et al.* 1999. Proliferation and apoptosis in the human adrenal cortex during the fetal and perinatal periods: implications for growth and remodeling. *J. Clin. Endocrinol. Metab.* **84:** 1110–1115.

133. Strobel, P., A. Murumagi, R. Klein, *et al.* 2007. Deficiency of the autoimmune regulator AIRE in thymomas is insufficient to elicit autoimmune polyendocrinopathy syndrome type 1 (APS-1). *J. Pathol.* **211:** 563–571.

134. Marx, A., P. Hohenberger, H. Hoffmann, *et al.* 2010. The autoimmune regulator AIRE in thymoma biology: autoimmunity and beyond. *J. Thorac. Oncol.* **5:** S266–S272.

135. Hill, M.E., H. Shiono, J. Newsom-Davis, *et al.* 2008. The myasthenia gravis thymus: a rare source of human autoantibody-secreting plasma cells for testing potential therapeutics. *J. Neuroimmunol.* **201–202:** 50–56.

136. Shiono, H., Y.L. Wong, I. Matthews, *et al.* 2003. Spontaneous production of anti-IFN-alpha and anti-IL-12 autoantibodies by thymoma cells from myasthenia gravis patients suggests autoimmunization in the tumor. *Int. Immunol.* **15:** 903–913.

Ann. N.Y. Acad. Sci. ISSN 0077-8923

ANNALS OF THE NEW YORK ACADEMY OF SCIENCES

Issue: *The Year in Human and Medical Genetics: Inborn Errors of Immunity*

Genetic lessons learned from X-linked Mendelian susceptibility to mycobacterial diseases

Jacinta Bustamante,[1,2] Capucine Picard,[1,2,3,4] Stéphanie Boisson-Dupuis,[1,2,5] Laurent Abel,[1,2,5] and Jean-Laurent Casanova[1,2,4,5]

[1]Laboratory of Human Genetics of Infectious Diseases, Necker Branch, Institut National de la Santé et de la Recherche Médicale, Paris, France. [2]Paris Descartes University, Necker Medical School, Paris, France. [3]Study Center of Primary Immunodeficiencies, [4]Pediatric Hematology-Immunology Unit, Necker Hospital, Paris, France. [5]St. Giles Laboratory of Human Genetics of Infectious Diseases, Rockefeller Branch, The Rockefeller University, New York, New York

Address for correspondence: Jacinta Bustamante, M.D., Ph.D., Laboratory of Human Genetics of Infectious Diseases, Necker Branch, Paris Descartes University, Necker Medical School, Paris, France 75015. jacinta.bustamante@inserm.fr

Mendelian susceptibility to mycobacterial disease (MSMD) is a rare syndrome conferring predisposition to clinical disease caused by weakly virulent mycobacteria, such as *Mycobacterium bovis* Bacille Calmette Guérin (BCG) vaccines and nontuberculous, environmental mycobacteria (EM). Since 1996, MSMD-causing mutations have been found in six autosomal genes involved in IL-12/23–dependent, IFN-γ–mediated immunity. The aim of this review is to provide the description of the two described forms of X-linked recessive (XR) MSMD. Germline mutations in two genes, *NEMO* and *CYBB,* have long been known to cause other human diseases—incontinentia pigmenti (IP) and anhidrotic ectodermal dysplasia with immunodeficiency (EDA-ID) (*NEMO/IKKG*), and X-linked chronic granulomatous disease (CGD) (*CYBB*)—but specific mutations in either of these two genes have recently been shown to cause XR-MSMD. NEMO is an essential component of several NF-κB–dependent signaling pathways. The MSMD-causing mutations in *NEMO* selectively affect the CD40-dependent induction of IL-12 in mononuclear cells. *CYBB* encodes gp91^{phox}, which is an essential component of the NADPH oxidase in phagocytes. The MSMD-causing mutation in *CYBB* selectively affects the respiratory burst in macrophages. Mutations in *NEMO* and *CYBB* may therefore cause MSMD by selectively exerting their deleterious impact on a single signaling pathway (CD40–IL-12, *NEMO*) or a single cell type (macrophages, *CYBB*). These experiments of Nature illustrate how specific germline mutations in pleiotropic genes can dissociate signaling pathways or cell lineages, thereby resulting in surprisingly narrow clinical phenotypes.

Keywords: mycobacteria; X-linked primary immunodeficiency; *NEMO*; *CYBB*; interleukin-12; interferon-γ; monocytes; macrophages

Introduction

Mendelian susceptibility to mycobacterial disease (MSMD) is a rare syndrome conferring predisposition to clinical disease caused by weakly virulent mycobacteria, such as *Mycobacterium bovis* Bacille Calmette Guérin (BCG) vaccines and nontuberculous, environmental mycobacteria (EM) (OMIM 209950).[1–3] It was recently found, as expected, that MSMD patients are also vulnerable to the more virulent *Mycobacterium tuberculosis*.[4–6] The syndrome was probably first reported in 1951, in an Alge-rian child with disseminated BCG disease,[7] and cases of "idiopathic" infections with BCG have since been reported worldwide.[8] Children with unexplained EM disease were also identified, once EM species had been described, with opportunistic EM, such as *Mycobacterium avium*, implicated most frequently. Typically, unlike patients with most conventional primary immunodeficiencies,[9] patients with MSMD are otherwise healthy and are not prone to other unusually severe infections, with the notable exception of systemic nontyphoidal salmonellosis, which is documented in about half

doi: 10.1111/j.1749-6632.2011.06273.x

the patients, including some without mycobacterial diseases.[10,11] However, other severe infectious diseases, as diverse as cytomegalovirus and varicella zoster virus diseases,[12] human herpes virus-8–associated Kaposi's sarcoma,[13] listeriosis,[14] klebsiellosis,[15] nocardiosis[16,17] histoplasmosis,[18] paracoccidioidomycosis,[19] coccidioidomycosis,[20,21] and leishmaniasis,[22] have been reported, mostly in single patients, raising the possibility that the clinical phenotype of MSMD may well extend beyond diseases caused by *Mycobacterium* or *Salmonella*. The original denomination of MSMD may therefore not accurately describe all patients, particularly if genetic etiologies common to various infectious phenotypes are described.

The syndrome of MSMD was long thought to be Mendelian, based on the large number of consanguineous and/or multiplex kindreds identified. The occurrence of MSMD in patients born to consanguineous parents and in siblings strongly suggested that most cases followed an autosomal recessive (AR) mode of inheritance.[2] Consistent with this hypothesis, six MSMD-causing genes identified were all found to be autosomal.[3,23] Since 1996, MSMD-causing mutations have been found in six autosomal genes—*IFNGR1*, *IFNGR2*, *STAT1*, *IL12B*, *IL12RB1*, and *IRF8*—all involved in IL-12/23–dependent,

IFN-γ–mediated immunity. Mutations in *IFNGR1* (encoding the ubiquitously expressed IFN-γ receptor ligand-binding chain, IFN-γ R1),[24–29] *IFNGR2* (IFN-γ R2),[30–34] and *STAT1* (STAT1)[35,36] impair cellular responses to IFN-γ, a cytokine produced by NK and T lymphocytes. Mutations in *IL12B* [16,37] and *IL12RB1*[38–40] impair the production of IFN-γ, by blocking the production of the p40 subunit of IL-12 and IL-23 (encoded by *IL12B*) or the response to IL-12 and IL-23 (*IL12RB1*, encoding the β1 chain of the IL-12 and IL-23 receptors) in phagocytes and dendritic cells (Fig. 1). IL-12 is a relatively specific, potent inducer of IFN-γ, whereas the newly described IL-23 is involved in the induction of IL-17 cytokines. Mutations in *IRF8*, an interferon regulatory factor inducible by IFN-γ, impair IL-12 secretion by monocytes and dendritic cells.[23] "MSMD" may therefore be described as a disorder of the IL-12–IFN-γ circuit, at least in patients bearing these defects. Interestingly, the genetic investigation of MSMD from this perspective has led to the description of the related, but different disorder of AR, complete STAT1 deficiency[41,42] and partial recessive STAT1 deficiency[43–45] in patients highly vulnerable to both mycobacteria and viruses. These patients have impaired responses to IFN-γ, accounting for mycobacterial diseases, and impaired responses to

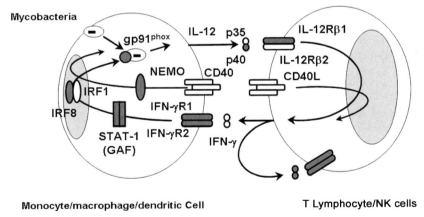

Figure 1. MSMD-causing gene products in the IL-12/23–IFN-γ circuit. Schematic representation of cytokine production and cooperation between monocytes/macrophages/dendritic cells and NK/T cells. Mutant molecules in patients with MSMD are indicated in gray. Allelic heterogeneity of the eight genes results in the definition of 15 genetic disorders. The IL-12–IFN-γ loop and the CD40L-activated CD40 pathway, mediating cooperation between T cells and monocyte/cells, are crucial for protective immunity to mycobacterial infection in humans. IRF8 is an IFN-γ–inducible transcription factor required for the induction of various target genes, including IL-12. The *NEMO* mutations in the LZ domain mostly impair CD40-NEMO–dependent pathways. The Q231P and T178P gp91*phox* mutations specifically abolish the respiratory burst in monocyte-derived macrophages; gp91*phox* induction might lead to release of IL-12 (for which, any evidence has not yet been demonstrated).

IFN-α/β and IFN-λ, accounting for overwhelming viral diseases.[46,47]

Moreover, the high level of allelic heterogeneity at these six loci accounted for the existence of 13 known distinct genetic disorders, depending on whether the alleles were null or hypomorphic, associated with a lack of protein expression, or the expression of an abnormal protein, in which case, depending on the molecular mechanism of disease, and more surprisingly, whether the alleles conferred recessive or dominant MSMD (Table 1). Indeed, whereas MSMD was first noticed to be inherited as an AR, and its first genetic etiologies were actually found to be AR, autosomal dominant (AD) MSMD, with both sporadic cases and multiplex kindreds with cases in several generations, has been found to be associated with specific *IFNGR1*, *STAT1*, and *IRF8* alleles.[23,26,35,36] A mutation in *IFNGR2* has even been found to be dominant in cells from a healthy individual, raising the possibility that there might be MSMD patients with dominant IFN-γR2 deficiency.[32] Four of the 13 known autosomal genetic etiologies of MSMD are AD, the others being AR. However, these known genetic etiologies account for no more than half the patients with MSMD, and probably even fewer of the patients with other unexplained infectious diseases, such as nontyphoidal salmonellosis. Interestingly, MSMD may also segregate as an X-linked recessive (XR) trait. We will herein review the two known forms of XR MSMD, due to mutations in *NEMO* and *CYBB*.

X-linked recessive MSMD type 1

The occurrence of mycobacterial disease in multiple, maternally related males in other kindreds suggested, as early as 1996, that there might be at least one XR form of MSMD.[48,49] Two patients from a kindred with X-linked MSMD were described clinically in 1991,[50] another patient related to these cases was identified in 1994,[51] and a fourth case relative with the same underlying genetic etiology was reported in 2006 (OMIM 300636).[52] Clinically, four maternally related males developed disseminated *Mycobacterium avium* complex infection but presented no other severe infectious diseases, with the exception of invasive *Haemophilus influenzae* type b infection in one patient and culture-proven, miliary tuberculosis in another. The known autosomal defects of the IL-12–IFN-γ circuit were ex-

Table 1. Genetic etiologies of MSMD

Gene	Inheritance	Defect	Protein
IL12B	AR	C	E−
IL12RB1	AR	C	E−
	AR	C	E+
IFNGR1	AR	C	E−
	AR	C	E+
	AR	P	E+
	AD	P	E++
IFNGR2	AR	C	E−
	AR	C	E+
	AR	P	E+
STAT1	AD	P	E+P−
	AD	P	E+P+B−
IRF8	AD	P	E+
NEMO	XR	P	E+
CYBB	XR	P	E+

Modes of inheritance are either autosomal dominant (AD), autosomal recessive (AR), or X-linked recessive (XR). The functional defects are either complete (C) or partial (P). The mutant proteins are either expressed (E+) or not (E−), being not phosphorylated (P−) or not binding DNA (P+ B−) upon IFN-γ stimulation.

cluded in these kindreds. However, a related immunological phenotype was identified by Frucht and Holland in 1996.[48] They reported low levels of IFN-γ and IL-12 production by the patients' mononuclear cells upon activation with phytohemaggutinin (PHA) or CD3-specific antibodies. The production of IL-12 in response to microbial stimulation, in the form of BCG, BCG plus IFN-γ, and LPS, was normal. Impaired IL-12 production by the patients' monocytes was shown to be the primary defect in assays in which autologous and heterologous monocytes and T cells were cocultured in the presence of PHA, resulting in a secondary defect in IFN-γ production. The monocyte defect was cell autonomous, but dependent on the presence of T cells, indicating a defect in the T cell-dependent monocyte activation pathway.

It was only later recognized that one of these four American patients had sparse teeth, leading to suspicion of a disorder related to anhidrotic ectodermal dysplasia (EDA) with immunodeficiency (EDA-ID). EDA-ID is a complex developmental and immunological syndrome caused by hypomorphic mutations in *NEMO/IKKG*, encoding a regulatory component of the IKK complex.[53–55] In its classical form, the EDA developmental syndrome is characterized by the lack of skin appendages, resulting in anodontia or hypodontia with conical incisors (decidual or permanent teeth), atrichosis or hypotrichosis (sparse hair, no eyebrows and eyelashes), and a lack of sweat glands (with heat intolerance). Most children with EDA do not suffer from any detectable immunodeficiency and carry mutations in the ectodysplasin pathway.[56] However, some children with EDA have been found to display severe infectious diseases and an impaired antibody response to glycan antigens—pneumococcal capsular antigens in particular—leading Abinun to coin the term EDA-ID.[57–59] No overt immunological abnormalities other than a poor inflammatory response have been identified in these patients. The range of infections varied considerably from case to case, with viral, bacterial, and fungal diseases observed, but most children suffered from invasive pneumococcal disease, which was by far the most frequent type of infection in these children. Some children have been found to have a much milder developmental phenotype, with conical incisors as the sole developmental abnormality.[60,61] Some children with hypomorphic mutations in *NEMO* have even been found to have no detectable developmental phenotype.[62–64]

The underlying genetic mutations in *NEMO* in children with EDA-ID were identified by serendipity, when two mothers with IP surprisingly gave birth at term to boys with EDA-ID,[65,66] after it had been shown that IP, an X-linked dominant disorder lethal *in utero* in boys, was associated with loss-of-function mutations in *NEMO*.[67,68] The two unrelated mothers were found to carry the same *NEMO* mutation, which, unlike the other IP-causing null mutations, was hypomorphic, indicating that there was a genotype–phenotype correlation in males, but not in females. Since 2001, up to 80 patients with hypomorphic mutations in *NEMO* have been reported[53–55,59–64,66,67,69–80] and many more have been diagnosed worldwide. For all mutations found (nonsense, frameshift, and missense), no obvious correlation between a given genotype and a particular infectious or immunological phenotype has been identified. However, the W420X mutation has been found to cosegregate with a severe phenotype of EDA-ID with osteopetrosis and lymphedema.[55,65,81,82]

Patients from the American kindred with XR-MSMD and impaired IL-12 production, by monocytes upon stimulation by PHA-activated T cells, were found to have the novel E315A *NEMO* mutation.[52] One boy in each of two other unrelated families, one from France and the other from Germany, developed infectious disease diagnosed as probable tuberculosis. The French patient presented very mild signs of EDA, limited to conical decidual incisors; he was vaccinated with BCG and, at the age of two years, had cervical lymphadenitis, fever, and a positive tuberculin skin test (TST). He was diagnosed with tuberculosis and treated for this disease. The German patient was not vaccinated with BCG, and at nine years of age, he was hospitalized for persistent fever and a strongly positive TST, suggestive of mycobacterial disease. This patient displayed no developmental abnormality. The same novel R319Q hemizygous mutation in *NEMO* was identified in these two kindreds.

The E315A and R319Q mutations were not mere polymorphisms, and were found to affect residues conserved in the *NEMO* genes of nine and six species (of nine studied). Moreover, residues E315 and R319 disrupt the formation of the salt bridge in the leucine zipper domain (LZD) of NEMO, suggesting that mutations in either of the amino acids may disturb the plasticity of the LZD-helix of NEMO, interfering with the CD40–NEMO–NF-κB signaling pathway. The folding defect of the E315A mutant is responsible for the defect in binding to ubiquitin chains.[83] These hypomorphic mutations in *NEMO* are associated with impaired NF-κB activation of c-Rel containing proteins in response to CD40. Not all CD40-dependent pathways are affected, as the induction of IL-12 in monocytes and dendritic cells is impaired, whereas that of the costimulatory molecules CD80 and CD86 is unaffected. The CD40–NF-κB pathway in B cells has also been shown to be intact. Moreover, these mutations do not affect NF-κB activation in response to classical activators, such as TNF-α, IL-1β, or lipopolysaccharide (LPS). The mutant NEMO protein was normally expressed in the hematopoietic and nonhematopoietic cells tested. The identification of these mutations therefore provided a molecular basis for XR-MSMD in the absence of other infections. Nonetheless, impairment of the CD40–IL-12 pathway cannot itself provide a full explanation for the predisposition to mycobacterial diseases, as CD40- and CD40L-deficient patients are prone to tuberculosis and regional "BCG-itis," but none has yet been shown to be particularly susceptible to *M. avium* disease or disseminated "BCG-osis." Other pathways affected by the *NEMO* mutations may also be involved. The key genetic feature of these two related mutations, found in six patients from three kindreds, is that they dissociate the multiple NEMO-dependent, NF-κB signaling pathways. By affecting the CD40–IL-12 pathway, while maintaining at least the other pathways tested, these two mutations result in a very narrow clinical phenotype, apparently restricted to MSMD, unlike other *NEMO* mutations, resulting in a much broader immunological and clinical phenotype.

X-linked recessive MSMD type 2

A second form of X-linked recessive MSMD has recently been reported (OMIM 3000645).[84] Four maternally related men from a large French kindred were identified as suffering from mycobacterial diseases.[85] The first patient, now aged 58 years, was not vaccinated with BCG in infancy but developed a clinical disease diagnosed as disseminated tuberculosis at the age of 34. The other three men, now aged 61, 56, and 37 years, suffered from disseminated BCG disease (BCG-osis) with lymph node involvement, or from recurrent regional BCG-itis, shortly after vaccination. Two of these men suffered relapses years later. Moreover, an obligate carrier from first kindred developed tuberculous salpingitis at the age of 29 years. Three maternally related men from another unrelated French kindred also displayed MSMD. The patients aged 37, 40, and 37 suffered from BCG-osis.[85] The seven patients did not suffer from any other infectious diseases. Other members of the two families were vaccinated with BCG, with no complications. The production of IL-12 and IFN-γ by the patients' cells in response to BCG was normal and, unlike patients with *NEMO* mutations (E315A and R319Q), these patients had an intact T cell–dependent pathway of monocyte IL-12 production. Moreover, CD40-dependent IL-12 production by monocytes and dendritic cells was normal. The involvement of *NEMO* was further excluded in theses kindreds by genetic means, including sequencing of the coding region and genetic linkage analysis. This linkage analysis identified two regions with a maximum LOD score

of 2.29, on the short and long arms of the X chromosome. The patients from the two kindreds therefore clearly displayed a new form of XR-MSMD.[85]

The sequencing of candidate genes in the intervals to which genes known to be associated with primary immunodeficiencies, including *CD40LG*, led to a specific mutation (Q231P) being identified in *CYBB* in the four male patients from the first family, and another specific mutation (T178P) identified in *CYBB* in the three male patients from the second family. This gene encodes gp91^{phox}, is located on the short arm of the X chromosome, and contains 13 exons. *CYBB* is expressed strongly in all phagocytic cells (including granulocytes, monocytes, and macrophages) and, to a lesser extent, in B cells. Germline mutations in *CYBB* are responsible for the most common form of chronic granulomatous disease (CGD) (OMIM 306400), a primary immunodeficiency disease in which phagocytic cells display little or no nicotinamide adenine dinucleotide phosphatase (NADPH) oxidase activity.[86–88] CGD patients suffer from recurrent life-threatening infections caused by multiple bacteria and fungi, *Staphylococcus* and *Aspergillus* in particular.[89] Mycobacterial diseases, caused by BCG and *M. tuberculosis*, are seen in about 30–40% of these patients, with a higher prevalence of tuberculosis in endemic countries.[90,91] A few rare cases have been reported of isolated mycobacterial disease, albeit in patients under the age of 17 years.[90] Patients also present steroid-sensitive granulomas, apparently not triggered by infectious agents. Three forms of X-linked CGD have been distinguished, based on X91 protein levels—X91^0 (no protein), X91$^-$ (low levels), and X91$^+$ (normal levels)—but there is no strict correlation with mutant gp91^{phoxn} function and the resulting clinical features.[89,92,93] Unlike the cells of CGD patients, neutrophils and monocytes from our seven patients displayed a perfectly functional respiratory burst, in terms of both superoxide production and hydroxide peroxide release after phorbol ester induction and the physiological stimuli.[85] Moreover, their granulocytes killed *Sthaphylococcus aureus* correctly, unlike granulocytes from CGD patients. This explains the lack of any of the common clinical features of CGD, whether infectious or granulomatous, in these seven adult patients, in the absence of any anti-infectious or immunosuppressive prophylaxis.

However, the hemizygous Q231P and T178P mutations were shown to affect respiratory burst function in monocyte-derived macrophages (MDMs) and EBV-transformed B cells. Indeed, when macrophages were activated with BCG, PPD, or IFN-γ and triggered with phorbol ester, the respiratory burst function was completely abolished.[85] Moreover, the growth of BCG in the patients' MDMs *in vitro* was enhanced. These alterations were documented *in vitro* and probably reflect the respiratory burst activity in tissue-resident macrophages *in vivo*. Indeed, B cells are known to play no substantial role in protective immunity to mycobacteria, as attested by the lack of mycobacterial diseases in B cell-deficient children.[94] This experiment of Nature therefore demonstrates that the respiratory burst in macrophages is essential for protective immunity to mycobacteria. These patients provide a cellular basis for the susceptibility to mycobacteria observed in CGD patients. The lack of environmental mycobacterial disease in patients with these mutations and the extreme rarity of such disease in CGD patients also indicate that the macrophage respiratory burst is not critical for the control of EM. The respiratory burst in granulocytes and monocytes also seems to be dispensable for protective immunity to mycobacteria. However, all six BCG-vaccinated patients in these kindreds had BCG disease (regional or disseminated forms), as do more than the 30–50% of vaccinated CGD patients. This may reflect the impact of modifier genes, or other unknown environmental factors. In any event, these data also strongly suggest that the macrophage respiratory burst is not involved in immunity to other bacteria and to fungi, consistent with the results obtained for patients with congenital or acquired neutropenia.[95] Immunity to these microbes principally involves the respiratory burst in granulocytes and monocytes.[96]

Why is the respiratory burst defective in macrophages (and B cells) but not in granulocytes or monocytes? The *CYBB* mutations are the germline mutations and were found in all cell types tested, including granulocytes and monocytes. However, the gp91^{phox} expression is different in all phagocytic cells, particularly in MDMs and EBV-B cells, correlating with the defect in the NADPH activity. Moreover, gp65^{phox}, a precursor of the mature gp91^{phox}, has been detected in the macrophages and EBV-B cells, indicating the impaired maturation of

gp65^{phox} to gp91^{phox} associated with impaired formation of the flavocytochrome b$_{558}$, the assembly and activation of which depend on a cell-specific threshold. Smaller amounts of gp91^{phox} protein can support flavocytochrome b$_{558}$ assembly and substantial oxidase activity in granulocytes and monocytes but not in B cells and macrophages. Additional experiments using Chinese hamster ovary (CHO) epithelial cell line and PLB-985 cell line found a small amount of gp91^{phox} and the presence of gp65 precursor by these two *CYBB* alleles.[85] The detailed biochemical mechanism underlying the selective, cell-specific impact of these germline mutations, which result in impaired flavocytochrome b$_{558}$ complex assembly required for NADPH activity, remains unknown.[85] The NADPH oxidase launches a series of biochemical reactions resulting in the successive production of multiple, short-lived reactive oxygen species (ROS).[96] In the *in vitro* and *ex vivo* assays, we determined the levels of only some of the ROS, such as superoxide and hydrogen peroxide, produced by cells extracted from their natural, physiological environment, and stimulated with artificial stimuli. For example, we determined hydrogen peroxide release by monocyte-derived macrophages. It is possible, although unlikely, that tissue macrophages *in vivo*, and perhaps even granulocytes or monocytes *in vivo*, have a phenotype different from that described in our study. Despite these hypothetical reservations, which are not yet possible to tackle experimentally in humans, these data strongly suggest that the Q231P and T178P *CYBB* mutations confer XR-MSMD because they selectively affect macrophages.

Conclusions

Elucidation of the molecular basis of the two forms of XR-MSMD was of immunological interest, as it indicated the role of the CD40–IL-12 pathway in monocyte-macrophages and dendritic cells (XR-MSMD type 1), and of the CYBB-dependent NADPH oxidase assembly and respiratory burst in macrophages (XR-MSMD type 2), in protective immunity to mycobacteria in humans. Mutations in *NEMO* are clearly connected with the IL-12–IFN-γ circuit, as CD40 stimulation leads to the induction of IL-12. The connection of the *CYBB* mutation with the previously identified mutations in autosomal genes controlling the IL-12–IFN-γ circuit is less clear. It may be that *CYBB* is controlled by IFN-γ, and the respiratory burst acts as an effector mechanism to destroy mycobacteria in macrophages. Alternatively, *CYBB* and the respiratory burst may be required for the optimal production of IL-12 by macrophages infected with mycobacteria. It is also possible that gp91^{phox} and the other MSMD-causing gene products are not directly connected but work independently to eliminate mycobacteria. These hypotheses are currently being tested *in vitro*. In any event, both *NEMO* and *CYBB* may be considered bona fide MSMD-causing genes, and MSMD is therefore allelic with two other XR primary immunodeficiencies: EDA-ID (*NEMO*) and CGD (*CYBB*) (Fig. 1).

These experiments of Nature are also of interest to the genetic community. Indeed, the two forms of XR-MSMD illustrate how subtle germline mutations in pleiotropic genes, involved in multiple signaling pathways (*NEMO*) and multiple cell types (*CYBB*), can impact on one pathway or one cell type, respectively. The XR-MSMD *NEMO* mutations do not impair *NEMO*-dependent NF-κB activation in response to most stimuli tested, accounting for the lack of associated EDA-ID developmental and infectious diseases—pyogenic bacterial diseases in particular. The XR-MSMD *CYBB* mutation does not impair the respiratory burst in granulocytes and monocytes, accounting for the lack of granulomas and infectious diseases seen in CGD—and of bacterial and fungal infections in particular. The MSMD-causing *NEMO* mutations thus seem to impair one pathway selectively, whereas the MSMD-causing *CYBB* mutation appears to impair one cell type selectively. From a genetic standpoint, these findings indicate that subtle mutations associated with a narrow phenotype may be found in genes, null mutations of which result in a broad phenotype, whether in mice or in humans.[97–100] Candidate genes should not be excluded *a priori* based solely on the phenotype associated with null alleles. The *NEMO* mutation, in particular, is reminiscent of the *STAT1* mutations previously found to affect one of the two signaling pathways involving STAT1.[35,36] As for *CYBB*, it now appears that germline mutations mimicking "conditional knockouts" in mice can be seen in humans. Candidate genes for subtle, narrow phenotypes should therefore not be excluded based solely on their involvement in multiple pathways or on the basis of their involvement in multiple cell types.

Acknowledgments

We thank all members of the two branches of the Laboratory of Human Genetics of Infectious Diseases for discussions. This work was supported by the *ANR*, the Rockefeller University Center for Clinical and Translational Science Grant number 5UL1RR024143, the Rockefeller University, and EU Grants HOMITB HEALTH-F3-2008-200732 and NEOTIM EEA05095KKA.

Conflicts of interest

The authors declare no conflicts of interest.

References

1. Hamosh, A. *et al.* 2005. Online Mendelian Inheritance in Man (OMIM), a knowledgebase of human genes and genetic disorders. *Nucleic Acids Res.* **33:** D514–517.
2. Casanova, J.L. & L. Abel. 2002. Genetic dissection of immunity to mycobacteria: the human model. *Annu. Rev. Immunol.* **20:** 581–620.
3. Filipe-Santos, O. *et al.* 2006. Inborn errors of IL-12/23- and IFN-gamma-mediated immunity: molecular, cellular, and clinical features. *Semin. Immunol.* **18:** 347–361.
4. Alcais, A. *et al.* 2005. Tuberculosis in children and adults: two distinct genetic diseases. *J. Exp. Med.* **202:** 1617–1621.
5. Boisson-Dupuis, S. *et al.* 2011. IL-12Rbeta1 deficiency in two of fifty children with severe tuberculosis from Iran, Morocco, and Turkey. *PLoS One* **6:** e18524.
6. Tabarsi, P. *et al.* 2011. Lethal tuberculosis in a previously healthy adult with IL-12 receptor deficiency. *J. Clin. Immunol.* **31:** 537–539.
7. Mimouni, J. 1951. Our experiences in three years of BCG vaccination at the center of the O.P.H.S. at Constantine; study of observed cases (25 cases of complications from BCG vaccination). *Alger. Medicale* **55:** 1138–1147.
8. Casanova, J.L. *et al.* 1996. Idiopathic disseminated bacillus Calmette–Guerin infection: a French national retrospective study. *Pediatric* **98:** 774–778.
9. Picard, C., J.L. Casanova & L. Abel. 2006. Mendelian traits that confer predisposition or resistance to specific infections in humans. *Curr. Opin. Immunol.* **18:** 383–390.
10. Bustamante, J. *et al.* 2008. Novel primary immunodeficiencies revealed by the investigation of paediatric infectious diseases. *Curr. Opin. Immunol.* **20:** 39–48.
11. Patel, S.Y. *et al.* 2008. Genetically determined susceptibility to mycobacterial infection. *J. Clin. Patho.* **61:** 1006–1012.
12. Dorman, S.E. *et al.* 1999. Viral infections in interferon-gamma receptor deficiency. *J. Pediatr.* **135:** 640–643.
13. Camcioglu, Y. *et al.* 2004. HHV-8-associated Kaposi sarcoma in a child with IFNgammaR1 deficiency. *J. Pediatr.* **144:** 519–523.
14. Roesler, J. *et al.* 1999. Listeria monocytogenes and recurrent mycobacterial infections in a child with complete interferon-gamma-receptor (IFNgammaR1) deficiency: mutational analysis and evaluation of therapeutic options. *Exp. Hematol* **27:** 1368–1374.

15. Pedraza, S. *et al.* 2010. Clinical disease caused by Klebsiella in 2 unrelated patients with interleukin 12 receptor beta1 deficiency. *Pediatrics* **126:** e971–e976.

16. Picard, C. *et al.* 2002. Inherited interleukin-12 deficiency: iL12B genotype and clinical phenotype of 13 patients from six kindreds. *Am. J. Hum. Genet.* **70:** 336–348.

17. Luangwedchakarn, V. *et al.* 2009. A novel mutation of the IL12RB1 gene in a child with nocardiosis, recurrent salmonellosis and neurofibromatosis type I: first case report from Thailand. *Asian Pac. J. Allergy Immunol.* **27:** 161–165.

18. Zerbe, C.S. & S.M. Holland. 2005. Disseminated histoplasmosis in persons with interferon-gamma receptor 1 deficiency. *Clin. Infect. Dis.* **41:** e38–e41.

19. Moraes-Vasconcelos, D. *et al.* 2005. Paracoccidioides brasiliensis disseminated disease in a patient with inherited deficiency in the beta1 subunit of the interleukin (IL)-12/IL-23 receptor. *Clin. Infect. Dis.* **41:** e31–e37.

20. Vinh, D.C. *et al.* 2009. Refractory disseminated coccidioidomycosis and mycobacteriosis in interferon-gamma receptor 1 deficiency. *Clin. Infect. Dis.* **49:** e62–e65.

21. Vinh, D.C. *et al.* 2011. Interleukin-12 receptor beta1 deficiency predisposing to disseminated coccidioidomycosis. *Clin. Infect. Dis.* **52:** e99-e102.

22. Sanal, O. *et al.* 2007. A case of interleukin-12 receptor beta-1 deficiency with recurrent leishmaniasis. *Pediatr. Infect. Dis. J.* **26:** 366–368.

23. Hambleton, S. *et al.* 2011. IRF8 mutations and human dendritic-cell immunodeficiency. *N. Engl. J. Med.* **365:** 127–138.

24. Newport, M.J. *et al.* 1996. A mutation in the interferon-gamma-receptor gene and susceptibility to mycobacterial infection. *N. Engl. J. Med.* **335:** 1941–1949.

25. Jouanguy, E. *et al.* 1996. Interferon-gamma-receptor deficiency in an infant with fatal bacille Calmette–Guerin infection. *N. Engl. J. Med.* **335:** 1956–1961.

26. Jouanguy, E. *et al.* 1999. A human IFNGR1 small deletion hotspot associated with dominant susceptibility to mycobacterial infection. *Nat. Genet.* **21:** 370–378.

27. Jouanguy, E. *et al.* 2000. In a novel form of IFN-gamma receptor 1 deficiency, cell surface receptors fail to bind IFN-gamma. *J. Clin. Invest.* **105:** 1429–1436.

28. Dorman, S.E. *et al.* 2004. Clinical features of dominant and recessive interferon gamma receptor 1 deficiencies. *Lancet* **364:** 2113–2121.

29. Kong, X.F. *et al.* 2010. A novel form of cell type-specific partial IFN-gammaR1 deficiency caused by a germ line mutation of the IFNGR1 initiation codon. *Hum. Mol. Genet.* **19:** 434–444.

30. Dorman, S.E. & S.M. Holland. 1998. Mutation in the signal-transducing chain of the interferon-gamma receptor and susceptibility to mycobacterial infection. *J. Clin .Invest.* **101:** 2364–2369.

31. Doffinger, R. *et al.* 2000. Partial interferon-gamma receptor signaling chain deficiency in a patient with bacille Calmette–Guerin and mycobacterium abscessus infection. *J. Infect. Dis.* **181:** 379–384.

32. Rosenzweig, S.D. *et al.* 2004. A novel mutation in IFN-gamma receptor 2 with dominant negative activity: biological consequences of homozygous and heterozygous states. *J. Immunol.* **173:** 4000–4008.

33. Vogt, G. *et al.* 2005. Gains of glycosylation comprise an unexpectedly large group of pathogenic mutations. *Nat. Genet.* **37:** 692–700.

34. Vogt, G. *et al.* 2008. Complementation of a pathogenic IFNGR2 misfolding mutation with modifiers of N-glycosylation. *J. Exp. Med.* **205:** 1729–1737.

35. Dupuis, S. *et al.* 2001. Impairment of mycobacterial but not viral immunity by a germline human STAT1 mutation. *Science* **293:** 300–303.

36. Chapgier, A. *et al.* 2006. Novel STAT1 alleles in otherwise healthy patients with mycobacterial disease. *PLoS. Genet.* **2:** e131.

37. Altare, F. *et al.* 1998. Inherited interleukin 12 deficiency in a child with bacille Calmette–Guerin and salmonella enteritidis disseminated infection. *J. Clin. Invest.* **102:** 2035–2040.

38. Fieschi, C. *et al.* 2003. Low penetrance, broad resistance, and favorable outcome of interleukin 12 receptor beta1 deficiency: medical and immunological implications. *J. Exp. Med.* **197:** 527–535.

39. Fieschi, C. *et al.* 2004. A novel form of complete IL-12/IL-23 receptor beta1 deficiency with cell surface-expressed nonfunctional receptors. *Blood* **104:** 2095–2101.

40. de Beaucoudrey, L. *et al.* 2010. Revisiting human IL-12Rbeta1 deficiency: a survey of 141 patients from 30 countries. *Medicine* **89:** 381–402.

41. Dupuis, S. *et al.* 2003. Impaired response to interferon-alpha/beta and lethal viral disease in human STAT1 deficiency. *Nat. Genet.* **33:** 388–391.

42. Chapgier, A. *et al.* 2006. Human complete STAT-1 deficiency is associated with defective type I and II IFN responses *in vitro* but immunity to some low virulence viruses *in vivo*. *J. Immunol.* **176:** 5078–5083.

43. Kong, X.F. *et al.* 2010. A novel form of human STAT1 deficiency impairing early but not late responses to interferons. *Blood* **116:** 5895–5906.

44. Chapgier, A. *et al.* 2009. A partial form of recessive STAT1 deficiency in humans. *J. Clin. Invest.* **119:** 1502–1514.

45. Vairo, D. *et al.* 2011. Severe impairment of IFN{gamma} and IFN{alpha} responses in cells of a patient with a novel STAT1 splicing mutation. *Blood* **118:** 1806–1817.

46. Jouanguy, E. *et al.* 2007. Human primary immunodeficiencies of type I interferons. *Biochimie* **89:** 878–883.

47. Zhang, S.Y. *et al.* 2008. Inborn errors of interferon (IFN)-mediated immunity in humans: insights into the respective roles of IFN-alpha/beta, IFN-gamma, and IFN-lambda in host defense. *Immunol. Rev.* **226:** 29–40.

48. Frucht, D.M. & S.M. Holland. 1996. Defective monocyte costimulation for IFN-gamma production in familial disseminated mycobacterium avium complex infection: abnormal IL-12 regulation. *J. Immunol.* **157:** 411–416.

49. Frucht, D.M. *et al.* 1999. IL-12-Independent costimulation pathways for interferon-gamma production in familial disseminated mycobacterium avium complex infection. *Clin. Immunol.* **91:** 234–241.

50. Nedorost, S.T. *et al.* 1991. Rosacea-like lesions due to familial mycobacterium avium-intracellulare infection. *Int. J. Dermatol.* **30:** 491–497.

51. Holland, S.M. *et al.* 1994. Treatment of refractory disseminated nontuberculous mycobacterial infection with interferon gamma. A preliminary report. *N. Engl. J Med.* **330:** 1348–1355.

52. Filipe-Santos, O. *et al.* 2006. X-linked susceptibility to mycobacteria is caused by mutations in NEMO impairing CD40-dependent IL-12 production. *J. Exp. Med.* **203:** 1745–1759.

53. Zonana, J. *et al.* 2000. A novel X-linked disorder of immune deficiency and hypohidrotic ectodermal dysplasia is allelic to incontinentia pigmenti and due to mutations in IKK-gamma (NEMO). *Am. J. Hum. Genet.* **67:** 1555–1562.

54. Jain, A. *et al.* 2001. Specific missense mutations in NEMO result in hyper-IgM syndrome with hypohydrotic ectodermal dysplasia. *Nat. Immunol.* **2:** 223–228.

55. Doffinger, R. *et al.* 2001. X-linked anhidrotic ectodermal dysplasia with immunodeficiency is caused by impaired NF-kappaB signaling. *Nat. Genet.* **27:** 277–285.

56. Priolo, M. & Lagana, C. 2001. Ectodermal dysplasias: a new clinical-genetic classification. *J. Med. Genet.* **38:** 579–585.

57. Abinun, M. 1995. Ectodermal dysplasia and immunodeficiency. *Arch. Dis. Child* **73:** 185.

58. Abinun, M. *et al.* 1996. Anhidrotic ectodermal dysplasia associated with specific antibody deficiency. *Eur. J. Pediatr.* **155:** 146–147.

59. Carrol, E.D. *et al.* 2003. Anhidrotic ectodermal dysplasia and immunodeficiency: the role of NEMO. *Arch. Dis. Child* **88:** 340–341.

60. Ku, C.L. *et al.* 2005. NEMO mutations in 2 unrelated boys with severe infections and conical teeth. *Pediatrics* **115:** e615–e619.

61. Hubeau, M. *et al.* 2011. A new mechanism of X-linked anhidrotic ectodermal dysplasia with immunodeficiency: impairment of ubiquitin binding despite normal folding of NEMO protein. *Blood* **118:** 926–935.

62. Puel, A. *et al.* 2006. The NEMO mutation creating the most-upstream premature stop codon is hypomorphic because of a reinitiation of translation. *Am. J. Hum. Genet.* **78:** 691–701.

63. Orange, J.S. *et al.* 2004. Human nuclear factor kappa B essential modulator mutation can result in immunodeficiency without ectodermal dysplasia. *J. Allergy Clin. Immunol.* **114:** 650–656.

64. Mooster, J.L. *et al.* 2010. Immune deficiency caused by impaired expression of nuclear factor-kappaB essential modifier (NEMO) because of a mutation in the 5' untranslated region of the NEMO gene. *J. Allergy Clin. Immunol.* **126:** 127–132 e7.

65. Mansour, S. *et al.* 2001. Incontinentia pigmenti in a surviving male is accompanied by hypohidrotic ectodermal dysplasia and recurrent infection. *Am. J. Med. Genet.* **99:** 172–177.

66. Dupuis-Girod, S. *et al.* 2002. Osteopetrosis, lymphedema, anhidrotic ectodermal dysplasia, and immunodeficiency in a boy and incontinentia pigmenti in his mother. *Pediatrics* **109:** e97.

67. Smahi, A. *et al.* 2000. Genomic rearrangement in NEMO impairs NF-kappaB activation and is a cause of incontinentia pigmenti. The International Incontinentia Pigmenti (IP) Consortium. *Nature* **405:** 466–472.

68. Smahi, A. *et al.* 2002. The NF-kappaB signalling pathway in human diseases: from incontinentia pigmenti to ectodermal dysplasias and immune-deficiency syndromes. *Hum. Mol. Genet.* **11:** 2371–2375.

69. Aradhya, S. *et al.* 2001. Atypical forms of incontinentia pigmenti in male individuals result from mutations of a cytosine tract in exon 10 of NEMO (IKK-gamma). *Am. J. Hum. Genet.* **68:** 765–771.

70. Kosaki, K. *et al.* 2001. Female patient showing hypohidrotic ectodermal dysplasia and immunodeficiency (HED-ID). *Am. J. Hum. Genet.* **69:** 664–666.

71. Nishikomori, R. *et al.* 2004. X-linked ectodermal dysplasia and immunodeficiency caused by reversion mosaicism of NEMO reveals a critical role for NEMO in human T-cell development and/or survival. *Blood* **103:** 4565–4572.

72. Jain, A. *et al.* 2004. Specific NEMO mutations impair CD40-mediated c-Rel activation and B cell terminal differentiation. *J. Clin. Invest.* **114:** 1593–1602.

73. Orstavik, K.H. *et al.* 2006. Novel splicing mutation in the NEMO (IKK-gamma) gene with severe immunodeficiency and heterogeneity of X-chromosome inactivation. *Am. J. Med. Genet. A* **140:** 31–39.

74. Lee, W.I. *et al.* 2005. Molecular analysis of a large cohort of patients with the hyper immunoglobulin M (IgM) syndrome. *Blood* **105:** 1881–1890.

75. Ku, C.L. *et al.* 2007. IRAK4 and NEMO mutations in otherwise healthy children with recurrent invasive pneumococcal disease. *J. Med. Genet.* **44:** 16–23.

76. Pachlopnik Schmid, J.M. *et al.* 2006. Transient hemophagocytosis with deficient cellular cytotoxicity, monoclonal immunoglobulin M gammopathy, increased T-cell numbers, and hypomorphic NEMO mutation. *Pediatrics* **117:** e1049—e1056.

77. Tono, C. *et al.* 2007. Correction of immunodeficiency associated with NEMO mutation by umbilical cord blood transplantation using a reduced-intensity conditioning regimen. *Bone Marrow Transplant* **39:** 801–804.

78. Hanson, E.P., L. Monaco-Shawver, L.A. Solt, *et al.* 2008. Hypomorphic nuclear factor-kappaB essential modulator mutation database and reconstitution system identifies phenotypic and immunologic diversity. *J. Allergy Clin. Immunol.* **122:** e1169–e1177.

79. Salt, B.H., J.E. Niemela, R. Pandey, *et al.* 2008. IKBKG (nuclear factor-kappa B essential modulator) mutation can be associated with opportunistic infection without impairing Toll-like receptor function. *J. Allergy Clin. Immunol.* **121:** 976–982.

80. Mancini, A.J., L.P. Lawley & G. Uzel. 2008. X-linked ectodermal dysplasia with immunodeficiency caused by NEMO mutation: early recognition and diagnosis. *Arch. Dermatol.* **144:** 342–346.

81. Dupuis-Girod, S. *et al.* 2006. Successful allogeneic hematopoietic stem cell transplantation in a child who had anhidrotic ectodermal dysplasia with immunodeficiency. *Pediatrics* **118:** e205–e211.

82. Roberts, C.M. *et al.* 2010. A novel NEMO gene mutation causing osteopetrosis, lymphoedema, hypohidrotic ectodermal dysplasia and immunodeficiency (OL-HED-ID). *Eur. J. Pediatr.* **169:** 1403–1407.

83. Lo, Y.C. *et al.* 2009. Structural basis for recognition of diubiquitins by NEMO. *Mol. Cell* **33:** 602–615.

84. Bustamante, J. *et al.* 2007. A novel X-linked recessive form of Mendelian susceptibility to mycobaterial disease. *J. Med. Genet,* **44:** e65.

85. Bustamante, J. *et al.* 2011. Germline CYBB mutations that selectively affect macrophages in kindreds with X-linked predisposition to tuberculous mycobacterial disease. *Nat. Immunol.* **12:** 213–221.

86. Royer-Pokora, B. *et al.* 1986. Cloning the gene for an inherited human disorder–chronic granulomatous disease–on the basis of its chromosomal location. *Nature* **322:** 32–38.

87. Dinauer, M.C. *et al.* 1987. The glycoprotein encoded by the X-linked chronic granulomatous disease locus is a component of the neutrophil cytochrome b complex. *Nature* **327:** 717–720.

88. Teahan, C. *et al.* 1987. The X-linked chronic granulomatous disease gene codes for the beta-chain of cytochrome b-245. *Nature* **327:** 720–721.

89. Roos, D., T.W. Kuijpers & J.T. Curnutte. 2007. Chronic granulomatous disease. In *Primary Immunodeficiency Diseases. A Molecular and Genetic Approach.* H.D. Ochs, C.I. Edvards Smith & J.M. Puch, Eds.: 525–549. Oxford University Press, New York.

90. Bustamante, J. *et al.* 2007. BCG-osis and tuberculosis in a child with chronic granulomatous disease. *J. Allergy Clin. Immunol.* **120:** 32–38.

91. Lee, P.P. *et al.* 2008. Susceptibility to mycobacterial infections in children with X-linked chronic granulomatous disease: a review of 17 patients living in a region endemic for tuberculosis. *Pediatr. Infect. Dis. J.* **27:** 224–230.

92. Holland, S.M. 2010. Chronic granulomatous disease. *Clin. Rev. Allergy Immunol.* **38:** 3–10.

93. Roos, D. *et al.* 2010. Hematologically important mutations: x-linked chronic granulomatous disease (third update). *Blood Cells Mol. Dis.* **45:** 246–265.

94. Conley, M.E., *et al.* 2009. Primary B cell immunodeficiencies: comparisons and contrasts. *Annu. Rev. Immunol.* **27:** 199–227.

95. Boztug, K. & C. Klein. 2009. Novel genetic etiologies of severe congenital neutropenia. *Curr. Opin. Immunol.* **21:** 472–480.

96. Segal, A.W. 2005. How neutrophils kill microbes. *Annu. Rev. Immunol.* **23:** 197–223.

97. Casanova, J.L. & L. Abel. 2007. Primary immunodeficiencies: a field in its infancy. *Science* **317:** 617–619.

98. Alcais, A., L. Abel & J.L. Casanova. 2009. Human genetics of infectious diseases: between proof of principle and paradigm. *J. Clin. Invest.* **119:** 2506–2514.

99. Notarangelo, L.D. & J.L. Casanova. 2009. Primary immunodeficiencies: increasing market share. *Curr. Opin. Immunol.* **21:** 461–465.

100. Alcais, A. *et al.* 2011. Life-threatening infectious diseases of childhood: single-gene inborn errors of immunity? *Ann. N.Y. Acad. Sci.* **1214:** 18–33.

Ann. N.Y. Acad. Sci. ISSN 0077-8923

ANNALS OF THE NEW YORK ACADEMY OF SCIENCES

Issue: *The Year in Human and Medical Genetics: Inborn Errors of Immunity*

IL-10 and IL-10 receptor defects in humans

Erik-Oliver Glocker,[1] Daniel Kotlarz,[2] Christoph Klein,[2] Neil Shah,[3] and Bodo Grimbacher[4,5]

[1]Institute of Medical Microbiology and Hygiene, University Hospital Freiburg, Germany. [2]Department of Pediatrics, Dr. von Hauner Children's Hospital, Ludwig-Maximilians-University, Munich, Germany. [3]Department of Paediatric Gastroenterology, Great Ormond Street Hospital, University College London, London, United Kingdom. [4]Department of Immunology, University College London Medical School (Royal Free Campus), London, United Kingdom. [5]Centre for Chronic Immune Deficiency, University Hospital Freiburg, Germany

Address for correspondence: Prof. Bodo Grimbacher, M.D., Department of Immunology and Molecular Pathology, Royal Free Hospital & University College London, Pond Street, London NW3 2QG, UK. b.grimbacher@ucl.ac.uk

Inflammatory bowel disease (IBD), which includes Crohn's disease (CD) and ulcerative colitis (UC), is chronic in nature and is characterized by abdominal pain, diarrhea, bleeding, and malabsorption. It is considered a complex multigenic and multifactorial disorder that results from disturbed interactions between the immune system and commensal bacteria of the gut. Recent work has demonstrated that IBD with an early-onset within the first months of life can be monogenic: mutations in IL-10 or its receptor lead to a loss of IL-10 function and cause severe intractable enterocolitis in infants and small children. Both IL-10 and IL-10 receptor deficiency can be successfully treated by hematopoietic stem cell transplantation.

Keywords: IL-10; IL-10 receptor; mutation; STAT3; inflammatory bowel disease

Introduction

Interleukin (IL)-10 may be considered the most important anti-inflammatory cytokine in humans. Secreted by a variety of cells including monocytes, macrophages, dendritic cells, T cells, B cells, granulocytes, epithelial cells, keratinocytes, and mast cells,[1] IL-10 limits secretion of pro-inflammatory cytokines such as TNF-α, IL-1, IL-6, and IL-12; it deactivates macrophages,[2] inhibits secretion of Th1 cytokines such as IL-2 and IFN-γ, and controls differentiation and proliferation of macrophages, T cells, and B cells.[1,3,4] By keeping pro-inflammatory events under control, it protects against excessive immune responses and tissue damage. Since IL-10 is a critical player in maintaining immune system balance, mutations in IL-10 or components of its signaling pathway that reduce or abolish their anti-inflammatory properties were thought to be involved in the pathogenesis of hyperinflammatory disorders such as rheumatoid arthritis or inflammatory bowel disease (IBD). IBD is relatively frequent, affecting about 1.4 million people in the United

States and 2.2 million in Europe.[5,6] Most often it manifests in the second or third decade of life, but IBD may also present in childhood with a severe and therapy-resistant course.[7,8]

Genome-wide linkage and association studies have emphasized the genetic complexity of IBD and identified a number of genes that may render individuals more susceptible to it;[9,10] for example, variations in genes involved in autophagy, in genes encoding proteins for intra- and extracellular pattern recognition receptors, in genes required for T helper 17 cell differentiation, in genes required for maintenance of the intestinal epithelium, and in genes required for shaping immune responses have been associated with susceptibility to IBD.

In contrast to the prevailing hypothesis that IBD is a multigenic disorder, recent work showed that certain variants of IBD or IL-10 and IL-10 receptor (IL-10R)-deficiency are monogenic autosomal recessive diseases. In this short review, we discuss the clinical phenotype and aspects of the pathogenesis of these novel entities and outline diagnostic procedures to confirm or rule-out these rare diseases.

doi: 10.1111/j.1749-6632.2011.06339.x

IL-10: a "shield" against hyperinflammation

To keep continuously ongoing pro-inflammatory events in the gut in check, a powerful countervailing activity capable of downregulating the immune system is required. The critical role of IL-10 as one such downregulator has been demonstrated in animal models; for example, mice deficient in IL-10 ($Il10^{-/-}$) or the IL-10R β-chain ($Il10rb^{-/-}$) develop severe enterocolitis.[11–13] Such murine phenotypes hint at a possible involvement of IL-10 signaling in the pathogenesis of human IBD. In support of that possibility, genetic variants of *IL10* in humans are associated with increased susceptibility to ulcerative colitis (UC);[14] and in patients suffering from Crohn's disease (CD), mutations in the leader sequence of IL-10 protein were shown to reduce its release from cells.[15] A frameshift insertion (3020insC) in the intracellular sensor molecule nucleotide-binding oligomerization domain containing 2 (NOD2), previously associated with CD, inhibits the ribonucleoprotein hnRNP-A1 and thereby actively blocks transcription of IL-10.[16]

Even though intestinal integrity is maintained by several factors, including the epithelial cell layer, mucus-secreting goblet cells, antimicrobial peptides-producing Paneth cells, IgA-releasing plasma cells, and gut-associated lymphoid tissue such as Peyer's patches, it is incontestable that IL-10 is the most relevant factor to protect against immunological imbalances.[17,18]

A main source of IL-10 in the gut are regulatory T (T_{reg}) cells, which tightly control chronic stimulation by resident intestinal flora and food antigens.[19] Scurfy mice lacking the T_{reg} cell lineage defining transcription factor forkhead box P3 (Foxp3) suffer from fatal multiorgan inflammation, and mice devoid of IL-10, a key cytokine of T_{reg} cells, die of wasting disease and colitis.[20–22] A similar phenotype occurs in humans; patients with mutations in *FOXP3*, located on the X chromosome, suffer from immunodysregulation, polyendocrinopathy, enteropathy, and X-linked (IPEX) syndrome, which is characterized by a lack of CD4$^+$ CD25$^+$ FOXP3$^+$ T_{reg} cells. Affected individuals develop autoimmune lymphoproliferation and multiple autoimmune disorders.[23–25] If not fatal in early childhood, patients with IPEX develop severe eczema, insulin-

dependent diabetes mellitus, hypo- or hyperthyroidism, and recurrent, sometimes severe, infections.[26–29] The predominant clinical feature, however, is an autoimmune enteropathy that starts as watery diarrhea and may turn slimy and bloody and mimic CD, UC, or celiac disease—all of which emphasize the indispensable role of IL-10 for intestinal homeostasis.[27,30]

The finding that loss-of-function mutations in either the IL-10 or IL-10R gene cause severe early-onset IBD in humans demonstrates the importance of IL-10 and shows that loss of IL-10 signaling significantly impairs life.[31,32] IL-10 appears to be of particular relevance for the integrity and homeostatis of the gut, which highlights the fact that the gut/bowel is highly vulnerable to disturbances of immunological balance.

IL-10 signaling pathway

To exert its actions, IL-10 dimerizes and binds to a cell-bound cytokine receptor made up of two molecules of the IL-10R α-chain (IL-10R1) and two molecules of the accessory IL-10R β-chain (IL-10R2).[1,4,33] Upon binding of IL-10 to the tetrameric receptor IL-10R complex, two members of the Janus kinase family—Janus kinase (JAK)1 and tyrosine kinase (Tyk)2—are activated and catalyze phosphorylation of themselves and then of IL-10R1 at specific intracellular tyrosine residues (tyrosine 446 and 496), thereby forming docking sites for STAT3.[33] STAT3 is then phosphorylated by JAK1 and Tyk2, which causes STAT3 dimerization and translocation to the nucleus where it induces expression of its target genes (summarized in Fig. 1).[33] In contrast to IL-10R1, which is unique to the IL-10R, IL-10R2 is shared by several other cytokines, including IL-22, IL-26, and the λ-interferons IL-28A/B and IL-29.[34,35] Both IL-10R1 and IL-10R2 are required for IL-10 signaling, as loss-of-function mutations in either one result in a complete signaling failure that cannot be compensated by any other pathway.

Clinical phenotypes of IL-10– and IL-10R–deficient patients

From investigations of two families with autosomal-recessive inherited enterocolitis, recent work has identified four patients with mutations in IL-10R: two patients carried homozygous missense mutations in *IL10RA* (encoding IL-10R1), resulting in

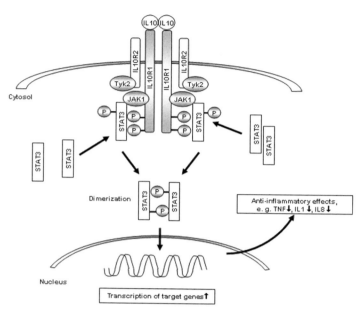

Figure 1. IL-10 signaling pathway.

amino acid exchanges at position 84 (Thr→Ile) or 141 (Gly→Arg); the other patients, two siblings, harbored a mutation affecting *IL10RB* (encoding IL-10R2), resulting in a premature stop codon (Try→Stop).[31] The patients presented within the first year of life with severe enterocolitis and perianal disease; subsequent formation of multiple abscesses and enterocutaneous fistula required several surgical interventions, eventually including complete colectomy. Histopathology revealed circumscribed, deep-set, thick, rolled-edged ulcers of the intestinal mucosa with inflammatory infiltrates of the epithelium, and the formation of abscesses extending to the *muscularis propria*. In addition, the patients suffered from chronic folliculitis and had a history of several recurring infections of their respiratory tract. The patients were treated with a wide spectrum of anti-inflammatory drugs, including steroids, methotrexate, thalidomide, and anti-TNF-α monoclonal antibodies, but none of these therapies induced sustained remission or long-term improvement.[31]

The discovery of the underlying genetic mutation opened novel therapeutic strategies. Since IL-10R1 and IL-10R2 double-deficiency described above has a very similar phenotype to severe colitis, it was hypothesized that severe colitis—the main clinical problem/phenotype in the above patients—was

due to defective IL-10 signaling in hematopoietic cells rather than defective IL-22, IL-26, and IFN-λ signaling in nonhematopoietic cells. In view of the life-threatening clinical course of the IL-10R mutations, allogeneic hematopoietic stem cell transplantation (HSCT) was proposed. The index patient with a loss-of-function mutation in IL-10R2 was successfully transplanted and showed sustained remission,[31] thus supporting the notion that IL-10 signaling in hematopoietic cells was critical to control hyperinflammation in the gut.

More recently, two other unrelated patients have been described with severe Crohn's-like colitis and the formation of perianal and rectovaginal fistulae, a phenotype resembling IL-10R deficiency.[32] Endoscopy and histopathology revealed extensive ulceration of the ileum and focal active colitis, with neutrophils infiltrating the surface epithelium. Both patients were found to have homozygous point mutations in *IL10* itself, leading to an amino acid change at codon 113 (Gly→Arg) that most likely changes the tertiary structure of the cytokine and results in impaired dimerization of IL-10. In contrast to wild-type IL-10, the mutated IL-10 failed to induce STAT3 phosphorylation or to inhibit lipopolysaccharide (LPS)-mediated TNF-α release in peripheral blood mononuclear cells (PBMCs).[32]

Ann. N.Y. Acad. Sci. 1246 (2011) 102–107 © 2011 New York Academy of Sciences.

Recently, Begue *et al.* investigated a cohort of 75 pediatric IBD patients for failures in IL-10 signaling.[36] They found one patient with a mutant IL-10R1 (Arg262Cys) and another patient with a mutant IL-10R2 (Glu141Stop). Both children presented with onset of symptoms at the first three months of life, including granuloma-positive colitis.[36] As anticipated, the patient harboring the IL-10R2 mutation showed impaired IL-22 signaling, whereas the patient with the IL-10R1 mutation (as well all other patients evaluated) did not. Also, typical for IL-10 and IL-10R deficiency, routine immunological work-up of the patients appeared to be normal.

Possible impact of defective IL-22, IL-26, and IFN-λ signaling

Since IL-10R2 is shared by the receptors for IL-22, IL-26 and λ-interferons and is expressed on various nonimmune cells, such as epithelial cells and keratinocytes,[35,37,38] one might presume that mutations in IL-10R2 result in more severe phenotypes than mutations in either IL-10R1 or IL-10. In particular, lack of IL-22 signaling may be additive to the phenotype of IL-10R2 deficiency because IL-22 protects against colitis and significantly improved colitis in a murine model of UC.[39,40] Among other activities, IL-22 upregulates expression of the antimicrobial proteins RegIII-β and RegIII-γ and enhances mucus production in murine colonic epithelial cells, which thereby maintains the epithelial barrier and prevents infection by intestinal bacterial pathogens.[39,41]

The folliculitis observed in IL-10R2–deficient patients may be at least in part attributed to impeded IL-22 signaling, which has been shown to control immunity of the skin by upregulating the expression of the β-defensins 2 and 3 and the antimicrobial heterodimer S100A8/9 in keratinocytes.[42–44] Furthermore, Nagalakshmi *et al.* demonstrated *in vitro* that IL-22 induces production of IL-10;[45] a similar activity was also found for IL-26.[46] In addition, IL-26 activates both STAT1 and STAT3, induces the release of IL-8 in colon epithelial cells, and keratinocytes, and increases the expression of intercellular cell adhesion molecule 1.[46] In murine lung epithelial cells, IL-22 regulates the innate immune defense by mediating expression of lipocalin-2, a protein capable of sequestering iron from Gram-negative bacteria and improving the killing of *Klebsiella pneumoniae*.[47] Recently, Celia *et al.* identified

a subset of natural killer cells that releases IL-22 and thereby controls inflammation and contributes to mucosal immunity.[48]

IL-28A, IL-28B, and IL-29 are primarily known to protect against viral infections,[49,50] but since other vital antiviral defense mechanisms—such as the IFN type I and II signaling pathways—are present, the antiviral activity of IL-28A, IL-28B, and IL-29 in general may be of minor importance. Further studies are required to properly assess their role and relevance in humans.

Diagnosis of IL-10 and IL-10R deficiency

Defects in the IL-10R may be easily tested by functional assays. PBMCs from healthy individuals show strong phosphorylation of STAT3 upon stimulation with IL-10, whereas PBMCs from IL-10R–deficient patients do not. In contrast to patients with IL-10R mutations, where administration of exogenous IL-10 has no effect at all, stimulation by IL-10 completely abrogates LPS-mediated TNF-α release in PBMCs from healthy controls.[2,11,31]

Of course, any functional abnormalities, such as the above, should always be confirmed by sequencing the IL10R genes *IL10RA* and *IL10RB*. Even though rarer and more challenging to rule out, lack of functional IL-10 should always be considered in cases of early-onset colitis with normal responses to exogenous IL-10. If sequencing of *IL10* reveals putative mutations, *in vitro* synthesis of the protein and subsequent functional testing, using STAT3 and/or TNF-α assays, should be carried out to prove that the observed mutation leads to a defective protein. Diagnostic procedures to confirm/rule out IL-10 and IL-10R mutations are summarized in Figure 2.

Conclusions

The functional consequences of IL-10 and IL-10R deficiency demonstrate the importance of IL-10 as a critical immunomodulatory factor that controls chronic stimulation by microbes in the intestine and keeps the immune system in balance; it also shows that in a subgroup of patients, IBD may be inherited as monogenic autosomal-recessive disease that is distinct from classical and more complex variants such as UC and CD. Allogeneic HSCT that restores IL-10 signaling in hematopoietic cells proved to be a promising therapeutic approach that may cure patients with IL-10 or IL-10R deficiency and sustain long-term remission. The progress in IBD research

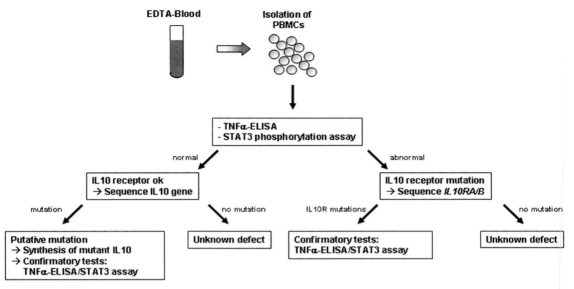

Figure 2. Diagnostic procedures to detect IL-10 and IL-10R mutations.

has broadened our knowledge of the mucosal immunity, the components that keep it in balance and genes that control susceptibility to IBD. However, there are still many unknown players that need to be identified to make us understand the complex immunity and ecosystem of the intestine.

Conflicts of interest

The authors declare no conflicts of interest.

References

1. Moore, K.W., R. de Waal Malefyt, R.L. Coffman & A. O'Garra. 2001. Interleukin-10 and the interleukin-10 receptor. *Annu. Rev. Immunol.* **19:** 683–765.
2. Bogdan, C., Y. Vodovotz & C. Nathan. 1991. Macrophage deactivation by interleukin 10. *J. Exp. Med.* **174:** 1549–1555.
3. de Waal Malefyt, R., J. Haanen, H. Spits, *et al.* 1991. Interleukin-10 (IL-10) and viral IL-10 strongly reduce antigen-specific human T cell proliferation by diminishing the antigen-presenting capacity of monocytes via down regulation of class II major histocompatibility complex expression. *J. Exp. Med.* **174:** 915–924.
4. Williams, L.M., G. Ricchetti, U. Sarma, *et al.* 2004. Interleukin-10 suppression of myeloid cell activation–a continuing puzzle. *Immunology* **113:** 281–292.
5. Carter, M.J., A.J. Lobo & S.P. Travis; IBD Section, British Society of Gastroenterology. 2004. Guidelines for the management of inflammatory bowel disease in adults. *Gut* **53**(Suppl 5): V1–V16.
6. Engel, M.A. & M.F. Neurath. 2010. New pathophysiological insights and modern treatment of IBD. *J. Gastroenterol.* **45:** 571–583.
7. Romano, C., A. Famiani, R. Gallizzi, *et al.* 2008. Indeterminate colitis: a distinctive clinical pattern of inflammatory bowel disease in children. *Pediatrics* **122:** e1278–e1281.
8. Xavier, R.J. & D.K. Podolsky. 2007. Unravelling the pathogenesis of inflammatory bowel disease. *Nature* **448:** 427–434.
9. Cho, J.H. 2008. The genetics and immunopathogenesis of inflammatory bowel disease. *Nat. Rev. Immunol.* **8:** 458–466.
10. Van Limbergen, J., D.C. Wilson & J. Satsangi. 2009. The genetics of Crohn's disease. *Annu. Rev. Genomics Hum. Genet.* **10:** 89–116.
11. Spencer, S.D., F. Di Marco, J. Hooley, *et al.* 1998. The orphan receptor CRF2–4 is an essential subunit of the interleukin 10 receptor. *J. Exp. Med.* **187:** 571–578.
12. Kühn, R., J. Lohler, D. Rennick, *et al.* 1993. Interleukin-10-deficient mice develop chronic enterocolitis. *Cell* **75:** 263–274.
13. Berg, D.J., R. Kühn, K. Rajewsky, *et al.* 1995. Interleukin-10 is a central regulator of the response to LPS in murine models of endotoxic shock and the Shwartzman reaction but not endotoxin tolerance. *J. Clin. Invest.* **96:** 2339–2347.
14. Franke, A., T. Balschun, T.H. Karlsen, *et al.* 2008. Sequence variants in *IL10, ARPC2* and multiple other loci contribute to ulcerative colitis susceptibility. *Nat. Genet.* **40:** 1319–1323.
15. van der Linde, K., P.P. Boor, L.A. Sandkuijl, *et al.* 2003. A Gly15Arg mutation in the interleukin-10 gene reduces secretion of interleukin-10 in Crohn disease. *Scand. J. Gastroenterol.* **38:** 611–617.
16. Noguchi, E., Y. Homma, X. Kang, *et al.* 2009. A Crohn's disease-associated NOD2 mutation suppresses transcription of human IL10 by inhibiting activity of the nuclear ribonucleoprotein hnRNP-A1. *Nat. Immunol.* **10:** 471–479.
17. Barnes, M. & F. Powrie. 2009. Regulatory T cells reinforce intestinal homeostasis. *Immunity* **31:** 401–411.

18. Artis, D. 2008. Epithelial-cell recognition of commensal bacteria and maintenance of immune homeostasis in the gut. *Nat. Rev. Immunol.* **8:** 411–420.

19. Boden, E.K. & S.B. Snapper. 2008. Regulatory T cells in inflammatory bowel disease. *Curr. Opin. Gastroenterol.* **24:** 733–741.

20. Fontenot, J.D., M.A. Gavin & A.Y. Rudensky. 2003. Foxp3 programs the development and function of CD4+CD25+ regulatory T cells. *Nat. Immunol.* **4:** 330–336.

21. Li, M.O., Y.Y. Wan & R.A. Flavell. 2007. T cell-produced transforming growth factor-beta1 controls T cell tolerance and regulates Th1- and Th17-cell differentiation. *Immunity* **26:** 579–591.

22. Rubtsov, Y.P., J.P. Rasmussen, E.Y. Chi, *et al.* 2008. Regulatory T cell-derived interleukin-10 limits inflammation at environmental interfaces. *Immunity* **28:** 546–558.

23. Bennett, C.L., R. Yoshioka, H. Kiyosawa, *et al.* 2000. X-Linked syndrome of polyendocrinopathy, immune dysfunction, and diarrhea maps to Xp11.23-Xq13.3. *Am. J. Hum. Genet.* **66:** 461–468.

24. Powell, B.R., N.R. Buist & P. Stenzel. 1982. An X-linked syndrome of diarrhea, polyendocrinopathy, and fatal infection in infancy. *J. Pediatr.* **100:** 731–737.

25. Ziegler, S.F. 2006. FOXP3: of mice and men. *Annu. Rev. Immunol.* **24:** 209–226.

26. Moraes-Vasconcelos, D., B.T. Costa-Carvalho, T.R. Torgerson & H.D. Ochs. 2008. Primary immune deficiency disorders presenting as autoimmune diseases: IPEX and APECED. *J. Clin. Immunol.* **28**(Suppl 1): S11–S19.

27. Gambineri, E., T.R. Torgerson & H.D. Ochs. 2003. Immune dysregulation, polyendocrinopathy, enteropathy, and X-linked inheritance (IPEX), a syndrome of systemic autoimmunity caused by mutations of FOXP3, a critical regulator of T-cell homeostasis. *Curr. Opin. Rheumatol.* **15:** 430–435.

28. Nieves, D.S., R.P. Phipps, S.J. Pollock, *et al.* 2004. Dermatologic and immunologic findings in the immune dysregulation, polyendocrinopathy, enteropathy, X-linked syndrome. *Arch. Dermatol.* **140:** 466–472.

29. Torgerson, T.R. & H.D. Ochs. 2007. Immune dysregulation, polyendocrinopathy, enteropathy, X-linked: forkhead box protein 3 mutations and lack of regulatory T cells. *J. Allergy Clin. Immunol.* **120:** 744–750.

30. Heltzer, M.L., J.K. Choi, H.D. Ochs, *et al.* 2007. A potential screening tool for IPEX syndrome. *Pediatr. Dev. Pathol.* **10:** 98–105.

31. Glocker, E.O., D. Kotlarz, K. Boztug, *et al.* 2009. Inflammatory bowel disease and mutations affecting the interleukin-10 receptor. *N. Engl. J. Med.* **361:** 2033–2045.

32. Glocker, E.O., N. Frede, M. Perro, *et al.* 2010. Infant colitis–it's in the genes. *Lancet* **376:** 1272.

33. Donnelly, R.P., H. Dickensheets & D.S. Finbloom. 1999. The interleukin-10 signal transduction pathway and regulation of gene expression in mononuclear phagocytes. *J. Interferon Cytokine Res.* **19:** 563–573.

34. O'Shea, J.J. & P.J. Murray. 2008. Cytokine signaling modules in inflammatory responses. *Immunity* **28:** 477–487.

35. Commins, S., J.W. Steinke & L. Borish. 2008. The extended IL-10 superfamily: IL-10, IL-19, IL-20, IL-22, IL-24, IL-26, IL-28, and IL-29. *J. Allergy Clin. Immunol.* **121:** 1108–1111.

36. Begue, B., J. Verdier, F. Rieux-Laucat, *et al.* 2011. Defective IL10 signaling defining a subgroup of patients with inflammatory bowel disease. *Am. J. Gastroenterol.* **106:** 1544–1555.

37. Wolk, K. & R. Sabat. 2006. Interleukin-22: a novel T- and NK-cell derived cytokine that regulates the biology of tissue cells. *Cytokine Growth Factor Rev.* **17:** 367–380.

38. Donnelly, R.P., F. Sheikh, S.V. Kotenko & H. Dickensheets. 2004. The expanded family of class II cytokines that share the IL-10 receptor-2(IL-10R2) chain. *J. Leukoc. Biol.* **76:** 314–321.

39. Sugimoto, K., A. Ogawa, E. Mizoguchi, *et al.* 2008. IL-22 ameliorates intestinal inflammation in a mouse model of ulcerative colitis. *J. Clin. Invest.* **118:** 534–544.

40. Zenewicz, L.A., G.D. Yancopoulos, D.M. Valenzuela, *et al.* 2008. Innate and adaptive interleukin-22 protects mice from inflammatory bowel disease. *Immunity* **29:** 947–957.

41. Zheng, Y., P.A. Valdez, D.M. Danilenko, *et al.* 2008. Interleukin-22 mediates early host defense against attaching and effacing bacterial pathogens. *Nat. Med.* **14:** 282–289.

42. Wolk, K., S. Kunz, E. Witte, *et al.* 2004. IL-22 increases the innate immunity of tissues. *Immunity* **21:** 241–254.

43. Wolk, K., E. Witte, E. Wallace, *et al.* 2006. IL-22 regulates the expression of genes responsible for antimicrobial defense, cellular differentiation, and mobility in keratinocytes: a potential role in psoriasis. *Eur. J. Immunol.* **36:** 1309–1323.

44. Kolls, J.K., P.B. McCray Jr. & Y.R. Chan. 2008. Cytokine-mediated regulation of antimicrobial proteins. *Nat. Rev. Immunol.* **8:** 829–835.

45. Nagalakshmi, M.L., A. Rascle, S. Zurawski, *et al.* 2004. Interleukin-22 activates STAT3 and induces IL-10 by colon epithelial cells. *Int. Immunopharmacol.* **4:** 679–691.

46. Hör, S., H. Pirzer, L. Dumoutier, *et al.* 2004. The T-cell lymphokine interleukin-26 targets epithelial cells through the interleukin-20 receptor 1 and interleukin-10 receptor 2 chains. *J. Biol. Chem.* **279:** 33343–33351.

47. Aujla, S.J., Y.R. Chan, M. Zheng, *et al.* 2008. IL-22 mediates mucosal host defense against Gram-negative bacterial pneumonia. *Nat. Med.* **14:** 275–281.

48. Cella, M., A. Fuchs, W. Vermi, *et al.* 2009. A human natural killer cell subset provides an innate source of IL-22 for mucosal immunity. *Nature* **457:** 722–725.

49. Kotenko, S.V., G. Gallagher, V.V. Baurin, *et al.* 2003. IFN-λs mediate antiviral protection through a distinct class II cytokine receptor complex. *Nat. Immunol.* **4:** 69–77.

50. Sheppard, P., W. Kindsvogel, W. Xu, *et al.* 2003. IL-28, IL-29 and their class II cytokine receptor IL-28R. *Nat. Immunol.* **4:** 63–68.

Ann. N.Y. Acad. Sci. ISSN 0077-8923

ANNALS OF THE NEW YORK ACADEMY OF SCIENCES

Issue: *The Year in Human and Medical Genetics: Inborn Errors of Immunity*

The case for newborn screening for severe combined immunodeficiency and related disorders

Jennifer M. Puck

Department of Pediatrics, University of California San Francisco, and UCSF Benioff Children's Hospital, San Francisco, California

Address for correspondence: Jennifer Puck, M.D., University of California, San Francisco, Box 0519, 513 Parnassus Avenue, HSE 301A, San Francisco, CA 94143-0519. puckj@peds.ucsf.edu

Early detection of primary immunodeficiency is recognized as important for avoiding infectious complications that compromise outcomes. In particular, severe combined immunodeficiency (SCID) is fatal in infancy unless affected infants can be diagnosed before the onset of devastating infections and provided with an immune system through allogenic hematopoietic cell transplantation, enzyme replacement, or gene therapy. A biomarker of normal T cell development, T cell receptor excision circles (TRECs), can be measured in DNA isolated from the dried blood spots routinely obtained for newborn screening; infants identified as lacking TRECs can thus receive confirmatory testing and prompt intervention. Early results of TREC testing of newborns in five states indicate that this addition to the newborn screening panel can be successfully integrated into state public health programs. A variety of cases with typical SCID genotypes and other T lymphocytopenic conditions have been detected in a timely manner and referred for appropriate early treatment.

Key words: primary immunodeficiency; T cell receptor excision circle (TREC); severe combined immunodeficiency (SCID); lymphocytopenia; dried blood spot; newborn screening

Introduction

Population-based newborn screening began with a test for phenylketonuria (PKU) developed by Robert Guthrie in 1963[1] following the demonstration that a phenylalanine restricted diet instituted early in life can prevent serious neurodevelopmental impairment in children lacking phenylalanine hydroxylase. PKU was identified in neonates by finding elevated phenylalanine levels in drops of infant blood obtained by heelstick and applied to filter paper. Dried blood spot testing needed to be done in standardized laboratories, and infants with abnormal tests had to be contacted promptly and directed to metabolic disease specialists for dietary management. In the United States these tasks have been instituted, supported, and directed by each state's public health program. Newborn screening efforts have grown as additional rare, but treatable conditions have been recognized that can be successfully identified by sensitive, specific, and inexpensive tests. Up to 50 or more metabolic disorders, hypothyroidism, and hemoglobinopathies have now been incorporated into dried blood spot testing of newborns in most states, and nursery-based tests to screen for deafness are also performed.[2]

Recently, severe combined immunodeficiency (SCID) has become the first genetic disorder of the immune system to be amenable to newborn screening. SCID and related conditions with low numbers of T lymphocytes can be identified by testing T cell receptor excision circles (TRECs), a DNA biomarker of normal T lymphocyte development, in dried blood spots routinely obtained for screening for other conditions. Coincidentally, the technology for SCID screening was developed at the same time as a new national oversight process was being rolled out to provide evidence-based assessments of new conditions proposed for addition to state newborn screening panels of tests. SCID became the first disease nominated to the national advisory committee that was reviewed and unanimously recommended for inclusion in the evidence-based uniform screening panel.[3] SCID is also the first newborn screening

doi: 10.1111/j.1749-6632.2011.06346.x

 Ann. N.Y. Acad. Sci. 1246 (2011) 108–117 © 2011 New York Academy of Sciences.

test for which the primary analyte is DNA. This review summarizes the current case for SCID newborn screening, presenting evidence available before it was undertaken and now that early results are available from statewide pilot programs, as well as future challenges that remain to be addressed.

Evidence for adding SCID to the panel of newborn screening tests

The U.S. Advisory Committee on Heritable Disorders in Newborns and Children was established in part to work toward uniform, evidence-based newborn screening in what has traditionally been a patchwork of individual state programs.[3] The Advisory Committee's mandate is to solicit nominations of conditions to be added to newborn screening; consideration of each nominated condition includes an independent review of evidence by public health experts and input from knowledgeable physicians and stakeholders such as family advocacy groups. Upon weighing the evidence and arriving at a determination, the Committee reports to the Department of Health and Human Services (DHHS) Secretary. SCID was first nominated in 2008, and evidence was assembled and reported in 2009 and again in 2010, at which time it was considered strong enough to merit a unanimous favorable recommendation.[4] Secretary of Health and Human Services Kathleen Sibelius accepted the recommendation and formally endorsed SCID screening in May 2010.

SCID is a collection of over 20 distinct genetic disorders characterized by profound defects in both cellular immunity and specific antibody production (Table 1). It is estimated to occur in 1 per 50,000 to 1 per 100,000 births, although true population incidence has been unknown prior to screening.[4–10] All SCID infants have absent or extremely low production of T lymphocytes from the thymus, while some also have deficiencies of B cells, NK cells or both. Although there are individual exceptions, SCID genotypes have characteristic profiles of lymphocyte impairment, as shown in Table 1, which also gives rough estimates of relative frequency. The combined defects of T and B cells, plus absent NK cells in some forms of SCID, severely compromise an infant's ability to resist infections, and the condition has thus been clinically defined since early descriptions by failure to thrive, thrush, *Pneumocystis jiroveci* pneumonia, and other bacterial, fungal, and viral infections.

The rationale for SCID newborn screening, outlined in Table 2, derives from our knowledge that SCID is potentially treatable, but is not recognized effectively prior to onset of devastating infections. Although treatment modalities have improved in the last four decades, SCID morbidity and mortality remain high. Affected infants do not survive unless provided with functional immunity, but this can be achieved by hematopoietic cell transplantation (HCT) from a healthy donor,[5] by enzyme replacement in cases of adenosine deaminase (ADA) deficiency,[6] and (although still experimental) by gene therapy for X-linked and ADA deficient SCID.[6,7] Infants with SCID are healthy at birth, initially protected by transplacentally derived maternal IgG antibodies; but persistent, severe, and opportunistic infections typically develop by age four to seven months. Repeated observations have shown superior outcomes in SCID infants diagnosed at a young age, particularly those fortunate enough to have an affected relative to alert health providers of the diagnosis.[5,8,11,12]

The first suggestion that screening infants for low lymphocytes could identify SCID in time for lifesaving treatment was by Buckley *et al.* in 1997.[8] Further retrospective analysis of cases treated by Buckley at Duke,[11] and recently in England,[12] have underlined the better survival of SCID infants diagnosed before developing infections. However, although these reports showed a clear benefit for early diagnosis, they were limited to the potentially biased population of SCID infants admitted to specialized immunodeficiency transplant centers. A family-based survey by the Immune Deficiency Foundation and Chan *et al.* found even more striking differences due to the higher mortality of SCID infants not recognized at birth; half of the deceased infants in this study were either not diagnosed pre-mortem or were too ill to be transferred to a center for specialized treatment.[13] Furthermore, confirmation that >80% of SCID infants were the first known to be affected in their family indicated that family history taking alone would not be sufficient to lead to identification of most SCID cases.

Mathematical modeling by two independent methods has also shown that a sensitive, specific, and economical newborn screening test for SCID would be likely to be cost effective.[14,15]

Another important development was the institution, beginning in 2006, of live attenuated

Table 1. Molecular causes of severe combined immunodeficiency

Gene defect	Defective protein, function, features	% SCID[a] cases	Lymphocyte profile		
			T[b]	B	NK
IL2RG (X-linked)	Common γ-chain (γc) of receptors for IL-2, -4, -7, -9, -15, and -21	45–50% (only males)	−	+	−
ADA	Adenosine deaminase enzyme	16%	−	+	−
IL7R	α-Chain of IL-7 receptor	9%	−	+	+
JAK3	Janus kinase 3, activated by γc	6%	−	+	−
RAG1, RAG2	Recombinase activating genes required for T and B cell antigen receptor gene rearrangement	5%	−	−	+
DCLRE1C (Artemis)	Part of T and B cell antigen receptor gene rearrangement complex, also required for DNA repair	< 5%	−	−	+
TCRD, TCRE, TCRZ	CD3 δ, ε, and ζ chains of the T cell receptor complex, required for T cell development	Rare	−/low	+	+
CD45	Protein tyrosine phosphatase receptor (PTPRC), required for T and B cell activation by antigen	Rare	−/low	+	+/low
LCK	Lymphocyte tyrosine kinase p56lck, required for T cell development and activation	Rare	−/low	+	+
PNP	Purine nucleoside phosphorylase enzyme, deficiency also causes neurological impairment	Rare	Low	Low	+/low
LIG4	DNA ligase IV required for antigen receptor gene rejoining	Rare	−	+	+
DNAPKCS	DNA protein kinase catalytic subunit, required for T and B cell antigen receptor rearrangement, and DNA repair	Rare	−	−	+
NHEJ1 (Cernunnos)	Nonhomologous end joining of DNA; deficiency also causes microcepahaly and radiation sensitivity	Rare	−	−	+
AK2	Adenylate kinase 2; deficiency causes reticular dysgenesis with granulocytopenia, lymphocytopenia, and deafness	Rare	−	−	−
FOXN1	Forkhead box N1, required for thymus and hair follicle development (ortholog of *nude* mouse)	Rare	−/low	+	+
STAT5a	Signal transducer and activator of transcription 5, phosphorylated after cytokine receptor engagement; deficiency also causes growth hormone–resistant growth failure	Rare	−/low	+	−
CORO1A	Coronin-1A, protein mediating lymphocyte migration and T cell emigration from the thymus	Rare	−/low	+	+
Currently unknown	Unknown defects, including SCID and congenital anomalies; SCID with multiple bowel atresias	∼10%	−/low	+/−	+/−

[a]Based on Buckley,[5] Lindegren *et al.*,[9] and unpublished estimates (J. Puck).
[b]Some patients have substantial numbers of maternally derived T cells at time of diagnosis; shown are autologous T cells.

Table 2. Rationale for newborn screening for SCID

Importance of early identification
    Establish diagnosis and institute immediate lifesaving treatment
    Avoid inefficient, costly, dangerous "diagnostic Odyssey"
    Provide families with genetic diagnosis and advice on reproductive risks
    Learn incidence and true spectrum of SCID
    Educate providers and public about SCID
    Permit multicenter collaborative trials to determine optimal treatments

Barriers to early diagnosis without screening
    SCID is rare
    Infections are common in all infants, not just those with SCID
    Over 80% of cases are sporadic, with no family history
    Family history can be missed, or nonspecific
    SCID infants are protected by maternal IgG for their first months of life
    Because both a gene defect and environmental exposure are required for overt disease, presentation is variable

vaccination of young infants against rotavirus infection, an important cause of infant diarrhea and dehydration leading to hospitalization and mortality. Infants receive two to three doses of rotavirus vaccine starting as early as six weeks to two months of age. Infants affected with SCID whose diagnosis had not been recognized and who unintentionally received the vaccination have developed severe diarrheal disease proven to be caused by the vaccine strain of rotavirus.[16,17] While the vaccine is specifically contraindicated in infants with immune compromise, there is no way to know whether a healthy-appearing infant at that age has SCID, other than by performing an immunological blood test. Newborn screening for SCID thus has become an important consideration to balance the public health benefit of protection from diarrhea against the harm of vaccine-strain rotavirus infection that occurs in rare infants lacking immunity.

The TREC test for SCID using newborn dried blood spots

A breakthrough for the actualization of population-based newborn screening for SCID was the development of a screening test that could be performed using the dried blood spot samples already collected by state screening laboratories for routine newborn screening for other conditions. Early proposed screening methods included absolute lymphocyte count (requiring a separate liquid blood sample),[8,11] IL-7 immunoassay,[10] bead-bound antibody-based detection of T cell proteins CD3, CD4, and the leukocyte marker CD5,[18] and gene resequencing microarrays.[19] However, to date the only assay with adequate sensitivity and specificity for dried blood spot use is the TREC assay, first published in 2005 by Chan and Puck.[20] Late in maturation, 70% of thymocytes that will ultimately express $\alpha\beta$ T cell receptors form a circular DNA TREC from the excised TCRδ gene that lies within the TCRα locus.[21] TRECs are stable because they lack free DNA ends to be attacked by DNA digesting enzymes, but because they have no origin of replication they do not increase in number when cells divide. Thus the TREC copy number, which can be measured by performing a quantitative PCR reaction across the joint of the circular TREC DNA, is an indicator of newly formed thymic emigrant T cells.

The frequency of TREC-bearing T cells in peripheral blood diminishes as newly formed T cells are diluted by T cells that have undergone mitosis. Normal newborns have a high rate of new T cell production, resulting in TREC numbers at about 10% of their total T cell numbers; in contrast older children and adults have progressively lower ratios of TRECs to T cells, reflecting peripheral T cell expansion.[21] Infants with SCID, sampled both at the time of their SCID diagnosis and upon recovery of neonatal dried blood spots obtained when they were in the nursery, have very low or undetectable TRECs (Fig. 1, Table 3).[20,22] Even maternal T cells present in the circulation of an infant with SCID do not falsely raise the TREC count to the normal range because maternal cells have very few TRECs. Thus, a normal

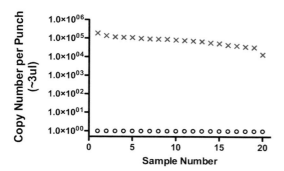

Figure 1. Copy number detected in actual nursery dried blood samples, recovered from state screening laboratories and tested by quantitative PCR of TRECs (o) and a control genomic DNA segment from the β-actin gene (×). Copy number is normalized to the amount of DNA isolated from a 3 mm punch from a dried blood filter, which is equivalent to about 3 μL of blood (J. Puck, unpublished data).

number of TRECs is an excellent biomarker for new autologous T cell production, provided the DNA is adequate for PCR (shown by amplification of a control, such as a segment of the β-actin gene).

Initiation of SCID screening programs

Although the TREC test in dried blood spots was a promising biomarker for insufficient T cell production, and retrospective analysis indicated that typical SCID cases would have been found by TREC screening had it been done in the past (Fig. 1), actual prospective tests in the field were required to establish clinical validity. The TREC test was first scaled up and adapted to a statewide newborn screening format by Baker *et al.* in Wisconsin.[23] Other states, including Massachusetts, devised their own adaptations of this assay.[24,25] Each state tailored its TREC screening according to individual program structure and requirements. A clinical study of TREC screening was also undertaken in selected hospitals on the Navajo Indian Reservation, because Navajo Native Americans are known to have a high rate of SCID (about 1 in 2,000 births) due to a founder mutation in the *DCLRE1C* (*Artemis*) gene.[26] The Centers for Disease Control and Prevention developed standards to be offered as unknowns for quality control and calibration purposes. Consideration of the performance of TREC newborn screening as well as available clinical data described above led to the recommendations for universal adoption of SCID newborn screening.

The Wisconsin program, which began in 2008, was recently described.[25] In the first year, in which 70,000 infants were screened, several were found with low T cell numbers, and one had a combined lymphocyte and granulocyte disorder, RAC2 deficiency, treated successfully by bone marrow transplantation.

Larger numbers of births and experience from additional state newborn screening programs would be needed to demonstrate clinical utility of SCID newborn screening. California, with over 500,000 births per year and a very diverse population, began its development program of statewide TREC screening in August 2010; a bill has now been passed and signed into law to make SCID a permanent addition to the California newborn screening panel. This state's SCID screening algorithm is shown in Figure 2. A TREC quantitative PCR similar to those of Chan and Puck and the Wisconsin program is followed by a β-actin gene PCR control only if the TREC number is inadequate. If both TREC and control DNA copy numbers are below cutoff values after two separate DNA extractions, the sample is considered a "DNA amplification failure" (DAF), and a second heel stick is requested from the baby. Preterm and ill infants in intensive care units have modified DAF cutoff values. All samples with undetectable or below cutoff TRECs and adequate control PCR are considered positive. Infants with a positive screening test result or two DAF samples require second tier testing with T cell enumeration.

An important feature of SCID screening in California is that a liquid blood sample following the positive screening result is an integral part of the program. Area service center staff work with providers and families so that blood is rapidly obtained at newborn blood drawing stations throughout the state that have been established for metabolic disease follow-up, and all samples are sent to a single central laboratory (Quest Nichols Institute, San Juan Capistrano, CA) for a complete blood count, differential count, and a specified flow cytometry panel of lymphocyte subset markers including naive and memory T cell markers. All results are interpreted by two designated immunodeficiency consultants for the program. In this centralized system infants receive a definitive diagnosis and are referred to a center of excellence for further management.

The performance of the TREC test in Wisconsin, Massachusetts, and California has been excellent to date, with no missed SCID cases that have come

Table 3. Summary of California TREC screening experience in the first year

- 507,000 births screened
- DNA amplification failures (DAF), <0.08%, requiring second heelstick[a]
    Comparable to other newborn screening assays
    56% were <1,500 g at birth
    44% had first sample drawn from an indwelling catheter, not a heelstick
    84% were in neonatal intensive care units at time of collection
- 50 positive tests, 0.01% of births, required CBC and lymphocyte flow cytometry
- 20 follow-up liquid blood samples, 40%, had low T cells confirmed by CBC and flow cytometry
- Diagnoses made:
    6 SCID[b]
        2 IL-7RA
        2 RAG1
        2 Common γ-chain
    1 Omenn syndrome[c] due to missense mutations of RAG2
    3 SCID variant with no known gene defect
    4 Syndromes with T lymphocytopenia
        3 DiGeorge (1 complete)
        1 Trisomy 21
    6 Secondary T lymphocytopenia
        2 Gastroschesis
        1 Gastrointestinal atresia
        3 Prematurity

[a]Since all non-SCID screening is done first in regional labs, with samples then forwarded to a central lab for TREC testing, most newborns were two weeks old when the TREC result was available. When a SCID-specific repeat heelstick was needed, older age usually resulted in a normal TREC value on redraw.
[b]Only one SCID case had a positive family history leading to testing at birth.
[c]Signs of Omenn syndrome in the first weeks of life had led to the diagnosis just before the TREC test was reported.

to light. The California experience is summarized in Table 3. There have been very few DAF samples necessitating a second heelstick, 1 per 1,250 births. Only 50 infants required a liquid blood sample (1 per 10,000 births); of these, 40% proved to have true T lymphocytopenia, indicating that TRECs recovered from blood spots are, as predicted, an excellent T cell biomarker. All infants with T lymphocytopenia were under the care of a primary immunodeficiency expert by one month of age (J. Puck and F. Lorey, unpublished information). The data in Table 3 suggest an incidence of typical SCID of 1 per 70,000 births, within the range of 1 per 50,000–100,000 estimated before screening began. Tracking of cases by race and ethnicity has suggested a somewhat higher rate than expected of T lymphocytopenia among Hispanics, and the large and diverse population of California will make possible assessment of rates between different ancestral groups. Compared to SCID and Omenn syndrome with seven cases, about twice

as many cases of non-SCID T lymphocytopenia have been found.

Conditions that may be detected by newborn screening

The states that perform SCID newborn screening have successfully identified a range of typical SCID and other T lymphocytopenic conditions that would not otherwise have been identified before the onset of serious infections (Tables 3). The first case of typical SCID due to JAK3 deficiency was reported from Massachusetts after screening 100,000 infants.[27] In addition to typical SCID, SCID-related disorders are increasingly appreciated, as reported by the early Wisconsin experience.[28] It is clear that more data will be needed to understand the full range of conditions detected. Not only the total incidence but also the relative incidence in different population subgroups remains to be defined. The conditions with low or absent TRECs fall into five categories

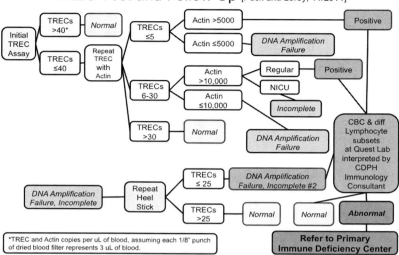

Figure 2. California algorithm for newborn screening and follow-up for SCID and related conditions. TREC and β-actin gene PCR adapted by PerkinElmer for the California Genetic Disease Screening Program. Values expressed as copies per 1 μL of blood (J. Puck, J. Church, and F. Lorey, unpublished data).

(Table 4):[28–31] (A) Typical SCID is defined by the Primary Immune Deficiency Treatment Consortium (PIDTC) as fewer than 300 autologous T cells/μL of peripheral blood (normal infants have 2,250 to 5,000/μL) and less than 10% of normal T cell proliferation to the mitogen PHA.[32,33] (B) Leaky SCID, which has no maternal engraftment and T cells ranging from 300–1,500/μL, may have a later age of onset of clinical symptoms or may present in infancy as Omenn syndrome (defined by erythroderma rash, adenopathy, and oligoclonal, poorly functioning T cells, due to hypomorphic mutations in *RAG1, RAG2* or other known SCID genes). (C) Variant SCID is defined as the absence of a known SCID gene defect and 300–1,500 autologous T cells/μL with impaired responses to mitogens. (D) Multisystem syndromes with T cell defects have a wide spectrum of T cell dysgenesis. Those with severely affected T cell production are expected to have positive TREC screens, while others with the same syndrome but more normal T cells will not be detected. In several instances infants with these syndromes have been found to have abnormally low TRECs (Table 4D). DiGeorge syndrome, usually associated with chromosome 22q.11 deletion; trisomy 21; and CHARGE syndrome (with ocular coloboma, heart defect, atresia of nasal choanae, retardation of growth and development, genitourinary abnormality, and ear abnormality) can all present with life-threatening infections in infancy due to T cell deficiency and have been identified by neonatal TREC screening.[28–30] In addition, RAC2 deficiency, previously known only as a granulocyte disorder, was diagnosed following newborn screening with low TRECs and T lymphocytopenia,[28] as was Jacobsen syndrome associated with terminal deletions of chromosome 11q24. Siblings affected with DOCK8 deficient hyper-IgE syndrome with lymphocytopenia had undetectable TRECs during childhood, though newborn samples have not yet been available.[31] Finally, (E) secondary T cell defects are characterized by acquired conditions with increased T cell loss. These include congenital heart defects, neonatal leukemia, lymphocyte loss by extravasation or third spacing, lymphangiectasia and possibly congenital HIV infection. Some of the secondary defects, such as lymphocytopenia associated with extreme low birthweight, may resolve over time. We expect that previously unrecognized conditions will come to light with screening. Furthermore, we recognize that many primary immunodeficiency diseases will not be detectable through TREC screening, and it is important to educate providers to remain alert for

Table 4. Conditions detected by low or absent TRECs

A. Typical SCID (see Table 1)

B. Leaky SCID, due to incomplete (hypomorphic) mutation(s) in a typical SCID gene

C. Variant SCID, with no known gene defect and persistence of 300–1,500 T cells/µL that have impaired function

D. Syndromes with variably affected cellular immunity that may be severe

    Complete DiGeorge syndrome[a]

    Partial DiGeorge syndrome with low T lymphocytes[a]

    CHARGE syndrome[a]

    Jacobsen syndrome[a]

    Trisomy 21[a]

    RAC2 dominant interfering mutation[a]

    DOCK8 deficient hyper-IgE syndrome[b]

    Cartilage hair hypoplasia

E. Secondary T lymphocytopenia

    Cardiac surgery with thymectomy[a]

    Neonatal leukemia[a]

    Gastroschesis[a]

    Third spacing[a]

    Extreme prematurity (resolves to normal with time)[a]

    HIV (severe prenatal infection with newborn lymphocytopenia, hypothesized)

[a]Observed to have low or absent TRECs upon newborn screening in one or more cases to date in U.S. pilot programs or published reports.

[b]Observed to have low or absent TRECs in one or more cases after diagnosis; newborn samples not available.

signs of these conditions in patients who have been screened.

Remaining challenges

Screening for SCID is a matter of fairness, access, and early awareness, designed to give all affected infants the advantages of early diagnosis and treatment that have previously been available primarily to families with means and second-born affected children. Parents in such families may have already lost an infant whose SCID diagnosis was delayed or unrecognized. However, in order for the case for newborn screening to be completely compelling, a seamless progression from prenatal education to screening to definitive diagnosis to optimal treatment must be established. This goal is challenging even for large states with centers of excellence in pediatric immunology and bone marrow transplantation; smaller states or those without such centers will have to consider regional collaborations and referrals of their SCID cases to treatment centers beyond their borders.

How best to perform HCT treatment in SCID to achieve maximum survival, minimal toxicity and B cell as well as T cell reconstitution remains controversial. In the absence of compelling data from well controlled multicenter trials, opinions remain divided as to whether cytoreductive or ablative versus no chemotherapy conditioning should be used, and what source of donor hematopoietic stem cells are best, among other questions.[32–34] Although HCT provides reliable T cell immunity for SCID, B cell recovery remains problematic, and some transplants may not be durable over many years. Pre-transplantation conditioning does not guarantee that B cell function will develop; therefore, one must decide whether there is justification for using agents that compromise innate immunity and have intrinsic toxicities to gain B cell immune reconstitution. Pharmacokinetic studies of chemotherapy drugs commonly used in older children and adults have not been done in infants, and risks judged acceptable for patients with lethal malignancies may not be prudent for young, healthy infants with SCID detected by newborn screening. The risks of delaying treatment and exposing infants to infection pending a search for a matched unrelated donor must be balanced against the option of performing a T cell–depleted haploidentical HCT from a parent. Even the laboratory workup essential for very small infants with SCID is controversial, since blood tests may cause anemia, requiring transfusions. Centers that perform HCT for children with malignant disease cannot be assumed to have the specialized knowledge and experience required for optimal success with HCT for SCID. Fortunately a national rare disease network, the PIDTC has been funded by the National Institutes of Health to conduct prospective studies of SCID treatments and outcomes, and eventually multicenter clinical treatment trials will identify the best approaches for each individual SCID genotype.[32,33]

Convincing states to add a disease to their newborn screening panel requires a coalition of immunologists, geneticists, parent advocates, nonprofit agencies, public health officials, and politicians. In times of financial restraint, state officials are asking for proof that SCID screening is cost effective. While it is widely believed that early diagnosis of SCID and related disorders through screening will save lives and also lead to savings in medical care dollars, population-based proof of better outcomes and lower costs through screening remains to be shown. Such proof will take time to acquire as states accumulate data from screening and outcome tracking. Beyond TREC testing for newborns states will need to have programs to assure that expert diagnostic follow-up and treatment are available to infants with positive screening results.

Finally, current controversies surrounding the collection, testing, storage, and use of dried blood spots from infants by state newborn screening programs highlight the need for better outreach and education regarding the public health benefits of newborn screening. States need to be sure that their policies are clear and consistent,[35] and better information needs to be transmitted to the public, perhaps by better linking of prenatal obstetrical care and counseling to postnatal newborn screening, particularly as DNA-based testing, started with TREC testing for SCID, becomes more widespread.[36] Raising public awareness of rare disorders, including primary immunodeficiencies, is also an important activity in support of early diagnosis through newborn screening.[37]

SCID screening is justified because early identification is associated with higher survival rate and better outcome. Newborn screening for SCID is being adopted by an increasing number of state public health programs following its successful initiation in Wisconsin, followed by Massachusetts, California, New York, Louisiana, and Puerto Rico. Colorado, Connecticut, and Michigan as well as additional states are beginning to screen infants for SCID. Classic SCID, leaky SCID, and Omenn syndrome as well as additional known disorders with T lymphocytopenia have been found, as well as cases with low T cell production of unknown cause. For the population as a whole and for groups of distinct ancestry or ethnicity, newborn screening will make it possible for the first time to determine the true incidence and spectrum of SCID and related disorders.

Acknowledgments

Thanks to Dr. Fred Lorey and colleagues at the California Department of Public Health and Genetic Disease Laboratory, and to Perkin Elmer and Quest Nichols Institute for design and conduct of testing; Drs. Joseph Church, Mort Cowan, Christopher Dvorak, Nina Kapoor, David Lewis, Sean McGhee, Ted Moore, E. R. Stiehm, Chu Ri Shin, and Ken Weinberg for helpful discussions; and agencies supporting this work: The Jeffrey Modell Foundation, NIH NIAID for support of PIDTC U54 AI082973, NICHD for RO3 HD 060311, NIAID for RO1 AI078248, and NCRR UL1 RR024131 for the UCSF CTSI.

Conflicts of interest

The author declares no conflicts of interest.

References

1. Guthrie, R. & I. Susi. 1963. A simple phenylalanine method for detecting phenylketonuria in large populations of newborn infants. *Pediatrics* **32:** 318–343.
2. Newborn Screening Status Report (updated 3/01/10). National Newborn Screening and Genetics Resource Center. Available at: http://genes-r-us.uthscsa.edu/nbsdisorders. pdf [Accessed Sept. 26, 2011].
3. Howell, R.R. & M.A. Lloyd-Puryear. 2010. From developing guidelines to implementing legislation: actions of the US Advisory Committee on Heritable Disorders in Newborns and Children toward advancing and improving newborn screening. *Semin Perinatol.* **34:** 121–124.
4. Lipstein, E.A., M.F. Browning, N.S. Green, *et al.* 2010. Systematic evidence review of newborn screening and treatment of severe combined immunodeficiency. *Pediatrics* **125:** 1226–1235.
5. Buckley, R.H. 2011. Transplantation of hematopoietic stem cells in human severe combined immunodeficiency: longterm outcomes. *Immunol. Res.* **49:** 25–43.

6. Gaspar, H.B, A. Aiuti, F. Porta, *et al.* 2009. How I treat ADA deficiency. *Blood* **114:** 3524–3532.

7. Fischer, A., S. Hacein-Bey-Abina & M. Cavazzana-Calvo. 2011. Gene therapy for primary adaptive immune deficiencies. *J. Allergy Clin. Immunol.* **127:** 1356–1359.

8. Buckley, R.H., R.I. Schiff, S.E. Schiff, *et al.* 1997. Human severe combined immunodeficiency: genetic, phenotypic and functional diversity in one hundred eight infants. *J. Pediatr.* **130:** 378–387.

9. Lindegren, M.L., L. Kobrynski, S.A. Rasmussen, *et al.* 2004. Applying public health strategies to primary immunodeficiency diseases: a potential approach to genetic disorders. *MMWR Recomm. Rep.* **53:** 1–29.

10. Puck, J.M. & Newborn Screening Working Group. 2007. SCID population-based newborn screening for severe combined immunodeficiency: steps toward implementation. *J. Allergy Clin. Immunol.* **120:** 760–768.

11. Myers, L.A., D.D. Patel, J.M. Puck & R.H. Buckley. 2002. Hematopoietic stem cell transplantation for severe combined immunodeficiency in the neonatal period leads to superior thymic output and improved survival. *Blood* **99:** 872–878.

12. Brown, L., J. Xu-Bayford, Z. Allwood, *et al.* 2011. Neonatal diagnosis of severe combined immunodeficiency leads to significantly improved survival outcome: the case for newborn screening. *Blood* **117:** 3243–3246.

13. Chan, A., C. Scalchunes, M. Boyle & J.M. Puck. 2011. Early vs. delayed diagnosis of severe combined immunodeficiency: a family perspective survey. *Clin. Immunol.* **138:** 3–8.

14. McGhee, S.A., E.R. Stiehm & E.R. McCabe. 2005. Potential costs and benefits of newborn screening for severe combined immunodeficiency. *J. Pediatr.* **147:** 603–608.

15. Chan, K., J. Davis, S.Y. Pai, *et al.* 2011. A Markov model to analyze cost-effectiveness of screening for severe combined immunodeficiency (SCID). *Mol. Genet. Metab.* Jul 12. [Epub ahead of print, PMID: 21810544]

16. Werther, R.L., N.W. Crawford, K. Boniface, *et al.* 2009. Rotavirus vaccine induced diarrhea in a child with severe combined immune deficiency. *J. Allergy Clin. Immunol.* **124:** 600.

17. Patel, N.C., P.M. Hertel, M.K. Estes, *et al.* 2010. Vaccine-acquired rotavirus in infants with severe combined immunodeficiency. *N. Engl. J. Med.* **362:** 314–319.

18. Janik, D.K., B. Lindau-Shepard, A.M. Comeau & K.A. Pass. 2010. A multiplex immunoassay using the Guthrie specimen to detect T-cell deficiencies including severe combined immunodeficiency disease. *Clin. Chem.* **56:** 1460–1465.

19. Lebet, T., R. Chiles, A.P. Hsu, *et al.* 2008. Mutations causing severe combined immunodeficiency: detection with a custom resequencing microarray. *Genet. Med.* **10:** 575–585.

20. Chan, K. & J.M. Puck. 2005. Development of population-based newborn screening for severe combined immunodeficiency. *J. Allergy Clin. Immunol.* **115:** 391–398.

21. Douek, D.C., R.D. McFarland, P.H. Keiser, *et al.* 1998. Changes in thymic function with age and during the treatment of HIV infection. *Nature* **396:** 690–695.

22. Morinishi Y., K. Imai, N. Nakagawa, *et al.* 2009. Identification of severe combined immunodeficiency by T-cell receptor excision circles quantification using neonatal Guthrie cards. *J. Pediatr.* **155:** 829–833.

23. Baker, M.W., W.J. Grossman, R.H. Laessig, *et al.* 2009. Development of a routine newborn screening protocol for severe combined immunodeficiency. *J. Allergy Clin. Immunol.* **124:** 522–527.

24. Gerstel-Thompson, J.L., J.C. Baptiste, J.S. Navas, *et al.* 2010. High-throughput multiplexed T-cell-receptor excision circle quantitative PCR assay with internal controls for detection of severe combined immunodeficiency in population-based newborn screening. *Clin. Chem.* **56:** 1466–1474.

25. Chase, N.M., J.W. Verbsky & J.M. Routes. 2010. Newborn screening for T-cell deficiency. *Curr. Opin. Allergy Clin. Immunol.* **10:** 521–525.

26. Li, L., D. Moshous, Y. Zhou, *et al.* 2002. A founder mutation in Artemis, an SNM1-like protein, causes SCID in Athabascan-speaking native Americans. *J. Immunol.* **168:** 6323–6329.

27. Hale, J.E., F.A. Bonilla, S.Y. Pai, *et al.* 2010. Identification of an infant with severe combined immunodeficiency by newborn screening. *J. Allergy Clin. Immunol.* **126:** 1073–1074.

28. Routes, J.M., J. Verbsky, R.H. Laessig, *et al.* 2009. Statewide newborn screening for severe T-cell lymphopenia. *JAMA* **302:** 2465–2470.

29. McDonald-McGinn, D.M. & K.E. Sullivan. 2011. Chromosome 22q11.2 deletion syndrome (DiGeorge syndrome/velocardiofacial syndrome). *Medicine* **90:** 1–18.

30. Ram, G. & J. Chinen. 2011. Infections and immunodeficiency in Down syndrome. *Clin. Exp. Immunol.* **164:** 9–16.

31. Dasouki, M., K.C. Okonkwo, A. Ray, *et al.* 2011. Deficient T cell receptor excision circles (TRECs) in autosomal recessive hyper IgE syndrome caused by DOCK8 mutation: implications for pathogenesis and potential detection by newborn screening. *Clin. Immunol.* **141:** 128–132.

32. Primary Immune Deficiency Treatment Consortium. Available at: http://rarediseasesnetwork.epi.usf.edu/PIDTC/SCID/index.htm [Accessed Sept. 30, 2011].

33. Griffith, L.M., M.J. Cowan, D.B. Kohn, *et al.* 2008. Allogeneic hematopoietic cell transplantation for primary immune deficiency diseases: current status and critical needs. *J. Allergy Clin. Immunol.* **122:** 1087–1096.

34. Buckley, R.H. 2010. B-cell function in severe combined immunodeficiency after stem cell or gene therapy: a review. *J. Allergy Clin. Immunol.* **125:** 790–797.

35. Therrell, B.L., Jr., W.H. Hannon, D.B. Bailey Jr., *et al.* 2011. Committee report: considerations and recommendations for national guidance regarding the retention and use of residual dried blood spot specimens after newborn screening. *Genet. Med.* **13:** 621–624.

36. Hiraki, S., & N.S. Green. 2010. Newborn screening for treatable genetic conditions: past, present and future. *Obstet. Gynecol. Clin. North Am.* **37:** 11–21.

37. Modell, F., D. Puente & V. Modell. 2009. From genotype to phenotype. Further studies measuring the impact of a Physician Education and Public Awareness Campaign on early diagnosis and management of primary immunodeficiencies. *Immunol. Res.* **44:** 132–149.

Ann. N.Y. Acad. Sci. ISSN 0077-8923

ANNALS OF THE NEW YORK ACADEMY OF SCIENCES

Issue: *The Year in Human and Medical Genetics: Inborn Errors of Immunity*

Newborn screening for primary immunodeficiencies: beyond SCID and XLA

Stephan Borte,[1,2,3] Ning Wang,[1] Sólveig Óskarsdóttir,[4] Ulrika von Döbeln,[5] and Lennart Hammarström[1]

[1]Division of Clinical Immunology and Transfusion Medicine, Department of Laboratory Medicine, Karolinska Institutet at Karolinska University Hospital Huddinge, Stockholm, Sweden. [2]Translational Centre for Regenerative Medicine (TRM), University of Leipzig, Germany. [3]Immuno Deficiency Center Leipzig (IDCL) at Hospital St. Georg gGmbH Leipzig, Jeffrey Modell Diagnostic and Research Center for Primary Immunodeficiencies, Leipzig, Germany. [4]The Queen Silvias Children's Hospital, Sahlgrenska University Hospital, Gothenburg, Sweden. [5]Division of Metabolic Diseases, Department of Laboratory Medicine, Karolinska Institutet at Karolinska University Hospital Huddinge, Stockholm, Sweden.

Address for correspondence: Lennart Hammarström, Division of Clinical Immunology F79, Karolinska Institutet at Karolinska University Hospital Huddinge, SE141-86 Stockholm, Sweden. Lennart.Hammarstrom@ki.se

Primary immunodeficiencies (PID) encompass more than 250 disease entities, including phagocytic disorders, complement deficiencies, T cell defects, and antibody deficiencies. While differing in clinical severity, early diagnosis and treatment is of considerable importance for all forms of PID to prevent organ damage and life-threatening infections. During the past few years, neonatal screening assays have been developed to detect diseases hallmarked by the absence of T or B lymphocytes, classically seen in severe combined immunodeficiencies (SCID) and X-linked agammaglobulinemia (XLA). As described in this review, a reduction or lack of T and B cells in newborns is also frequently found in several other forms of PID, requiring supplemental investigation and involving the development of additional technical platforms in order to help classify abnormal screening results.

Keywords: TREC; KREC; SCID; XLA; ataxia telangiectasia; DiGeorge syndrome

Introduction

The purpose of neonatal screening programs is the early recognition of treatable genetic diseases that manifest with a high rate of morbidity and mortality.[1] While the implementation of newborn screening tests for metabolic disorders traces back to the mid-1960s, suitable technologies to identify severe inborn errors of immune function have emerged only in recent years.[2] The estimated incidence of primary immunodeficiency diseases (PID) that would require immediate treatment ranges from 2 to 8 per 100,000 live births, making high demands on the effectiveness and availability of screening tests.[3–5] In comparison with metabolic diseases, the identification of sensitive and traceable biomarkers poses a challenge due to the genetic diversity of pediatric PID patients. Furthermore, and to be applicable as a first-tier test in newborn screening, the specificity of a given assay is pivotal, as it critically affects the

false-positive rate, dictating repeat testing and the overall costs of the method.[6] So far, the best promise to fulfill these criteria has been to use methods measuring T cell receptor excision circles (TRECs) and kappa-deleting recombination excision circles (KRECs) as markers for T or B lymphopenia at birth, indicative of severe combined immunodeficiencies (SCID) and X-linked agammaglobulinemia (XLA), respectively.[7,8] The ability of the TREC assay to detect clinically relevant diseases other than SCID, based on low T cell numbers, has been noted previously.[9] Here, we sought to determine the overlap of such disorders when applying the design of a novel multiplexed TREC/KREC screening assay.[10] Moreover, technologies for proteome-based early detection of various primary immunodeficiencies as well as the perspective of whole-transcriptome screening approaches and their potential for supplemental testing will be discussed.

doi: 10.1111/j.1749-6632.2011.06350.x

The era of functional genomics in newborn screening

The exclusion of genetic diseases by performing a systematic diagnostic test is commonly referred to as genetic screening, regardless of whether metabolites or cellular intermediates are measured. The implementation of molecular screening programs for cystic fibrosis, initiated in several European countries and the United States during the last decade, opened the floodgates to apply the concept of functional genomics in newborn screening in order to connect the dynamic aspects of gene transcription, protein function, and disease pathogenesis.[11] The next step was the proposal to use excision products of DNA-editing processes, such as the recombination of the T cell receptor variable α and β chains or the B cell receptor genes after Vα-Jα rearrangement, to serve as screening markers for lymphocyte development.[2,12] This diagnostic strategy proved to be fruitful for genetic disorders caused by mutations in genes being of critical importance for the development of T or B cells, including recombination activating genes (*RAG1/2*) and the Bruton agammaglobulinemia tyrosine kinase (*BTK*).[7,8] Similarly, inherent defects abrogating the maturation of T and B lymphocytes, as exemplified by mutations in cytokine or antigen receptors, are amenable for detection by excision circle assays. The observation that disease-causing mutations in lymphocyte-specific genes differently shape the peripheral immunophenotype in PID patients lead to an established classification based on the presence of T, B, and NK cells, which can also be interpreted by means of TREC and KREC copy numbers in newborn screening assays. Combining the measurement of T and B cell excision circles not only reduces the assay costs and improves the test performance rate, but may also narrow down candidate genes for distinct SCID immunophenotypes.[10] Moreover, simultaneous detection of TRECs and KRECs in neonatal samples seems to be advantageous when aiming for a coherent screening program targeting the whole range of primary immunodeficiencies that present with T or B lymphopenia in early childhood (Table 1). Such disease entities are likely to encompass a major portion of chromosomal instability syndromes with signs of immunodeficiency, represented by diseases such as Ataxia-telangiectasia (AT) and the Nijmegen breakage syndrome (NBS), exhibiting increased leukocyte apoptosis due to defects in DNA damage recognition, response, and repair.[58] Other disorders that can potentially be identified by TREC assays originate from structural defects of thymic embryogenesis or function, frequently seen in DiGeorge syndrome (DGS) and Down syndrome, as well as aberrations of the thymic homing microenvironment required for thymocyte maturation (extracellular matrix network defects).[59–61] The enumeration of KREC copy numbers as a supplement could be helpful to elucidate disorders of telomere maintenance, that seem to affect B cell homeostasis in particular, as illustrated by the various manifestations of dyskeratosis congenita.[62] Moreover, metabolic defects like the branched-chain organic acidurias might limit early lymphocyte development by accumulation of toxic compounds, notably observed in propionic acidemia, thus potentially returning abnormal screening results in excision circle assays.[63] Other mechanisms to explain T or B lymphopenia in newborns include developmental immaturity of the adaptive immunity in premature infants, or pleural effusions with lymphocyte extravasation as frequently seen in the nonimmune hydrops fetalis.[64] In contrast to "false positive" screening results with regard to the target diseases SCID and XLA, one has to keep in mind that patients with severe defects in lymphocyte activation, for example, due to mutations affecting the function of Ca^{2+} release activated Ca^{2+} channels (CRAC) directly or via stimulatory Ca^{2+} sensors (STIM1), or the tyrosine phosphatase CD45, are likely to present with normal T and B lymphocyte counts and normal TREC and KREC copy numbers, respectively.[65,66] Future research and retrospective analysis of screening results from excision circle assays will be guiding if additional screening of biomarkers—given their availability and helpfulness—are required to identify patients with severe "functional" immunodeficiencies in spite of having normal lymphocyte counts.

Immunophenotype in premature newborns

Infants born before 37 weeks of gestation may suffer from a variety of cardiovascular, neurological, metabolic, and gastrointestinal complications, in addition to an increased susceptibility to respiratory and urinary tract infections.[67] Although many risk factors have been linked to preterm birth, the multifactorial causes remain unresolved in most of the

Table 1. Genetic disorders besides well-characterized SCID entities or XLA with an immunophenotype that can resemble T or B lymphopenia in early life

Disease	Genetic defect	Heredity	Estimated incidence	Early life immunophenotype	Reference
Cartilage hair hypoplasia	RMRP	AR	1/20,000*Finland	T⁻ B^low	13
Idiopathic CD4 lymphocytopenia	Unknown		Unknown	T⁻ B^low	14, 15
Down syndrome	Chr 21		1/600–900	T^low B^low	16
Ataxia-telangiectasia	ATM	AR	1/50,000	T^low B^low	17
Shwachman-Diamond syndrome	SBDS	AR	1/50,000	T^low B^low	18, 19
Vici syndrome	Unknown		Unknown	T^low B^low	20, 21
TAR syndrome	Chr 1		1/200,000	T^low B^low	22
Ataxia-telangiectasia-like disease (ATLD)	MRE11	AR	Unknown	T^low B^low	23
Nijmegen breakage syndrome-like disorder (NBSLD)	RAD50	AR	Unknown	T^low B^low	24
Barth syndrome	TAZ	XL	1/300,000	T^low B^low	25
Dyskeratosis congenita (Hoyeraal-Hreidarsson syndrome)	DKC1	XL	1/1,000,000	T^low Bl^ow	26
	TERT, NOP10, NHP2	AR	1/1,000,000	T^low B^low	27
Combined immunodeficiency due to DOCK8 deficiency	DOCK8	AR	1/1,000,000	T^low B^low	28, 29
LAD with Rac2 GTPase deficiency	Rac2	AD	Unknown	T^low B^low	30, 31
Complete DiGeorge syndrome	del22q11.2	AD	1/15,000	T⁻ B⁺	32
CHARGE association	CHD7	AD	1/10,000	T⁻ B⁺	33, 34
VACTERL association	Chr 16		1/7,000	T⁻ B⁺	35
Winged helix deficiency (WHN)	WHN	AR	Unknown	T⁻ B⁺	36
EEC syndrome	Chr 19		Unknown	T^low B⁺	37
STAT5b deficiency	STAT5b	AR	Unknown	T^low B⁺	38
ITK deficiency	ITK	AR	Unknown	T^low B⁺	39
MAGT1 deficiency	MAGT1	XL	Unknown	T^low B⁺	40
Schimke immuno-osseous dysplasia	SMARCAL1	AR	1/1,000,000	T^low B⁺	41
Jacobsen syndrome	del11q23	PI	1/100,000	T^low B⁻	42
Dyskeratosis congenita	TERC, TINF2, DCLRE1B	AD	1/1,000,000	T⁺ B⁻	43, 44
Agammaglobulinemia due to LRRC8 deficiency	LRRC8		Unknown	T⁺ B⁻	45
Congenital pancytopenia due to Ikaros deficiency	IKZF1		Unknown	T⁺ B⁻	46, 47
WHIM syndrome	CXCR4	AD	Unknown	T⁺ B⁻	48, 49
Hoffman syndrome	Unknown		Unknown	T⁺ B⁻	50, 51
Nijmegen breakage syndrome	NBS1	AR	1/40,000* Slavic	T⁺ B^low	52, 53
Propionic acidemia (PCCD)	PCCA, PCCB	AR	1/35,000	T⁺ B^low	54, 55
IPEX syndrome	FOXP3	XL	Unknown	T⁺ B^low	56
GATA2 deficiency	GATA-2	AD	Unknown	T⁺ B^low	57

AD, autosomal dominant; AR, autosomal recessive; CHARGE, coloboma, heart defect, atresia choanae, retarded growth and development, genital hypoplasia, ear anomalies/deafness; EEC, ectrodactyly-ectodermal dysplasia-cleft; IPEX, immune dysregulation, polyendocrinopathy, enteropathy, X-linked syndrome; LAD, leukocyte adhesion defect; LRRC8, leucine rich repeat containing 8 family; PI, paternal imprinting; TAR, thrombocytopenia with absent radius; VACTERL, vertebral anomalies, anal atresia, cardiovascular anomalies, tracheoesophageal fistula, esophageal atresia, renal anomalies, and limb defects; WHIM, warts, hypogammaglobulinemia, infections, and myelokathexis; XL, X-linked.
*Representative only in populations of selected descent.

affected infants, limiting the availability of effective interventions.[68] In developed countries, the birth rate of premature newborns is about 5–12% with a tendency to rise, posing a significant concern for newborn screening programs in particular and for public healthcare systems in general.[69] Thus, if dried blood spot samples are taken before the 32nd week of gestation, a second analysis later on for newborn screening tests of metabolic disorders to distinguish abnormal results of genetic origin from physiological immaturity is often required. If transferring this concept to the field of newborn screening for PID, it might be difficult to define the best time for retesting, as the immaturity of immune function is likely to be maintained for several months.

A higher rate of abnormal test results for preterm infants has previously been observed in the TREC assay.[9,70] In this context, the immaturity of the immune system as a temporal effect of the gestational age may well be distinguished from specific factors related to the medical condition of preterm newborns. These factors are likely to include congenital anomalies, infectious complications, and disturbed metabolic and endocrinologic conditions that may contribute to thymic stress and reduced output of recent thymic emigrants.[70] Still, no data on reference ranges for TREC and KREC copy numbers have been published for premature infants, which results in different practices for repeat testing of samples and referral of patients.[71] Reflecting the authors' experience in the field, reference samples of anonymized premature newborns from the Swedish neonatal screening center were used to correlate the rate of abnormal TREC or KREC screening results with absolute counts of lymphocyte subpopulations that determine the occurrence of TRECs and KRECs (Table 2). In groups of premature newborns sorted by gestational age in weeks, analysis of TREC and KREC copy numbers tended to be consistent until 28 weeks age of gestation, though outliers with the detected frequencies would have an impact in regular newborn screening programs. Infants below 28 weeks of gestational age presented with an increased rate of abnormal TREC copy numbers, paralleling the diminished absolute counts of $CD45RA^+ CD4^+$ T lymphocytes in this period (Table 2).[72] Notably, a trend for reduced KREC copy numbers was seen not in the youngest infants but rather in the 32–34 weeks range of gestation. It is intriguing that TREC copy numbers have been shown to decline with increas-

ing age, caused by involution and subsequent loss of thymic function.[73] However, this paradigm does not apply for B cell homeostasis, and it is questionable if KREC copy numbers follow an undulating course dependent upon the effects of stromal growth factors, adhesion molecules, and cytokines that determine bone marrow output.[74,75] The interaction of these factors in early childhood and in prematurity in particular is poorly understood and deserves further attention to correctly evaluate excision circle copy numbers in infants. However, samples from premature infants are basically eligible to be analyzed by excision circle assays and might not have to be retested at a later stage if cutoff values to exclude SCID and XLA have been exceeded initially.

The spectrum of 22q11 deletion syndromes

Genetic alterations in the chromosomal 22q11 region account for the morphogenesis of different disorders, characterized by congenital malformations, developmental delay, speech abnormalities, and a varying degree of immunodeficiency. Velo-cardio-facial syndrome (VCFS) and DGS are the two most common disorders associated with the locus and show a highly variable penetrance and clinical spectrum.[76] The anomaly resembling DGS, originally described in 1965 by the pediatric endocrinologist Angelo DiGeorge, can be perceived as the severe end of a spectrum of clinical characteristics, including thymus hypoplasia, conotruncal heart malformations, hypocalcemia—owing to hypoparathyroidism that can lead to neonatal tetany—a characteristic facial appearance, and many additional features. The overlap between VCFS and DGS constitutes the most common genetic disorder in humans that directly affects the development of T cell immunity.[29] Therefore, a fraction of patients with VCFS/DGS might be identified using TREC-based assays, and the clinical anomalies should also be borne in mind when evaluating abnormal screening results of the excision circle assays.[9] It has previously been shown in children and adolescents with 22q11 deletion syndromes of clinical significance that approximately one-third of the patients present with low TREC copy numbers irrespective of individual age and without a clinical course that would have resembled a SCID-like immunodeficiency.[77] This observation matches results obtained from the Swedish reference sample set of patients with VCFS/DGS

Table 2. Correlation of the gestational age with absolute counts of T and B lymphocytes and the frequency of abnormal results of the TREC/KREC copy number assay in premature newborns (10 prematures per age group, $n = 120$)[a]

Gestational age	37–35 weeks	34–32 weeks	31–29 weeks	<28 weeks
Absolute counts of CD45RA$^+$ CD4$^+$ T lymphocytes [70]	2×10^9/L	1.5×10^9/L	0.9×10^9/L	$<0.5 \times 10^9$/L
Absolute counts of IgD$^+$ CD27$^-$ B lymphocytes [70]	0.8×10^9/L	0.6×10^9/L	0.5×10^9/L	$<0.4 \times 10^9$/L
TREC copy numbers < 15/μl of whole blood	1 * / 10	1 / 10	1 * / 10	2 / 10
KREC copy numbers < 10/μl of whole blood	1 * / 10	2 / 10	1 * / 10	1 / 10

[a]The lower range of TREC and KREC copy numbers was compared to established cutoff ranges for the detection of patients with SCID or XLA, based on the aim of increasing the sensitivity to 1.0 at expense of the specificity. Asterisks indicate patients with concomitant reduction of TREC and KREC copy numbers. The general methodology used to measure TREC or KREC copy numbers has been described previously.[7,8]

who actually required medical treatment by pediatric cardiologists, infectiologists and immunologists, or neuropediatricians (Fig. 1). In this context, it is of importance to mention that the observed frequency of abnormal newborn screening TREC results, for patients to be diagnosed with the DGS, is much lower, owing to the poor genotype/phenotype correlation of 22q11 deletion syndromes, and given that only a portion of these patients ultimately requires medical care. Still, it could be helpful to have confirmatory screening methods available that can be multiplexed with TREC assays, such as copy number analysis of genes encoded within the 22q11 cluster, to quickly differentiate disorders that exhibit low TREC copy numbers in early life from the target disease SCID (Table 1).[78]

In summary, a fraction of the patients with VCFS or DGS without a "SCID-resembling" immunodeficiency might be detected when screening for SCID patients; yet, employing molecular tests for 22q11 deletions will be of value for confirmatory testing and might additionally serve as an independent screening program for patients with the DGS.

Genome instability syndromes

The maintenance of chromosomal integrity is permanently challenged by environmental and autologous genotoxic stressors. Damage responses to DNA double-strand breaks (DSB) and chromosome-end protecting telomerase function are essential to cope with the terrestrial ionizing radiation and solar UV radiation, as well as oxidative stress arising during cell replication and aging, to prevent formation of malignant diseases and bone marrow failure.[79,80] Telomere-mediated diseases and DNA repair disorders are, furthermore, likely to affect the maturation

and lifespan of rapidly dividing cells such as leukocytes, putatively leading to a T or B lymphopenia that could be detected during newborn screening using excision circle assays (Table 1).

We have previously shown that low TREC and KREC copy numbers can be observed in patients with AT, a syndrome caused by mutations in the *ATM* kinase gene, thereby disrupting the stabilization of DSB in lymphocytes and limiting their developmental capacity.[10] Following DSB sensing, ATM associates with the MRE11-RAD50-NBS1 complex, of which two members have been linked to other chromosome instability disorders, namely the Nijmegen breakage syndrome (NBS) (*NBN* gene) and the Ataxia-telangiectasia-like disease (ATLD) (*MRE11A* gene).[81] In patients with NBS, a profound lymphopenia in early life has been reported that mainly affects the absolute numbers of B lymphocytes, but might also expand to a reduction in the number of NK and T cells.[82,83] Upon analysis with excision circle assays, such patients of Slavic and southeast German descent will most likely present solely with reduced KREC copy numbers (TREC copies are normal) in contrast to patients with AT (Fig. 1).[10] The discrepancy in the results of the TREC/KREC assays agrees well with the observation that NBS patients suffer from a precursor B cell differentiation defect due to unresolved breaks in the immunoglobulin locus, while both T and B lineages are affected in AT patients because of defects in coding joint formation during V(D)J recombination.[84,85] Collectively, these results suggest that excision circle assays for target diseases SCID and XLA might also be helpful to identify AT and NBS patients, thus posing the question of whether these chromosome instability syndromes should be

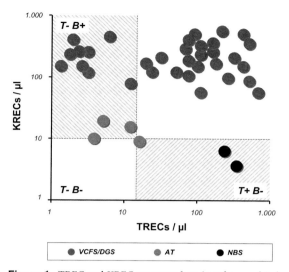

Figure 1. TREC and KREC copy numbers in reference dried blood spot samples from patients diagnosed with Velo-Cardio-Facial syndrome/DiGeorge syndrome (VCFS/DGS, $n = 33$), Ataxia telangiectasia (AT, $n = 4$), and Nijmegen breakage syndrome (NBS, $n = 2$). Dashed lines represent established cutoff values of the multiplex TREC/KREC assay validated for classification of SCID and XLA patients.[10]

included into newborn screening programs. Given that considerable progress has been made during the recent years to improve the therapeutic perspective for AT and NBS patients, earliest-as-possible diagnosis of these diseases would be a major clinical goal to fully exert the beneficial effects of antioxidants, PARP inhibitors, immunoglobulins and read-through compounds in order to slow down the progress of neurodegeneration, to tackle associated malignancies and to treat the associated immunodeficiency.[17,86] It is also evident that both AT and NBS would fulfill the main criteria to be eligible as target diseases in neonatal screening, including (i) a poor outcome due to malignancies, progressive neurodegeneration, and immunodeficiency[87,88]; (ii) a healthy appearance upon initial pediatric examination[83,87]; (iii) existence of genetic confirmatory tests[87,88]; (iv) availability of therapeutic options such as hematopoietic stem cell transplantation, immunoglobulin substitution therapy, or treatment with antioxidants[17,89,90]; and (v) evidence that early treatment does improve the survival and the overall quality of life.[88,89] It has been known for decades that serum levels of alpha fetoprotein (AFP) are elevated in children with AT but not in patients with NBS, and AFP has therefore

been suggested to serve as a diagnostic marker using dried blood spot specimens.[91,92] However, the specificity of serum AFP is low, as elevated levels are also observed in neural tube defects, duodenal and esophageal atresia, newborn hypothyroidism, and some viral infections.[93] Thus, the potential of excision circle assays for detection of children with AT and NBS needs to be explored further.

Proteome screening for complement and antibody disorders

The use of excision circle assays has not proven to be helpful for early detection of antibody deficiencies, such as common variable immunodeficiency (CVID), hyper-IgM syndromes (HIGM), or selective IgA deficiency (IgAD), nor would these assays be expected to identify patients with complement deficiencies.[10] Moreover, disorders that are detected only partially by TREC/KREC assays will require alternative screening approaches to be eligible for preventive programs.

The beneficial effects of diagnosis at the earliest possible for patients with antibody deficiency diseases is exemplified by XLA, which is one of the primary antibody deficiencies that can initially manifest with nonspecific clinical aspects, such as arthritis or skin manifestations, that can lead to misdiagnosis and inappropriate medical treatment.[94] More commonly, delayed diagnosis results in irrevocable organ damage such as bronchiectasis, which predisposes patients to increased progression of lung disease that affects long-term global health.[28] Thus, prompt treatment strategies for XLA besides providing protective immunoglobulin substitutions, has been proven through clinical experience over the past 20 years, can be designated a state-of-the-art therapeutic goal today.[28,95] Besides clinical aspects, delayed diagnosis of XLA can result in frequent hospitalization due to bacterial infections, such as pneumonia, sepsis, or meningitis, and disproportional increases healthcare expenditures, compared to immunoglobulin treatment costs.[96]

To overcome the difficulties to find common delineators for PID screening, it might be useful to develop assays that measure disease-specific biomarkers. A variety of potential biomarkers is summarized in Table 3, setting the frame for proteome-based methods that may be applied in future newborn screening. To cover the extensive

Table 3. Comparison of protein candidate levels in serum or plasma samples for proteome-based newborn screening

Disease	Genetic defect	Clinical features	Estimated incidence	Normal protein concentration	Reference
Antibody deficiencies					
XHIM-CD40 L deficiency	CD40 ligand (*CD40LG*)	Opportunistic infections	1/200,000	>125 pg/mL	97
Neutrophil disorders					
Myeloperoxidase deficiency	Myeloperoxidase (*MPO*)	Disseminated candidiasis	1/2,000	>30 ng/mL	98
Alternative complement pathway					
Factor D deficiency	Complement fD (*CFD*)	Neisserial infections	Unknown	>1 µg/mL	99
Properdin deficiency	Properdin (*CFP*)	Neisserial infections	Unknown	>25 µg/mL	100
Factor B deficiency	Complement fB (*CFB*)	Atypic HUS	Unknown	>200 µg/mL	101
C3 deficiency	C3 complement (*C3*)	Pyogenic infections, SLE-like disease	Unknown	>900 µg/mL	102
Classical component pathway					
C2 deficiency	C2 complement (*C2*)	Pyogenic infections, SLE-like disease	1/20,000* Europe	>20 µg/mL	103
C1r and C1s deficiency	C1 esterases (*C1R, C1S*)	Recurrent infections, SLE-like disease	Unknown	>50 µg/mL	104
C1q deficiency	C1q complement (*C1QA-C*)	Recurrent infections, SLE-like disease	Unknown	>150 µg/mL	105
C4 deficiency	C4 complement (*C4A, C4B*)	Bacterial meningitis, SLE-like disease	Unknown	>300 µg/mL	104
Lectin pathway					
MBL deficiency	Mannose binding lectin (*MBL2*)	Pyogenic infections	1/500	>50 ng/mL	106
MASP-2 deficiency	*MASP2*	Pyogenic infections	Unknown	>2 µg/mL	107
Terminal pathway					
C6 deficiency	C6 complement (*C6*)	Neisserial infections	Unknown	>45 µg/mL	104
C8 deficiency	C8 complement (*C8A, B, G*)	Neisserial infections	Unknown	>55 µg/mL	104
C9 deficiency	C9 complement (*C9*)	Neisserial infections	1/5,000* Japan	>60 µg/mL	104
C5 deficiency	C5 complement (*C5*)	Neisserial infections	Unknown	>80 µg/mL	125
C7 deficiency	C7 complement (*C7*)	Neisserial infections	Unknown	>90 µg/mL	125
Complement control proteins					
Factor I deficiency	Complement fI (*CFI*)	Pyogenic infections, HUS, SLE	Unknown	>20 µg/mL	108
Factor H deficiency	Complement fH (*CFH*)	HUS, MPGN	Unknown	>280 µg/mL	109

HUS, hemolytic-uremic syndrome; MPGN, membrano-proliferative glomerulonephritis; SLE; systemic lupus erythematodes.
*Representative only in populations of selected descent.

magnitude of protein levels and to be able to analyze several biomarkers in a complex sample, new technological platforms, and nanomaterials for immunoassays and enzyme activity assays need to be developed and benchmarked. The bead-based flowmetric Luminex® xMAP technology has been shown to offer versatility for multianalyte measurement in a high-throughput manner, but the sensitivity to intracellular protein concentrations might be a limiting factor for PID screening (Table 3).[110]

Bead-based technologies for protein detection in clinical samples (serum, whole blood, liquor, or body fluid aspirates) commonly rely on chemical surface modification or antibody immobilization on defined microspheres to capture the analyte of interest. Detection and absolute quantitation can be achieved using fluorescence labeling or by size in-/exclusion on high-throughput platforms such as flow cytometry analyzers.

Our group has previously demonstrated that analyzing a multitude of serum protein levels is also feasible using reverse phase protein microarrays, a technique that can be adapted for the screening of C3 complement deficiency in eluted dried blood spot cards and might also be expanded on low abundance complement factor deficiencies (Table 3).[111,112] Such microarrays are designed to absorb all protein compounds contained in a serum or cell lysis sample in a defined spot area and are usually combined with detection antibodies to identify one or several target biomarkers. Combining this protein microarray platform with digital microfluidics has furthermore the potential to markedly reduce the amount of reagents and time consumed.[113]

One of the technologies that could be employed in future newborn screening is based on proximity ligation of unique nucleic acid "flags" that can be attached to diagnostic antibodies or designed to capture bacterial or viral recognition sequences directly.[114] The proximity ligation assay (PLA) offers a possibility for multiplex analysis and quantitation of proteins in nanoliter volumes of crude sample mixtures with a sensitivity reaching the picomolar range.[115] Modifying the dynamic range of PLA by using asymmetric connector hybridization would transfer the assay into direct applicability for the newborn screening of antibody deficiencies and complement disorders (Table 3).[116] However, the availability of diagnostic antibodies with a given specificity for proteins, possibly structurally altered in a disease, may be a limiting hurdle for routine diagnostics. It would be of importance to command sensitive technologies for protein discrimination and relative quantitation, which do not depend on highly specific antibodies, but can be operated satisfactorily following pre-enrichment based on broadly available and cost-efficient polyclonal antibodies.

The process of immunoaffinity enrichment might be optimized using nanoscale polymer networks on surfaces that serve as sample carriers for matrix-assisted laser-desorption/ionization time-of-flight mass spectrometry (MALDI-TOF).[117] These polymer networks would facilitate the structural recognition of native-folded protein analytes in defined three-dimensional spaces, thereby concentrating the samples when dried up for MALDI-TOF analysis, which requires a plain matrix target. Such MALDI-TOF analyses allow discrimination of the molecular weight of proteins, and might therefore be of particular interest in diseases that are associated with the occurrence of protein variants, as exemplified by the NBS. In Eastern and Central Europe, about 90% of the NBS patients are affected by the c.657del5 founder mutation that truncates the p95-Nibrin, resulting in a *c*-terminal p70-Nibrin variant (Fig. 2A). Two other mutations observed in the syndrome, c.835del4 and c.900del25, also produce variant proteins of lower molecular weights by an alternative translation mechanism.[118] The absence of the *N*-terminus is believed to account for the loss of cell-cycle checkpoint control of the truncated Nibrin variants, while the remaining *C*-terminus preserves the function of the MRE11-RAD50-NBS1 DNA repair complex, justifying the observation that NBS patients with residual p70-Nibrin expression are at lower risk to develop lymphomas (Fig. 2B).[119] It remains to be seen if this aspect of disease recognition, coupled with predictive risk assessment, can also be established in screening tests for other primary immunodeficiencies.

The economical evaluation of the cost-effectiveness of novel technologies for neonatal screening is a challenging mission, as various factors—which may also underlie regional or country-specific characteristics—determine the outcome of such analyses. If intending to enhance the quality of life and to reduce the mortality and comorbidity of patients with PID by recognition of these diseases already at birth, one has to balance the estimated treatment costs, that accumulate upon a delayed diagnosis, and the virtual equivalent for the loss of quality adjusted life years (QALYs) in comparison with the expenditures for technical screening instrumentation, staff training, and the actual assay costs per sample. For the setting of neonatal SCID screening in the United States, a Markov model-based approach has recently shown that, besides technical factors such as specificity and sensitivity of the assay, the savings of earlier stem cell

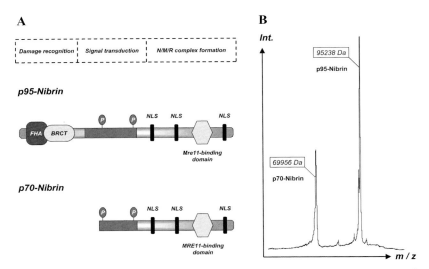

Figure 2. Determination of Nibrin protein configuration in NBS. (A) Structural topology of wild-type p95-Nibrin and truncated p70-Nibrin. BRCT, breast cancer *C*-terminal domain; FHA, forkhead-associated domain; Mre11, DNA double-strand break repair protein; NLS, nuclear localizing signal sequences. (B) Typical result of reflectron MALDI-TOF analysis of immunoaffinity-enriched Nibrin protein fractions from an NBS patient with confirmed c.657del5 founder mutation of the *NBN* gene and a healthy volunteer. Int., peak intensity; *m/z*, mass-to-charge ratio.

therapy and the value that a society intends to admit for one QALY per identified patient are fundamental factors for cost-effectiveness of neonatal screening programs.[120] When transferring these conclusions to PID other than SCID, the value of QALYs might be the crucial determinate in diseases where life-long supportive treatment is preferred over experimental curative therapies (e.g., in antibody deficiencies).

Next-generation screening

Expanding possibilities of genome- and transcriptome-wide analysis have not just entered the field of life science research in the past years, but also point to an application in preventive medicine. Contemporary concepts of research ethics with a focus on personalized genomics, as well as state laws, may restrict the transfer of high-throughput DNA and RNA sequencing into the field of nationwide newborn screening.[121] Besides second-generation resequencing strategies for candidate genes involved in the pathogenesis of defined diseases, advanced nanoscale platforms may be used to sequence whole genomes within hours.[122] Although these novel high-throughput platforms allow the generation of massive amounts of sequence data, less progress has been made in sequence analysis, which is still consuming considerable time and human resources. It may thus be

reasonable to limit the complexity and coverage of genomic starting material, figuratively by retracting to transcriptome analysis using RNA sequencing or microarray technologies.[123] The feasibility of acquiring expression profiles in a genome-wide manner from dried blood spot punches has recently been reported, yielding a comprehensive range of about 9,000 differently regulated gene signatures from stored Guthrie card samples.[124] Examining these RNA transcripts could also constitute a rapid and cost-effective approach to detect mutations in very large genes with mutations scattered all over their length, for example, in the Marfan syndrome with about 600 mutations spread throughout the 65-exon spanning *fibrillin-1* gene.[125] The genetic diagnosis of several other cardiovascular long-range gene disorders, including Long QT syndrome and hypertrophic cardiomyopathy, has previously confirmed the usefulness of transcriptome analysis to detect mutations, deletions, transpositions, and even alternative splice events.[126] Storage, transport, and analysis of whole-blood RNA samples have also been facilitated during the past years and now largely conforms to clinical routine demands due to the introduction of RNA-stabilizing methods based on fluid solutions (PAXgene® system, Catrimox-14™) or solid layers (FTA® paper).[127,128] Such preservation methods do indeed favor the retention of sample material, potentially to be used in order to improve the quality of existing assays or to develop novel newborn screening tests. However, storing and analyzing samples for functional genomics purposes are complicated by bioethical considerations.

The dilemma is perhaps best exemplified by the report on massively parallel DNA sequencing of the complete genome of the Noble Prize winner James D. Watson, in 2008, that was accompanied by a section on ethical concerns, public disclosure of the data, and subject protection.[129] In this particular case, obtaining informed consent and returning research results was quite understandable in the light of the expertise of Dr. Watson in the field of research. However, informed consent relies on knowledge about the dimensions and impact of genome analysis and furthermore on the ability of physicians and geneticists to explain this context to their patients. In this regard, it remains indistinct how informed consent should be obtained for newborns, as genetic discrimination by third parties may occur later in life given the long-lasting impact of the obtained genomic results.[130]

Summary

Newborn screening programs for SCID have come of age during the past few years and have paved the way for testing of additional forms of PID. Excision circle assays, preferably combining TREC and KREC measurements, are still prompting further research and prospective studies to correctly classify the screening results and to compile guidelines for subsequent follow-up. The influence of abnormal results originating from children born prematurely and patients with aberrations in the 22q11 region should be considered in the light of the rare PID forms that are similarly detected using TREC/KREC testing. With regard to PID that are currently not covered by the excision circle strategy, novel assays are needed to screen for various antibody disorders and complement deficiencies. Future research will also have to tackle questions arising from contemporary views on the research ethics of newborn screening in the functional genomics era.

Acknowledgments

The authors are indebted to Kerstin Krist for genomic sequence analysis and to Peter Ahnert for excellent technical guidance on MALDI-TOF analysis. We thank all the included patients and their families for their support and participation. This work was supported in part by the Swedish Research Council, the German Federal Ministry of Education and Research (BMBF, PtJ-Bio, 0315883), the Saxon State Ministry of Social Affairs (SMS), and the Jeffrey Modell Foundation.

Conflicts of interest

The authors declare no conflicts of interest.

References

1. Fernhoff, P.M. 2009. Newborn screening for genetic disorders. *Pediatr. Clin. North Am.* **56:** 505–513.
2. Chan, K. & J.M. Puck. 2005. Development of population-based newborn screening for severe combined immunodeficiency. *J. Allergy Clin. Immunol.* **115:** 391–398.
3. Fasth, A. 1982. Primary immunodeficiency disorders in Sweden: cases among children, 1974–1979. *J. Clin. Immunol.* **2:** 86–92.
4. Lim, D.L. 2003. Primary immunodeficiency diseases in Singapore—the last 11 years. *Singapore Med. J.* **44:** 579–586.
5. Joshi, A.Y. 2009. Incidence and temporal trends of primary immunodeficiency: a population-based cohort study. *Mayo Clin. Proc.* **84:** 16–22.
6. McGhee, S.A., E.R. Stiehm & E.R. McCabe. 2005. Potential costs and benefits of newborn screening for severe combined immunodeficiency. *J. Pediatr.* **147:** 603–608.
7. Baker, M.W. 2009. Development of a routine newborn screening protocol for severe combined immunodeficiency. *J. Allergy Clin. Immunol.* **124:** 522–527.
8. Nakagawa, N. 2011. Quantification of κ-deleting recombination excision circles in Guthrie cards for the identification of early B-cell maturation defects. *J. Allergy Clin. Immunol.* **128:** 223–225.
9. Routes, J.M. 2009. Statewide newborn screening for severe T-cell lymphopenia. *JAMA* **302:** 2465–2470.
10. Borte, S. 2011. Neonatal screening for severe primary immunodeficiency diseases using high-throughput triplex real-time PCR. *Blood* DOI: 10.1182/blood-2011-08-371021.
11. Castellani, C. & J. Massie. 2010. Emerging issues in cystic fibrosis newborn screening. *Curr. Opin. Pulm. Med.* **16:** 584–590.
12. van Zelm, M.C. 2007. Replication history of B lymphocytes reveals homeostatic proliferation and extensive antigen-induced B cell expansion. *J. Exp. Med.* **204:** 645–655.
13. Rider, N.L. 2009. Immunologic and clinical features of 25 Amish patients with RMRP 70 A—>G cartilage hair hypoplasia. *Clin. Immunol.* **131:** 119–128.
14. Walker, U.A. & K. Warnatz. 2006. Idiopathic CD4 lymphocytopenia. *Curr. Opin. Rheumatol.* **18:** 389–395.
15. Kuijpers, T.W. 2011. Idiopathic CD4+ T lymphopenia without autoimmunity or granulomatous disease in the slipstream of RAG mutations. *Blood* **117:** 5892–5896.

16. Ram, G. & J. Chinen. 2011. Infections and immunodeficiency in Down syndrome. *Clin. Exp. Immunol.* **164:** 9–16.

17. Lavin, M.F. 2007. Current and potential therapeutic strategies for the treatment of ataxia-telangiectasia. *Br. Med. Bull.* **81-82:** 129–147.

18. Dror, Y. 2001. Immune function in patients with Shwachman–Diamond syndrome. *Br. J. Haematol.* **114:** 712–717.

19. Burroughs, L., A. Woolfrey A & A. Shimamura. 2009. Shwachman-Diamond syndrome: a review of the clinical presentation, molecular pathogenesis, diagnosis, and treatment. *Hematol. Oncol. Clin. North Am.* **23:** 233–248.

20. Vici, C.D. 1988. Agenesis of the corpus callosum, combined immunodeficiency, bilateral cataract, and hypopigmentation in two brothers. *Am. J. Med. Genet.* **29:** 1–8.

21. Al-Owain, M. 2010. Vici syndrome associated with unilateral lung hypoplasia and myopathy. *Am. J. Med. Genet A.* **152:** 1849–1853.

22. Bonsi, L. 2009. Thrombocytopenia with absent radii (TAR) syndrome: from hemopoietic progenitor to mesenchymal stromal cell disease? *Exp. Hematol.* **37:** 1–7.

23. Taylor, A.M., A. Groom & P.J. Byrd. 2004. Ataxia-telangiectasia-like disorder (ATLD)-its clinical presentation and molecular basis. *DNA Repair* **3:** 1219–1225.

24. Waltes, R. 2009. Human RAD50 deficiency in a Nijmegen breakage syndrome-like disorder. *Am. J. Hum. Genet.* **84:** 605–616.

25. Yen, T.Y. 2008. Acute metabolic decompensation and sudden death in Barth syndrome: report of a family and a literature review. *Eur. J. Pediatr.* **167:** 941–944.

26. Gupta, V. & A. Kumar. 2010. Dyskeratosis congenita. *Adv. Exp. Med. Biol.* **685:** 215–219.

27. Aspesi, A. 2010. Compound heterozygosity for two new TERT mutations in a patient with aplastic anemia. *Pediatr. Blood Can.* **55:** 550–553.

28. Quinti, I. 2011. Effectiveness of immunoglobulin replacement therapy on clinical outcome in patients with primary antibody deficiencies: results from a multicenter prospective cohort study. *J. Clin. Immunol.* **31:** 315–322.

29. Su, H.C. 2010. Dedicator of cytokinesis 8 (DOCK8) deficiency. *Curr. Opin. Allergy Clin. Immunol.* **10:** 515–520.

30. Williams, D.A. 2000. Dominant negative mutation of the hematopoietic-specific Rho GTPase, Rac2, is associated with a human phagocyte immunodeficiency. *Blood* **96:** 1646–1654.

31. Accetta, D. 2011. Human phagocyte defect caused by a Rac2 mutation detected by means of neonatal screening for T-cell lymphopenia. *J. Allergy Clin. Immunol.* **127:** 535–538.

32. Buckley, R.H. 2002. Primary cellular immunodeficiencies. *J. Allergy Clin. Immunol.* **109:** 747–757.

33. Chopra, C. 2009. T-cell immunodeficiency in CHARGE syndrome. *Acta Paediatr.* **98:** 408–410.

34. Jyonouchi, S. 2009. CHARGE (coloboma, heart defect, atresia choanae, retarded growth and development, genital hypoplasia, ear anomalies/deafness) syndrome and chromosome 22q11.2 deletion syndrome: a comparison of immunologic and nonimmunologic phenotypic features. *Pediatrics* **123:** 871–877.

35. Shaw-Smith, C. 2010. Genetic factors in esophageal atresia, tracheo-esophageal fistula and the VACTERL association: roles for FOXF1 and the 16q24.1 FOX transcription factor gene cluster, and review of the literature. *Eur. J. Med. Genet.* **53:** 6–13.

36. Pignata, C., A. Fusco & S. Amorosi. 2009. Human clinical phenotype associated with FOXN1 mutations. *Adv. Exp. Med. Biol.* **665:** 195–206.

37. Roelfsema, N.M. & J.M. Cobben. 1996. The EEC syndrome: a literature study. *Clin. Dysmorphol.* **5:** 115–127.

38. Hwa, V. 2011. STAT5b deficiency: lessons from STAT5b gene mutations. *Best Pract. Res. Clin. Endocrinol. Metab.* **25:** 61–75.

39. Huck, K. 2009. Girls homozygous for an IL-2-inducible T cell kinase mutation that leads to protein deficiency develop fatal EBV-associated lymphoproliferation. *J. Clin. Invest.* **119:** 1350–1358.

40. Li, F.Y. 2011. Second messenger role for Mg2+ revealed by human T-cell immunodeficiency. *Nature* **475:** 471–476.

41. Saraiva, J.M. 1999. Schimke immuno-osseous dysplasia: case report and review of 25 patients. *J. Med. Genet.* **36:** 786–789.

42. Fernández-San José, C. 2011. Hypogammaglobulinemia in a 12-year-old patient with Jacobsen syndrome. *J. Paediatr. Child Health* **47:** 485–486.

43. Knudson, M. 2005. Association of immune abnormalities with telomere shortening in autosomal-dominant dyskeratosis congenita. *Blood* **105:** 682–688.

44. Touzot, F. 2010. Function of Apollo (SNM1B) at telomere highlighted by a splice variant identified in a patient with Hoyeraal–Hreidarsson syndrome. *Proc. Natl. Acad. Sci. USA* **107:** 10097–10102.

45. Sawada, A. 2003. A congenital mutation of the novel gene LRRC8 causes agammaglobulinemia in humans. *J. Clin. Invest.* **112:** 1707–1713.

46. Kirstetter, P. 2002. Ikaros is critical for B cell differentiation and function. *Eur. J. Immunol.* **32:** 720–730.

47. Goldman, F.D. 2011. Congenital pancytopenia and absence of B lymphocytes in a neonate with a mutation in the ikaros gene. *Pediatr. Blood Can.* DOI: 10.1002/pbc.23160.

48. Kawai, T. & H.L. Malech. 2009. WHIM syndrome: congenital immune deficiency disease. *Curr. Opin. Hematol.* **16:** 20–26.

49. Mc Guire, P.J. 2010. Oligoclonality, impaired class switch and B-cell memory responses in WHIM syndrome. *Clin. Immunol.* **135:** 412–421.

50. Hoffman, H.M, J.F. Bastian & L.M. Bird. 2001. Humoral immunodeficiency with facial dysmorphology and limb anomalies: a new syndrome. *Clin. Dysmorphol.* **10:** 1–8.

51. Hügle, B. 2011. Hoffman syndrome: new patients, new insights. *Am. J. Med. Genet A.* **155:** 149–153.

52. Michałkiewicz, J. 2003. Abnormalities in the T and NK lymphocyte phenotype in patients with Nijmegen breakage syndrome. *Clin. Exp. Immunol.* **134:** 482–490.

53. Gregorek, H. 2010. Nijmegen breakage syndrome: long-term monitoring of viral and immunological biomarkers in peripheral blood before development of malignancy. *Clin. Immunol.* **135:** 440–447.

54. Raby, R.B., J.C. Ward & H.G. Herrod. 1994. Propionic acidaemia and immunodeficiency. *J. Inherit. Metab. Dis.* **17:** 250–251.

55. Kuhara, T. 2002. Gas chromatographic-mass spectrometric newborn screening for propionic acidaemia by targeting methylcitrate in dried filter-paper urine samples. *J. Inherit. Metab. Dis.* **25:** 98–106.

56. Bakke, A.C., M.Z. Purtzer & R.S. Wildin. 2004. Prospective immunological profiling in a case of immune dysregulation, polyendocrinopathy, enteropathy, X-linked syndrome (IPEX). *Clin. Exp. Immunol.* **137:** 373–378.

57. Hsu, A.P. 2011. Mutations in GATA2 are associated with the autosomal dominant and sporadic monocytopenia and mycobacterial infection (MonoMAC) syndrome. *Blood* **118:** 2653–2655.

58. Gennery, A.R. 2000. Primary immunodeficiency syndromes associated with defective DNA double-strand break repair. *Br. Med. Bull.* **77-78:** 71–85.

59. Prada, N. 2005. Direct analysis of thymic function in children with Down's syndrome. *Immun. Ageing* **2:** 4.

60. Lima, K. 2010. Low thymic output in the 22q11.2 deletion syndrome measured by CCR9+CD45RA+ T cell counts and T cell receptor rearrangement excision circles. *Clin. Exp. Immunol.* **161:** 98–107.

61. Savino, W. 2010. Intrathymic T cell migration is a multivectorial process under a complex neuroendocrine control. *Neuroimmunomodulation* **17:** 142–145.

62. Wenig, N.P. 2008. Telomere and adaptive immunity. *Mech. Ageing Dev.* **129:** 60–66.

63. Wajner, M. 1999. Inhibition of mitogen-activated proliferation of human peripheral lymphocytes in vitro by propionic acid. *Clin. Sci.* **96:** 99–103.

64. Caserío, S. 2010. Congenital chylothorax: from foetal life to adolescence. *Acta Paediatr.* **99:** 1571–1577.

65. Feske, S. 2010. CRAC channelopathies. *Pflugers Arch* **460:** 417–435.

66. Kung, C. 2000. Mutations in the tyrosine phosphatase CD45 gene in a child with severe combined immunodeficiency disease. *Nat. Med.* **6:** 343–345.

67. Strunk, T. 2011. Innate immunity in human newborn infants: prematurity means more than immaturity. *J. Matern. Fetal Neonatal Med.* **24:** 25–31.

68. Simmons, L.E. 2010. Preventing preterm birth and neonatal mortality: exploring the epidemiology, causes, and interventions. *Semin. Perinatol.* **34:** 408–415.

69. Goldenberg, R.L. 2008. Epidemiology and causes of preterm birth. *Lancet* **371:** 75–84.

70. Accetta, D.J. 2011. Cause of death in neonates with inconclusive or abnormal T-cell receptor excision circle assays on newborn screening. *J. Clin. Immunol.* **31:** 962–967.

71. Puck, J.M. 2011. Expert commentary: practical issues in newborn screening for severe combined immune deficiency (SCID). *J. Clin. Immunol.* DOI: 10.1007/s10875-011-9598-3.

72. Walker, J.C. 2011. Development of lymphocyte subpopulations in preterm infants. *Scand. J. Immunol.* **73:** 53–58.

73. Zubakov, D. 2010. Estimating human age from T-cell DNA rearrangements. *Curr. Biol.* **20:** 970–971.

74. Serana, F. 2011. Thymic and bone marrow output in patients with common variable immunodeficiency. *J. Clin. Immunol.* **31:** 540–549.

75. Min, H., E. Montecino-Rodriguez & K. Dorshkind. 2005. Effects of aging on early B- and T-cell development. *Immunol. Rev.* **205:** 7–17.

76. Hong, R. 2001. The DiGeorge anomaly. *Clin. Rev. Allergy Immunol.* **20:** 43–60.

77. Lima, K. 2010. Low thymic output in the 22q11.2 deletion syndrome measured by CCR9+CD45RA+ T cell counts and T cell receptor rearrangement excision circles. *Clin. Exp. Immunol.* **161:** 98–107.

78. Tomita-Mitchell, A. 2010. Multiplexed quantitative real-time PCR to detect 22q11.2 deletion in patients with congenital heart disease. *Physiol. Genomics* **42:** 52–60.

79. Taylor, A.M. 2001. Chromosome instability syndromes. *Best Pract. Res. Clin. Haematol.* **14:** 631–644.

80. Armanios, M. 2009. Syndromes of telomere shortening. *Annu. Rev. Genom. Hum. Genet.* **10:** 45–61.

81. Carson, C.T. 2003. The Mre11 complex is required for ATM activation and the G2/M checkpoint. *EMBO J.* **22:** 6610–6620.

82. Varon, R. 2000. Clinical ascertainment of Nijmegen breakage syndrome (NBS) and prevalence of the major mutation, 657del5, in three Slav populations. *Eur. J. Hum. Genet.* **8:** 900–902.

83. Maurer, M.H. 2010. High prevalence of the NBN gene mutation c.657-661del5 in Southeast Germany. *J. Appl. Genet.* **51:** 211–214.

84. van der Burg, M. 2010. Loss of juxtaposition of RAG-induced immunoglobulin DNA ends is implicated in the precursor B-cell differentiation defect in NBS patients. *Blood* **115:** 4770–4777.

85. Huang, C.Y. 2007. Defects in coding joint formation in vivo in developing ATM-deficient B and T lymphocytes. *J. Exp. Med.* **204:** 1371–1381.

86. Hu, H. & R.A. Gatti. 2008. New approaches to treatment of primary immunodeficiencies: fixing mutations with chemicals. *Curr. Opin. Allergy Clin. Immunol.* **8:** 540–546.

87. Perlman, S., S. Becker-Catania & R.A. Gatti. 2003. Ataxia-telangiectasia: diagnosis and treatment. *Semin. Pediatr. Neurol.* **10:** 173–182.

88. Demuth, I. & M. Digweed. 2007. The clinical manifestation of a defective response to DNA double-strand breaks as exemplified by Nijmegen breakage syndrome. *Oncogene* **26:** 7792–7798.

89. Albert, M.H. 2010. Successful SCT for Nijmegen breakage syndrome. *Bone Marrow Transplant.* **45:** 622–626.

90. Claret Teruel, G. 2005. Variability of immunodeficiency associated with ataxia telangiectasia and clinical evolution in 12 affected patients. *Pediatr. Allergy Immunol.* **16:** 615–618.

91. Stray-Pedersen, A. 2007. Alpha fetoprotein is increasing with age in ataxia-telangiectasia. *Eur. J. Paediatr. Neurol.* **11:** 375–380.

92. Chrzanowska, K.H. 1995. Eleven Polish patients with microcephaly, immunodeficiency, and chromosomal instability: the Nijmegen breakage syndrome. *Am. J. Med. Genet.* **57:** 462–471.

93. Mizejewski, G.J. 2003. Levels of alpha-fetoprotein during pregnancy and early infancy in normal and disease states. *Obstet. Gynecol. Surv.* **58:** 804–826.

94. Conley, M.E. & V.C. Howard. 2009. X-linked agammaglobulinemia. In *GeneReviews.* Pagon, R.A., T.D. Bird, C.R. Dolan & K. Stephens, Eds. GeneReviews at Genetests: Medical Genetics Information Resource. University of Washington, Seattle. 1997-2009. Available at: http://www.genetests.org.

95. Kaveri, S.V. 2011. Intravenous immunoglobulins in immunodeficiencies: more than mere replacement therapy. *Clin. Exp. Immunol.* **164:** 2–5.

96. Högy, B., H.O. Keinecke & M. Borte. 2005. Pharmacoeconomic evaluation of immunoglobulin treatment in patients with antibody deficiencies from the perspective of the German statutory health insurance. *Eur. J. Health Econ.* **6:** 24–29.

97. Davies, E.G. & A.J. Thrasher. 2010. Update on the hyper immunoglobulin M syndromes. *Br. J. Haematol.* **149:** 167–180.

98. Nauseef, W.M. 2004. Lessons from MPO deficiency about functionally important structural features. *Jpn. J. Infect. Dis.* **57:** 4–5.

99. Sprong, T. 2006. Deficient alternative complement pathway activation due to factor D deficiency by 2 novel mutations in the complement factor D gene in a family with meningococcal infections. *Blood* **107:** 4865–4870.

100. Linton, S.M. & B.P. Morgan. 1999. Properdin deficiency and meningococcal disease—identifying those most at risk. *Clin. Exp. Immunol.* **118:** 189–191.

101. Dehoorne, J. 2008. Complement factor B deficiency associated with recurrent aseptic meningitis. *Pediatric Rheumatol.* **6:** P266.

102. Botto, M. 2009. Complement in human diseases: lessons from complement deficiencies. *Mol. Immunol.* **46:** 2774–2783.

103. Sjöholm, A.G. 2006. Complement deficiency and disease: an update. *Mol. Immunol.* **43:** 78–85.

104. Barilla-LaBarca, M.L. & J.P. Atkinson. 2003. Rheumatic syndromes associated with complement deficiency. *Curr. Opin. Rheumatol.* **15:** 55–60.

105. Schejbel, L. 2011. Molecular basis of hereditary C1q deficiency-revisited: identification of several novel disease-causing mutations. *Genes Immun.* DOI: 10.1038/gene.2011.39.

106. Tsutsumi, A., R. Takahashi & T. Sumida. 2005. Mannose binding lectin: genetics and autoimmune disease. *Autoimmun. Rev.* **4:** 364–372.

107. Sørensen, R., S. Thiel & J.C. Jensenius. 2005. Mannan-binding-lectin-associated serine proteases, characteristics and disease associations. *Springer Semin. Immunopathol.* **27:** 299–319.

108. Nilsson, S.C. 2011. Complement factor I in health and disease. *Mol. Immunol.* **48:** 1611–1620.

109. Buhé, V. 2010. Updating the physiology, exploration and disease relevance of complement factor H. *Int. J. Immunopathol. Pharmacol.* **23:** 397–404.

110. Skogstrand, K. 2005. Simultaneous measurement of 25 inflammatory markers and neurotrophins in neonatal dried blood spots by immunoassay with xMAP technology. *Clin. Chem.* **51:** 1854–1866.

111. Janzi, M. 2005. Serum microarrays for large scale screening of protein levels. *Mol. Cell. Proteomics* **4:** 1942–1947.

112. Janzi, M. 2009. Screening for C3 deficiency in newborns using microarrays. *PLoS One.* **4:** e5321.

113. Millington, D.S. 2010. Digital microfluidics: a future technology in the newborn screening laboratory? *Semin. Perinatol.* **34:** 163–169.

114. Blokzijl, A. 2010. Profiling protein expression and interactions: proximity ligation as a tool for personalized medicine. *J. Intern. Med.* **268:** 232–245.

115. Lundberg, M. 2011. Multiplexed homogeneous proximity ligation assays for high-throughput protein biomarker research in serological material. *Mol. Cell. Proteomics.* **10:** M110.004978 1–10.

116. Kim, J. 2010. Improvement of sensitivity and dynamic range in proximity ligation assays by asymmetric connector hybridization. *Anal. Chem.* **82:** 6976–6982.

117. Pippig, F. & A. Holländer. 2010. Hydrogel nanofilms for biomedical applications: synthesis via polycondensation reactions. *Macromol. Biosci.* **10:** 1093–1105.

118. Antoccia, A. 2006. Nijmegen breakage syndrome and functions of the responsible protein, NBS1. *Genome. Dyn.* **1:** 191–205.

119. Krüger, L. 2007. Cancer incidence in Nijmegen breakage syndrome is modulated by the amount of a variant NBS protein. *Carcinogenesis* **28:** 107–111.

120. Chan, K. 2011. A Markov model to analyze cost-effectiveness of screening for severe combined immunodeficiency (SCID). *Mol. Genet. Metab.* **104:** 383–389.

121. Clayton, E.W. 2010. Currents in contemporary ethics. State run newborn screening in the genomic era, or how to avoid drowning when drinking from a fire hose. *J. Law Med. Ethics* **38:** 697–700.

122. Pareek, C.S., R. Smoczynski & A. Tretyn. 2011. Sequencing technologies and genome sequencing. *J. Appl. Genet.* **52:** 413–435.

123. Ozsolak, F. & P.M. Milos. 2011. RNA sequencing: advances, challenges and opportunities. *Nat. Rev. Genet.* **12:** 87–98.

124. Khoo, S.K. 2011. Acquiring genome-wide gene expression profiles in Guthrie card blood spots using microarrays. *Pathol. Int.* **61:** 1–6.

125. Boileau, C. 2005. Molecular genetics of Marfan syndrome. *Curr. Opin. Cardiol.* **20:** 194–200.

126. Miller, T.E. 2007. Whole blood RNA offers a rapid, comprehensive approach to genetic diagnosis of cardiovascular diseases. *Genet. Med.* **9:** 23–33.

127. Debey-Pascher, S., D. Eggle & J.L. Schultze. 2009. RNA stabilization of peripheral blood and profiling by bead chip analysis. *Methods Mol. Biol.* **496:** 175–210.

128. Rogers, C.D. & L.A. Burgoyne. 2000. Reverse transcription of an RNA genome from databasing paper (FTA(R)). *Biotechnol. Appl. Biochem.* **31:** 219–224.

129. Wheeler, D.A. 2008. The complete genome of an individual by massively parallel DNA sequencing. *Nature* **452:** 872–876.

130. Dhondt, J.L. 2010. Expanded newborn screening: social and ethical issues. *J. Inherit. Metab. Dis.* **33:** 211–217.

Ann. N.Y. Acad. Sci. ISSN 0077-8923

Homologous recombination-based gene therapy for the primary immunodeficiencies

Matthew Porteus

Department of Pediatrics, Divisions of Cancer Biology, Hematology/Oncology, Human Gene Therapy, Stanford University, Stanford, California

Address for correspondence: Matthew Porteus, Department of Pediatrics, Divisions of Cancer Biology, Hematology/Oncology, Human Gene Therapy, Stanford University, Stanford, CA 94305. mporteus@stanford.edu

The devastating nature of primary immunodeficiencies, the ability to cure primary immunodeficiencies by bone marrow transplantation, the ability of a small number of gene-corrected cells to reconstitute the immune system, and the overall suboptimal results of bone marrow transplantation for most patients with primary immunodeficiencies make the development of gene therapy for this class of diseases important. While there has been clear clinical benefit for a number of patients from viral-based gene therapy strategies, there have also been a significant number of serious adverse events, including the development of leukemia, from the approach. In this review, I discuss the development of nuclease-stimulated, homologous recombination-based approaches as a novel gene therapy strategy for the primary immunodeficiencies.

Keywords: gene targeting; homologous recombination; zinc finger nuclease; severe combined immunodeficiency; TAL effector nuclease

Introduction

The primary immunodeficiencies (PIDs) are a diverse set of genetic disorders that result in the development of a dysfunctional immune system. The severe combined immunodeficiencies (SCIDs) are among the most severe form of PID and are the consequence of single gene mutations such that T cells are unable to develop. Since T cells regulate and activate multiple arms of the immune system, the lack of T cells leads to a profound immunodeficiency that, without treatment, results in death in the first years of life. The only current curative therapy for SCID is allogeneic bone marrow transplantation. While there remain disagreements about the details of how such transplantation should be performed in different patients, in general, the cure rate using matched sibling donors is greater than 90%.[1,2] Most patients with SCID, however, do not have an HLA-matched sibling donor, and the cure rate using alternative donors is lower. The cure rate using parental haploidentical donors, for example, is 60–65%.[1,2]

The curative nature of bone marrow transplantation suggested that gene modification of autologous hematopoietic stem cells (gene therapy) could potentially be curative for these diseases. An important experiment of nature demonstrated that just a single corrected cell might be sufficient to functionally correct the immunodeficiency.[3] In this example, a patient was born with a point mutation in the interleukin 2 receptor subunit gamma (IL-2RG) gene (*IL2RG*) causing X-linked severe combined immunodeficiency (SCID-X1). Surprisingly, at one year of age, he was found to have a normal number of T cells but remained hypogammaglobulinemic and without NK cells. Molecular analysis demonstrated that he had a point mutation changing thymidine to cytosine causing a C115R amino acid change in the IL-2RG protein in his B cells, neutrophils, and monocytes, consistent with a diagnosis of SCID-X1. The patient's CD3$^+$ cells (which were determined to be autologous by karyotype analysis), however, were found to have a revertant mutation such that the cytosine was changed back to a thymidine creating the wild-type amino acid sequence. The revertant

doi: 10.1111/j.1749-6632.2011.06314.x

mutation must have occurred in a T cell precursor after separation from the NK cell and B cell lineages because of the lack of NK cells and the lack of the reversion mutation in B cells. Analysis of the patient's T cell repertoire showed that a diverse and functional T cell repertoire developed from this single T cell precursor and that this repertoire seemed to be stable for at least five years.[4,5] It will be extremely interesting and important to determine if the repertoire is maintained over decades. If the immune repertoire were not maintained, it would suggest that to maintain long-term immune reconstitution either an earlier precursor cell needs to be corrected or that more precursor cells need to be corrected. Overall, this amazing result demonstrates that a small number of autologous gene-corrected precursor cells, perhaps as few as one, might be sufficient as a general approach to curing patients of SCID.

The gene therapy approach that has advanced farthest is based on phenotypic correction by uncontrolled gene addition, rather than direct gene correction, using retroviral vectors to introduce the wild-type transgene into hematopoietic stem/progenitor cells (HSPCs). This approach has entered phase I/II clinical trials for a number of PIDs including SCID-X1, ADA-SCID, Wiskott–Aldrich syndrome (WAS), and chronic granulomatous disease (CGD).[6–11] These trials have reflected the yin/yang of the gene therapy field. In ADA-SCID, 31 patients have safely received the gene modified HSPCs without serious adverse events and 21 of those have developed functional immune systems without the need for enzyme replacement therapy after years of follow-up. For SCID-X1 (20 patients) and WAS (10 patients), most of the patients developed functional immune systems after receiving retrovirally modified HSPCs but a significant fraction (~10–20%) have also developed leukemias from the insertion of the retrovirus near a proto-oncogene thereby activating it. The activation of the proto-oncogene is probably not sufficient to cause leukemia, as patients who have not developed leukemia in these trials and in the ADA-SCID trial have identifiable clones in which the retrovirus also inserted near the same proto-oncogene. The insertion is a major contributing factor, however. Finally, in the CGD gene therapy trials, while patients did develop some transient clinical benefit from the transduced cells, 100% of the patients have developed myelodysplasia or leukemia from the insertional activation of proto-oncogenes. Overall, while the risk of developing leukemia from retroviral insertion seems to be disease specific, the general short-term risk seems to be on the order of 10–20% (5/20 in SCID-X1, 1/10 in WAS, and 3/3 in CGD). The longer-term risk remains to be determined. Clinically, it is reassuring that 5/6 of the patients who developed leukemia in the SCID-X1 and WAS trials have been cured of their leukemia and have not lost their immune system in the process of curing their leukemia. It is also important that researchers are developing improved next-generation viral vectors that include self-inactivating long terminal repeats (LTRs) and transgenes driven by internal promoters. Comparison of these next-generation vectors with the first-generation vector in preclinical studies demonstrated a decreased level of genotoxicity. Recently initiated clinical trials with these new vectors will determine if the reduced genotoxicity in preclinical studies results in a decreased incidence of leukemia in humans.

Gene targeting by homologous recombination in somatic cells

An alternative strategy to using uncontrolled viral-mediated gene addition to phenotypically correct cells is to use homologous recombination to precisely modify the genome. In this way, disease-causing mutations could either be directly corrected at the nucleotide level, disease-causing genomic loci modified in more sophisticated ways, or transgenes introduced into specific locations in the genome (Fig. 1). Homologous recombination-mediated genome modification (hereafter called "gene targeting") has been used experimentally for decades in yeast. Its use in mammalian cells was limited by its low spontaneous rate (10^{-6}).[12,13] That is, when a DNA fragment is introduced into mammalian somatic cells, the frequency that its sequence information is incorporated into the genome in a homologous fashion is 10^{-6} (or one recombinant per one million cells). Nonetheless, gene targeting has been harnessed as an extremely important tool in murine embryonic stem cells. Smithies et al. and Capecchi et al. have both developed sophisticated positive and negative selection strategies to identify single clones that had undergone gene targeting events in mouse embryonic stem cells.[14,15]

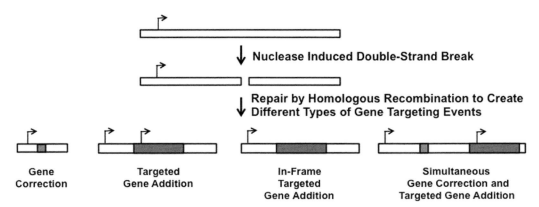

Figure 1. Alternative genome modifications that can be generated by homologous recombination-based gene targeting. By designing the donor/targeting vector in different ways, a variety of different targeted genome modifications can be created, of which four examples are depicted here. These include small changes of one or a few nucleotides ("gene correction") or the targeted addition of a full gene containing its own promoter. Another possible modification includes targeting a gene or cDNA in frame such that its expression is driven by the endogenous promoter ("in-frame–targeted gene addition"). Finally, one can simultaneously both perform gene correction and insert another gene downstream (such as in an intron of the gene). In this example, the downstream gene that is inserted is driven by its own promoter. This downstream gene could be designed such that cells that have undergone gene targeting are given a selective advantage over unmodified cells.

These modified embryonic stem cells could then be injected into a preimplantation mouse blastocyst, implanted into the uterus, and offspring derived from the gene-targeted ES cells can be derived. For this work, they were awarded the Noble Prize in medicine in 2007 and using this strategy thousands of mouse models have been derived. Moreover, Smithies also showed that human somatic cells that have undergone gene targeting, in this example at the beta-globin locus, could also be identified with sophisticated selection strategies and extensive screening.[16] Similar strategies were used by Sedivy *et al.* to generate primary fibroblast lines to better understand the ontogeny of cancer.[17] But in all cases of using gene targeting in mammalian cells, the absolute rate of gene targeting was far too low to be considered a viable gene therapy approach.

In the mid-1990s, several groups, including those led by Maria Jasin, made a critical discovery using the I-SceI homing endonuclease.[18–21] They found that if a DNA double-strand break is created within a genomic target gene, the frequency of gene targeting increased by three orders of magnitude. Under optimized conditions, the stimulation of gene targeting could reach almost five orders of magnitude, such that 3–5% of cells without selection were targeted.[13] I-SceI and the family of homing endonucleases are also known as meganucleases. These endonucleases, in contrast to well-known restriction enzymes that

have recognition sites of 4, 6, or 8 basepairs, have recognition sites of 18 basepairs or longer.[22,23] In the above experiments, an I-SceI recognition site was embedded within a reporter gene, producing a modified, nonfunctional reporter gene that was then inserted as a single copy into the genome to create a cell line. The frequency of gene targeting can then be measured by the genetic correction of the integrated, mutated reporter gene. For example, when a donor/targeting plasmid engineered to correct the mutated reporter gene was transfected into the reporter cell line alone, the frequency of gene targeting was found to be 10^{-6}. But when the donor/targeting plasmid was cotransfected along with an expression plasmid for the I-SceI nuclease—thereby creating a DNA double-strand break within the reporter gene—the frequency of gene targeting increased 3–5 orders of magnitude (0.1–5% depending on the cell line and experimental conditions). In principle, therefore, with the use of I-SceI nuclease, gene-targeting frequencies could be increased to levels that might be therapeutically useful, and there was no intrinsic barrier in mammalian cells to achieving such frequencies, as might have been surmised by earlier studies of gene targeting in mammalian cells.

The mechanism of gene-targeting stimulation by a DNA double-strand break is that double-strand breaks are naturally repaired by homologous recombination.[24] Double-strand breaks are particularly problematic DNA lesions for maintaining genome integrity because they can create point mutations, insertions/deletions, translocations, and chromosomal loss.[25] Moreover, double-strand breaks are relatively common lesions because they can be generated naturally by reactive oxygen species.

It is believed that ~50 double-strand breaks are generated per cell per cell cycle as the result of natural cellular metabolism.[26] There are two major cellular mechanisms for the repair of DNA double-strand breaks (Fig. 2). One of these is homologous recombination. In homologous recombination repair of a double-strand break in mitotic cells, an undamaged template is used to make a copy of the region surrounding the break and then "pastes" this copy over the break, thereby repairing it. In such a case, there is transfer of information from the donor/template to the broken strands but not a physical exchange of DNA molecules. The lack of physical exchange during the repair of double-strand breaks in mitotic cells contrasts with some types of meiotic homologous recombination in which there is actual physical exchange of DNA molecules between homologous chromosomes to generate genetic diversity and to promote faithful chromosomal segregation.[27] In the normal repair of a DNA double-strand break by homologous recombination, the undamaged template used by the homologous recombination machinery is the undamaged sister-chromatid. For reasons that remain unclear, in gene targeting, the homologous recombination machinery uses the exogenous donor plasmid as a template for the repair of the nuclease-induced double-strand break.

In summary, the high frequency of gene targeting after the induction of a gene-specific DNA double-strand break results from harnessing the cell's endogenous homologous recombination machinery to create precise genome modifications.

Zinc finger nucleases

Although experiments with I-SceI demonstrated that gene-targeting frequencies in mammalian cells could be increased to therapeutically useful levels, these experiments were limited in scope because the target site for the nuclease had to be inserted into the reporter gene that was then inserted into the genome, a feature that obviously precluded using I-SceI to target endogenous genes. The challenge thus became one of engineering a nuclease to recognize a target site within an endogenous gene.

One strategy has been to re-engineer homing endonucleases to recognize new target sites, and sophisticated protein engineering and screening protocols have been developed toward this end.[22,23] The strategy that has advanced furthest for the PIDs is the use of zinc finger nucleases (ZFNs) (Fig. 3). ZFNs are engineered proteins first developed by Chandrasegaran et al. and then in conjunction with Carroll et al., in which a zinc finger DNA-binding domain is fused to the nuclease domain derived from the type IIS FokI restriction endonuclease.[28,29] The FokI nuclease domain cuts DNA as a dimer; thus ZFNs cut DNA most efficiently when arranged in the orientation shown in Figure 2, in which one ZFN is bound to the lower strand and the other is bound to the upper strand, and the two ZFNs are separated by 5–7 basepairs. The key feature of ZFNs is that the zinc finger DNA-binding domain, the most common domain in the mammalian genome and the domain that mediates DNA recognition for a large number of transcription factors, can be re-engineered through a variety of different methods to recognize a wide variety of new (endogenous) target sequences.[30–33]

Gene targeting with ZFNs

ZFNs were found to be as effective as I-SceI in stimulating gene targeting in mammalian cells.[13] In these experiments, a ZFN recognition site was inserted adjacent to an I-SceI recognition site within a mutated reporter gene and a stable cell line was made with the reporter gene. Correction of the mutated reporter gene by gene targeting was the same using either the I-SceI endonuclease to create the double-strand break or a defined (i.e., target-specific) ZFN. Moreover, a new ZFN, made de novo from a previously characterized zinc finger DNA-binding domain, could also stimulate gene targeting in the reporter gene.

In the I-SceI/ZFN comparison experiments, target sites for each endonuclease were embedded in the reporter gene. Subsequently, ZFNs were engineered to recognize target sites within the natural sequence of the reporter gene itself.[33,34] Just as for sites embedded within the target gene, the ZFNs that recognize natural reporter gene sequences were able to stimulate gene targeting by greater than three orders of magnitude. In these experiments, alternative targeting vectors were used rather than just simply correcting small mutations, and more complex targeted

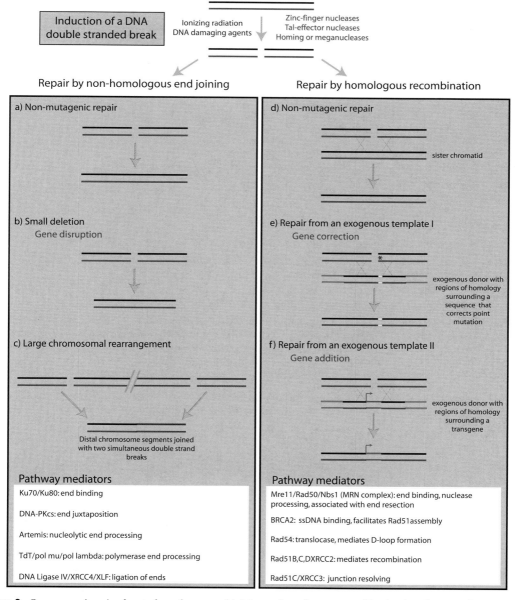

Figure 2. Genome engineering by nonhomologous end-joining or homologous recombination-based repair of double-strand breaks. Double-strand breaks can be generated in multiple different ways. A double-strand break can be repaired by two primary mechanisms: nonhomologous end-joining (shown on the left) and homologous recombination (shown on the right). Depicted are three possible genome modifications if the double-strand break is repaired by either nonhomologous end-joining or homologous recombination. At the bottom of each is a partial list and a brief overview of the genes involved in each repair pathway.

genome modifications were generated (schematized in Fig. 1). For example, a full transgene cassette in which a second gene was precisely inserted by gene targeting into a defined locus was demonstrated.[33] A more sophisticated targeted genome modification involved simultaneously correcting a mutation at one site while inserting a downstream selectable marker at another site. In this way, cells that had undergone gene targeting could be given a selective advantage and thus enriched by using the selectable marker.[33] While the efficiency of simultaneous modifications was lower than simple gene correction, the

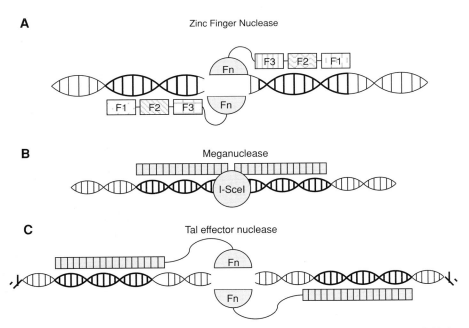

Figure 3. Alternative nuclease platforms for genome engineering. There are three current platforms or scaffolds for engineering nucleases for targeted genome modification. ZFNs create double-strand breaks as dimers, and each nuclease binds to a target site of between 9 (shown here for a three finger protein) and 18 basepairs. The total binding length of the two binding sites is between 18 and 36 basepairs. The optimal spacer length between the two zinc finger nuclease binding sites is 5–7 basepairs. Homing endonucleases bind and cut DNA as monomers and recognized binding sites that are longer than 18 basepairs in length. TAL effector nucleases also create double-strand breaks through the *Fok*I nuclease domain ("Fn") as dimers. Each nuclease binds to a target site between 12 and 24 basepairs. The total length of the combined binding sites can range from 24 to 48 basepairs. The optimal spacer length between the two binding sites is 12–20 basepairs. Statistically, a binding site of 17 basepairs or greater should be unique in the mammalian genome.

selectable marker gave a method to enrich for targeted cells by a thousand-fold. In the setting of many PIDs where gene-corrected cells have a natural selective advantage over uncorrected cells, such a strategy may not be necessary. But in other settings where the gene-corrected cells may not have a selective advantage or only a minimal selective advantage, this strategy could be very useful in enriching targeted cells to a level that might provide therapeutic benefit.

Gene targeting with ZFNs at the *IL2RG* locus

The first demonstration of nuclease-mediated genome modification of an endogenous mammalian gene was for exon 5 of the *IL2RG*.[34] Exon 5 is a hotspot for mutations that cause SCID-X1.[35] A series of ZFNs were engineered and optimized using a combination of *in vitro* and cell-based reporter assays to identify a ZFN pair that had optimal activity for an exon 5 target site. This optimal pair was then tested in K562 cells, a human erythroleukemia cell line, and primary human T cells. In K562 cells, 17% of alleles had targeted genome modification, with 6% of cells having modification of both alleles of *IL2RG*. Moreover, in a series of experiments, the ZFNs were used to generate a clone in which a nonsense mutation was introduced into both exon 5 alleles creating a K562 cell line that was null for *IL2RG* expression, thus mimicking a human SCID-X1 patient. This cell line was then retargeted using the ZFNs, and cells with either a single allele or both alleles could be easily identified in which the mutation had been corrected to form a functional *IL2RG* gene, thus mimicking what might be done in SCID-X1 patient-derived hematopoietic cells. In primary T cells, the overall frequency of allele modification was lower than in K562 but still within a potentially therapeutic range (~4%). Overall, this work demonstrated both the potential of homologous recombination as a possible therapy for patients with PIDs and the possibility of engineered nucleases, such as ZFNs, to mediate this strategy.

In addition to using exon 5 *IL2RG*–directed ZFNs for gene correction changes, the same ZFNs were used to target gene addition to the locus in K562 cells.[36] Interestingly, in K562 cells the frequency of targeted gene addition by homologous recombination was not significantly different from the creation of single nucleotide changes by homologous recombination. The demonstration of similar frequencies of gene modification by homologous recombination for both small and large changes meant that one could consider more sophisticated gene modifications without compromising on the overall frequency.

The method of delivery and range of cell types for targeting exon 5 of *IL2RG* was expanded by using integration-deficient lentivirus (IDLV) to target both gene correction events and gene addition events in human lymphoblastoid cell lines.[37] The gene correction frequencies using IDLV in K562 cells or EBV-transformed lymphoblastoid cells were similar to the gene modification frequencies found using nonviral electroporation-based methods of gene delivery techniques. Similarly, the gene addition frequencies in K562 cells using IDLV were similar to the frequencies obtained using nonviral electroporation-based methods. There are challenges in using IDLV vectors, however, including obtaining high levels of transduction of the target cell, low expression of the nuclease from the vector, and the difficulty of producing high-titer IDLV preparations.[38]

An important finding from such IDLV studies was a much lower frequency of gene targeting in human CD34[+] cells than in other cell types.[37] Whether the lower frequency of targeting in CD34[+] cells is an intrinsic property of that cell type or a reflection of the specific experimental conditions used (using IDLV to deliver IL-2RG ZFNs to human CD34[+] cells under specific culture conditions) is an area of active investigation and a critically important problem if the nuclease-mediated homologous recombination approach is to be translated to the clinic.

Targeted gene addition to a "safe harbor"

While there is intrinsic appeal of a patient-specific gene correction approach, a more general approach

might be to use gene targeting by homologous recombination to target the therapeutic transgene to a specific genomic location, a so-called safe harbor. While targeting a gene to a safe and specific genomic location would mean that it is not expressed from the endogenous promoter, the risk of insertional oncogenesis, as a result of uncontrolled integration, would be eliminated.

The principle of targeted-transgene addition by nuclease-mediated homologous recombination was first described in 2006.[33] Subsequently, targeting of transgenes to the *IL2RG, CCR5,* and *PPP1R12C* genes has been described.[36,37,39] Whether these loci are the best "safe harbors" to use clinically remains to be determined. The concept that one might use one set of nucleases to target a single locus with multiple different transgenes, however, has great appeal because it does not require the generation and characterization of clinical grade nucleases for each patient.

Minimizing off-target effects of ZFNs

With the first report of using ZFNs for mammalian cell-targeted genome modification came the recognition that expression of ZFNs could have cellular cytotoxicity.[13] The presumed mechanism of cellular cytotoxicity is that the ZFNs are creating off-target double-strand breaks, as the degree of cytotoxicity is directly correlated with the number of extra double-strand breaks that are being created.[40,41] An increasing understanding of the nature of these off-target sites has been gained by using both *in vitro* and *in vivo* assays to identify these sites.[42,43] There have been several different approaches to minimizing the off-target effects.

The first has been to improve the specificity of the zinc finger DNA-binding domain. For example, using more sophisticated design strategies results in ZFNs that have both improved on-target activity and reduced off-target activity.[41] The second has been to create what are called "obligate heterodimer" ZFNs.[44–46] Since ZFNs only efficiently create double-strand breaks as dimers, the nuclease domain has been re-engineered to prevent homodimers of ZFNs from cutting DNA. This modification would be expected to reduce off-target double-strand breaks by 50%. But, interestingly, these modifications seem to reduce off-target breaks by a greater extent, and while the mechanism is not known, it may be the result of weakening the dimer interface even between heterodimers, thereby decreasing the probability of cutting at off-target sites that the ZFNs only weakly bind to. The third modification is to add domains to the ZFNs that destabilize the protein in the absence of a small molecule.[40] Using this method the duration of ZFN expression can be regulated tightly such that it is present for only a short, critical window of time. In this way, significant reductions in off-target DSBs and cytotoxicity can be obtained without compromising on-target gene targeting activity.

The development of TAL effector nucleases

An exciting new discovery in the nuclease-mediated genome engineering field is the development of a new nuclease platform called *TAL effector nucleases* (TALENS) (Fig. 3).[47–49] TAL effector proteins are transcription factors from a bacterial plant[48] pathogen whose DNA-binding domain consists of repeating subunits with a two amino acid variable domain in each repeat called the RVD. In 2009, two groups broke the TAL effector code and determined that each repeat code for the recognition of a single nucleotide and the two amino acid RVD determines the nucleotide recognized.[50] Several groups have now used modular assembly-based techniques to generate new TAL-effector DNA binding domains to recognize novel target sequences and then fuse these new DNA binding domains to the *Fok*I nuclease domain to create TALENs.[47,48] In comparison with ZFNs, TALENs seem to have an excellent profile of activity and specificity. TALENs made to target *IL2RG* have less cytotoxicity than the corresponding *IL2RG* ZFNs and ~30–50% of the on-target gene modification activity.[51] Overall, the ease of assembling new TALENs, in contrast to the difficult methods for generating highly active ZFNs and the favorable activity and specificity profiles for TALENs, make this a promising new nuclease platform for genome engineering including for the PIDs.

Nuclease-mediated gene targeting in induced pluripotent cells

Although this review has focused on using gene targeting in mammalian somatic cells, an alternative approach is to use gene targeting to correct disease-causing mutations in induced pluripotent cells (iPSCs), followed by conversion of these gene-corrected cells into transplantable immune or immune precursor and then transplantation of these cells into the patient.[52] A variety of patient-derived iPS cells have now been generated as a first stop in the process.[53] While nuclease-mediated gene correction of disease-causing mutations in PID-derived iPS cells has not been published yet, the general approach of using nucleases to perform gene targeting in iPS cells has been reported.[54–56] The major limitation to this approach is likely to be deriving sufficient numbers of transplantable hematopoietic cells, either HSCs or a broad repertoire of T cells, from the gene-corrected iPS cells that can then be transplanted in a safe fashion. Direct derivation of T cells from ES cells has been described,[53] but HSCs that give rise to definitive hematopoiesis derived from hES or hIPS cells have not.

Overall, the use of homologous recombination-based gene therapy strategies is extremely promising because of the tremendous selective advantage of gene-corrected cells in PIDs combined with the precision of homologous recombination. There has been important progress toward developing this approach for patients with SCID. The remaining major challenge will be to demonstrate that sufficient numbers of gene-corrected hematopoietic precursor cells can be generated in this way. Once this problem is solved, it is hoped that clinical trials using a homologous recombination-based strategy will be initiated within the next several years.

Acknowledgments

I thank the Burroughs-Wellcome fund, the NIH/Nanomedicine Development Program (PN2EY018244), the Amon Carter Fund, and the Laurie Kraus Lacob Faculty Scholar Fund for their ongoing support to my lab and my work.

Conflicts of interest

The author declares no conflicts of interest.

References

1. Buckley, R.H. 2000. Advances in the understanding and treatment of human severe combined immunodeficiency. *Immunol. Res.* **22:** 237–251.
2. Gennery, A.R. *et al.* 2010. Transplantation of hematopoietic stem cells and long-term survival for primary immunodeficiencies in Europe: entering a new century, do we do better? *J. Allergy Clin. Immunol.* **126:** 602–610 e601–e611.
3. Stephan, V. *et al.* 1996. Atypical X-linked severe combined immunodeficiency due to possible spontaneous reversion of the genetic defect in T cells. *N. Engl. J. Med.* **335:** 1563–1567.

4. Bousso, P. *et al.* 2000. Diversity, functionality, and stability of the T cell repertoire derived *in vivo* from a single human T cell precursor. *Proc. Natl. Acad. Sci. USA* **97:** 274–278.

5. Fischer, A. *et al.* 2002. Gene therapy for human severe combined immunodeficiencies. *Isr. Med. Assoc. J.* **4:** 51–54.

6. Fischer, A., S. Hacein-Bey-Abina & M. Cavazzana-Calvo. 2010. 20 years of gene therapy for SCID. *Nat. Immunol.* **11:** 457–460.

7. Cavazzana-Calvo, M. *et al.* 2005. Gene therapy for severe combined immunodeficiency. *Annu Rev. Med.* **56:** 585–602.

8. Aiuti, A. *et al.* 2009. Gene therapy for immunodeficiency due to adenosine deaminase deficiency. *N. Engl. J. Med.* **360:** 447–458.

9. Boztug, K. *et al.* 2010. Stem-cell gene therapy for the Wiskott–Aldrich syndrome. *N. Engl. J. Med.* **363:** 1918–1927.

10. Ott, M.G. *et al.* 2006. Correction of X-linked chronic granulomatous disease by gene therapy, augmented by insertional activation of MDS1-EVI1, PRDM16 or SETBP1. *Nat. Med.* **12:** 401–409.

11. Stein, S. *et al.* 2010. Genomic instability and myelodysplasia with monosomy 7 consequent to EVI1 activation after gene therapy for chronic granulomatous disease. *Nat. Med.* **16:** 198–204.

12. Sedivy, J.M. & P.A. Sharp. 1989. Positive genetic selection for gene disruption in mammalian cells by homologous recombination. *Proc. Natl. Acad. Sci. USA* **86:** 227–231.

13. Porteus, M.H. & D. Baltimore. 2003. Chimeric nucleases stimulate gene targeting in human cells. *Science* **300:** 763.

14. Doetschman, T., N. Maeda & O. Smithies. 1988. Targeted mutation of the Hprt gene in mouse embryonic stem cells. *Proc. Natl. Acad. Sci. USA* **85:** 8583–8587.

15. Thomas, K.R. & M.R. Capecchi. 1987. Site-directed mutagenesis by gene targeting in mouse embryo-derived stem cells. *Cell* **51:** 503–512.

16. Smithies, O. *et al.* 1985. Insertion of DNA sequences into the human chromosomal beta-globin locus by homologous recombination. *Nature* **317:** 230–234.

17. Sedivy, J.M. & A. Dutriaux. 1999. Gene targeting and somatic cell genetics—a rebirth or a coming of age? *Trends Genet.* **15:** 88–90.

18. Jasin, M. 1996. Genetic manipulation of genomes with rare-cutting endonucleases. *Trends Genet.* **12:** 224–228.

19. Rouet, P., F. Smih & M. Jasin. 1994. Expression of a site-specific endonuclease stimulates homologous recombination in mammalian cells. *Proc. Natl. Acad. Sci. USA* **91:** 6064–6068.

20. Sargent, R.G., M.A. Brenneman & J.H. Wilson. 1997. Repair of site-specific double-strand breaks in a mammalian chromosome by homologous and illegitimate recombination. *Mol. Cell. Biol.* **17:** 267–277.

21. Choulika, A. *et al.* 1995. Induction of homologous recombination in mammalian chromosomes by using the I-SceI system of Saccaromyces cerevisiae. *Mol. Cell. Biol.* **15:** 1968–1973.

22. Stoddard, B.L. 2011. Homing endonucleases: from microbial genetic invaders to reagents for targeted DNA modification. *Structure* **19:** 7–15.

23. Paques, F. & P. Duchateau. 2007. Meganucleases and DNA double-strand break-induced recombination: perspectives for gene therapy. *Curr. Gene. Ther.* **7:** 49–66.

24. Wyman, C., D. Ristic & R. Kanaar. 2004. Homologous recombination-mediated double-strand break repair. *DNA Repair* **3:** 827–833.

25. Weinstock, D.M. *et al.* 2006. Modeling oncogenic translocations: distinct roles for double-strand break repair pathways in translocation formation in mammalian cells. *DNA Repair* **5:** 1065–1074.

26. Vilenchik, M.M. & A.G. Knudson. 2003. Endogenous DNA double-strand breaks: production, fidelity of repair, and induction of cancer. *Proc. Natl. Acad. Sci. USA* **100:** 12871–12876.

27. Neale, M.J. & S. Keeney. 2006. Clarifying the mechanics of DNA strand exchange in meiotic recombination. *Nature* **442:** 153–158.

28. Kim, Y.G., J. Cha & S. Chandrasegaran. 1996. Hybrid restriction enzymes: zinc finger fusions to Fok I cleavage domain. *Proc. Natl. Acad. Sci. USA* **93:** 1156–1160.

29. Smith, J. *et al.* 2000. Requirements for double-strand cleavage by chimeric restriction enzymes with zinc finger DNA-recognition domains. *Nucleic Acids Res.* **28:** 3361–3369.

30. Wolfe, S.A., L. Nekludova & C.O. Pabo. 2000. DNA recognition by Cys2His2 zinc finger proteins. *Annu. Rev. Biophys. Biomol. Struct.* **29:** 183–212.

31. Jamieson, A.C., J.C. Miller & C.O. Pabo. 2003. Drug discovery with engineered zinc-finger proteins. *Nat. Rev. Drug. Discov.* **2:** 361–368.

32. Pabo, C.O., E. Peisach & R.A. Grant. 2001. Design and selection of novel Cys2His2 zinc finger proteins. *Annu. Rev. Biochem.* **70:** 313–340.

33. Porteus, M.H. 2006. Mammalian gene targeting with designed zinc finger nucleases. *Mol. Ther.* **13:** 438–446.

34. Urnov, F.D. *et al.* 2005. Highly efficient endogenous human gene correction using designed zinc-finger nucleases. *Nature* **435:** 646–651.

35. Notarangelo, L.D. *et al.* 2000. Combined immunodeficiencies due to defects in signal transduction: defects of the gammac-JAK3 signaling pathway as a model. *Immunobiology.* **202:** 106–119.

36. Moehle, E.A. *et al.* 2007. Targeted gene addition into a specified location in the human genome using designed zinc finger nucleases. *Proc. Natl. Acad. Sci. USA* **104:** 3055–3060.

37. Lombardo, A. *et al.* 2007. Gene editing in human stem cells using zinc finger nucleases and integrase-defective lentiviral vector delivery. *Nat. Biotechnol.* **25:** 1298–1306.

38. Banasik, M.B. & P.B. McCray, Jr. 2010. Integrase-defective lentiviral vectors: progress and applications. *Gene Ther.* **17:** 150–157.

39. DeKelver, R.C. *et al.* 2010. Functional genomics, proteomics, and regulatory DNA analysis in isogenic settings using zinc finger nuclease-driven transgenesis into a safe harbor locus in the human genome. *Genome Res.* **20:** 1133–1142.

40. Pruett-Miller, S.M. *et al.* 2009. Attenuation of zinc finger nuclease toxicity by small-molecule regulation of protein levels. *PLoS Genet.* **5:** e1000376.

41. Pruett-Miller, S.M. *et al.* 2008. Comparison of zinc finger nucleases for use in gene targeting in mammalian cells. *Mol. Ther.* **16:** 707–717.

42. Gabriel, R. *et al.* 2011. An unbiased genome-wide analysis of zinc-finger nuclease specificity. *Nat. Biotechnol.* **29:** 816–823.

43. Pattanayak, V. *et al.* 2011. Revealing off-target cleavage specificities of zinc-finger nucleases by in vitro selection. *Nat. Methods* **8:** 765–770.

44. Doyon, Y. *et al.* 2011. Enhancing zinc-finger-nuclease activity with improved obligate heterodimeric architectures. *Nat. Methods* **8:** 74–79.

45. Miller, J.C. *et al.* 2007. An improved zinc-finger nuclease architecture for highly specific genome editing. *Nat Biotechnol.* **25:** 778–785.

46. Szczepek, M. *et al.* 2007. Structure-based redesign of the dimerization interface reduces the toxicity of zinc-finger nucleases. *Nat. Biotechnol.* **25:** 786–793.

47. Miller, J.C. *et al.* 2011. A TALE nuclease architecture for efficient genome editing. *Nat. Biotechnol.* **29:** 143–148.

48. Cermak, T. *et al.* 2011. Efficient design and assembly of custom TALEN and other TAL effector-based constructs for DNA targeting. *Nucleic Acids Res.* **39:** e82.

49. Christian, M. *et al.* 2010. Targeting DNA double-strand breaks with TAL effector nucleases. *Genetics* **186:** 757–761.

50. Moscou, M.J. & A.J. Bogdanove. 2009. A simple cipher governs DNA recognition by TAL effectors. *Science* **326:** 1501.

51. Mussolino, C. *et al.* 2011. A novel TALE nuclease scaffold enables high genome editing activity in combination with low toxicity. *Nucleic Acids Res.* **39:** 9283–9293.

52. Pessach, I.M. & L.D. Notarangelo. 2011. Gene therapy for primary immunodeficiencies: looking ahead, toward gene correction. *J. Allergy Clin. Immunol.* **127:** 1344–1350.

53. Pessach, I.M. *et al.* 2011. Induced pluripotent stem cells: a novel frontier in the study of human primary immunodeficiencies. *J. Allergy Clin. Immunol.* **127:** 1400–1407 e1404.

54. Zou, J. *et al.* 2009. Gene targeting of a disease-related gene in human induced pluripotent stem and embryonic stem cells. *Cell. Stem. Cell.* **5:** 97–110.

55. Hockemeyer, D. *et al.* 2009. Efficient targeting of expressed and silent genes in human ESCs and iPSCs using zinc-finger nucleases. *Nat. Biotechnol.* **27:** 851–857.

56. Hockemeyer, D. *et al.* 2011. Genetic engineering of human pluripotent cells using TALE nucleases. *Nat. Biotechnol.* **29:** 731–734.

Ann. N.Y. Acad. Sci. ISSN 0077-8923

Corrigendum for Ann. N.Y. Acad. Sci. 1238: 106–121

Marsh, R.A. & A.H. Filipovich. 2011. Familial hemophagocytic lymphohistiocytosis and X-linked lymphoproliferative disease. *Ann. N.Y. Acad. Sci.* **1238:** 106–121.

The second complete paragraph on page 109 should read as follows:

Mutations in IL-2–inducible T cell kinase (ITK) can also be associated with HLH, and will be discussed later due to its association with lymphoma.[43]

The first sentence of the last paragraph on page 110 should read as follows:

Most recently, mutations in the *ITK* gene have been observed to cause an autosomal recessive XLP-like disorder.[43,99]

doi: 10.1111/j.1749-6632.2011.06406.x